New Technology in Urologic Surgery

Guest Editor

MIHIR M. DESAI, MD

UROLOGIC CLINICS OF NORTH AMERICA

www.urologic.theclinics.com

May 2009 • Volume 36 • Number 2

SAUNDERS an imprint of ELSEVIER, Inc.

W.B. SAUNDERS COMPANY
A Division of Elsevier Inc.

1600 John F. Kennedy Blvd. ● Suite 1800 ● Philadelphia, PA 19103-2899

http://www.theclinics.com

UROLOGIC CLINICS OF NORTH AMERICA Volume 36, Number 2
May 2009 ISSN 0094-0143, ISBN-13: 978-1-4377-0555-3, ISBN-10: 1-4377-0555-3

Editor: Kerry Holland
Developmental Editor: Donald Mumford

Urologic Clinics of North America (ISSN 0094-0143) is published quarterly by Elsevier Inc., 360 Park Avenue South, New York, NY 10010-1710. Months of issue are February, May, August, and November. Business and Editorial Offices: 1600 John F. Kennedy Blvd., Suite 1800, Philadelphia, PA 19103-2899. Periodicals postage paid at New York, NY and additional mailing offices. Subscription prices are $269.00 per year (US individuals), $429.00 per year (US institutions), $308.00 per year (Canadian individuals), $526.00 per year (Canadian institutions), $383.00 per year (foreign individuals), and $526.00 per year (foreign institutions). Foreign air speed delivery is included in all *Clinics* subscription prices. All prices are subject to change without notice. **POSTMASTER:** Send address changes to *Urologic Clinics of North America*, Elsevier Periodicals Customer Service, 11830 Westline Industrial Drive, St. Louis, MO 63146. Customer Service: 1-800-654-2452 (US). From outside the United States, call 1-314-453-7041. Fax: 1-314-453-5170. E-mail: JournalsCustomerService-usa@elsevier.com (for print support) and JournalsOnlineSupport-usa@elsevier.com (for online support).

Reprints. For copies of 100 or more, of articles in this publication, please contact the Commercial Reprints Department, Elsevier Inc., 360 Park Avenue South, New York, New York 10010-1710. Tel.: 212-633-3813; Fax: 212-462-1935; E-mail: reprints@elsevier.com.

Urologic Clinics of North America is covered in *MEDLINE/PubMed* (*Index Medicus*), *Excerpta Medica, Current Contents/ Clinical Medicine, Science Citation Index,* and *ISI/BIOMED.*

Printed and bound in the United Kingdom
Transferred to Digital Print 2011

Contributors

GUEST EDITOR

MIHIR M. DESAI, MD
Associate Professor of Surgery; and Director,
Stevan B. Streem Center for Endourology,
Glickman Urological and Kidney Institute,
Cleveland Clinic, Cleveland, Ohio

AUTHORS

MONISH ARON, MD
Department of Urology, Glickman Urological
and Kidney Institute, Cleveland Clinic
Foundation, Cleveland, Ohio

ANTHONY ATALA, MD
W. Boyce Professor and Chair, Department
of Urology; and Director, Wake Forest Institute
for Regenerative Medicine, Wake Forest
University School of Medicine, Winston-Salem,
North Carolina

SHELBY L. BUETTNER, BS
Research Associate, Minimally Invasive
and Robotic Surgery, University of Nebraska
Medical Center, Omaha, Nebraska

JEFFREY A. CADEDDU, MD
Professor of Urology; Ralph C. Smith, M.D.
Distinguished Chair in Minimally Invasive
Urologic Surgery; and Director, Clinical Center
for Minimally Invasive Urologic Cancer
Treatment, University of Texas Southwestern
Medical Center, Dallas, Texas

JEAN DE LA ROSETTE, MD, PhD
Department of Urology, Academic Medical
Center, University of Amsterdam, Amsterdam,
The Netherlands

THEODOR DE REIJKE, MD, PhD
Department of Urology, Academic Medical
Center, University of Amsterdam, Amsterdam,
The Netherlands

MIHIR M. DESAI, MD
Associate Professor of Surgery; and Director,
Stevan B. Streem Center for Endourology,
Glickman Urological and Kidney Institute,
Cleveland Clinic, Cleveland, Ohio

MARK J. DOERR, MD
Department of Urology, Mayo Clinic,
Rochester, Minnesota

SHANE M. FARRITOR, PhD
Associate Professor, Department
of Mechanical Engineering, University
of Nebraska, Lincoln, Nebraska

MICHAEL S. GEE, MD, PhD
Instructor in Radiology, Harvard Medical
School; and Assistant Radiologist,
Massachusetts General Hospital, Boston,
Massachusetts

MATTHEW GETTMAN, MD
Associate Professor of Urology, Department
of Urology, Mayo Clinic, Rochester, Minnesota

TROY R.J. GIANDUZZO, MBBS, FRACS (Urol)
Department of Urology, Royal Brisbane and Women's Hospital; and Department of Urology, Wesley Medical Centre, Brisbane, Australia

INDERBIR S. GILL, MD
Professor and Chairman, USC Institute of Urology; and Associate Dean for Clinical Innovation, Keck School of Medicine, University of Southern California, Los Angeles, California

RAJ K. GOEL, MD, FRCSC
Clinical Fellow, Glickman Urological and Kidney Institute, Cleveland Clinic Foundation, Cleveland, Ohio

STAVROS GRAVAS, MD, PhD
Department of Urology, University of Thessaly, School of Medicine, Larissa, Greece

GEORGES-PASCAL HABER, MD
Section of Laparoscopic and Robotic Urologic Surgery, Glickman Urological and Kidney Institute, Cleveland Clinic, Cleveland, Ohio

MUKESH G. HARISINGHANI, MD
Associate Professor of Radiology, Harvard Medical School; and Director, Abdominal MRI, Massachusetts General Hospital, Boston, Massachusetts

BRIAN H. IRWIN, MD
Department of Urology, Stevan B. Streem Center for Endourology; and Center for Laparoscopic and Robotic Surgery, Glickman Urological and Kidney Institute, Cleveland Clinic, Cleveland, Ohio

SHIHUA JIN, MD
Postdoctoral Research Fellow, Department of Biomedical Engineering, Lerner Research Institute, Cleveland Clinic, Cleveland, Ohio

JIHAD H. KAOUK, MD
Director, Center for Advanced Laparoscopic and Robotic Surgery, Glickman Urological and Kidney Institute, Cleveland Clinic Foundation, Cleveland, Ohio

VINOD LABHASETWAR, PhD
Professor and Staff, Department of Biomedical Engineering, Lerner Research Institute, Cleveland Clinic; and Taussig Cancer Center, Cleveland Clinic, Cleveland, Ohio

JASON LEE, MBBS, MClinEpid
Department of Urology, Royal Brisbane and Women's Hospital, Brisbane, Australia

AMY C. LEHMAN, MS
Research Fellow, Department of Mechanical Engineering, University of Nebraska, Lincoln, Nebraska

CHARALAMPOS MAMOULAKIS, MD, MSc, PhD
Department of Urology, Academic Medical Center, University of Amsterdam, Amsterdam, The Netherlands

DMITRY OLEYNIKOV, MD, FACS
Associate Professor, Department of Surgery; and Director, Center for Advanced Surgical Technology, University of Nebraska Medical Center, Omaha, Nebraska

SIJO PAREKATTIL, MD
Assistant Professor of Urology; and Co-Director for Robotic and Minimally Invasive Urologic Surgery, Department of Urology, University of Florida, Gainesville, Florida

LEE E. PONSKY, MD
Assistant Professor of Urology; Chief, Division of Urologic Oncology; and Director, Center for Urologic Oncology and Minimally Invasive Therapies, Department of Urology, University Hospitals Case Medical Center, Cleveland, Ohio

PRADEEP P. RAO, MD
Mamata Hospital, Dombivli East, Mumbai, India

JORGE RIOJA, MD, PhD
Department of Urology, Academic Medical Center, University of Amsterdam, Amsterdam, The Netherlands

BHAVIN C. SHAH, MD
Research Fellow, Minimally Invasive
and Robotic Surgery, Department of Surgery,
University of Nebraska Medical Center,
Omaha, Nebraska

ROBERT J. STEIN, MD
Department of Urology, Stevan B. Streem
Center for Endourology; and Center for
Laparoscopic and Robotic Surgery, Glickman
Urological and Kidney Institute, Cleveland
Clinic, Cleveland, Ohio

LI-MING SU, MD
David A. Cofrin Professor of Urology;
and Chief, Division of Robotic and Minimally
Invasive Urologic Surgery, Department
of Urology, University of Florida, Gainesville,
Florida

SHAHIN TABATABAEI, MD
Assistant Professor of Surgery, Harvard
Medical School; and Department of Urology,
Massachusetts General Hospital, Boston,
Massachusetts

**GERALD Y. TAN, MBChB, MRCSEd,
MMed, FAMS**
Ferdinand C. Valentine Fellow, Brady
Foundation Department of Urology, Weill
Medical College of Cornell University; Clinical
Fellow, Lefrak Institute of Robotic Surgery,
New York Presbyterian Hospital, New York,
New York; and Associate Consultant,
Department of Urology, Tan Tock Seng
Hospital, Singapore

ASHUTOSH K. TEWARI, MD, MCh
Ronald P. Lynch Associate Professor
of Urologic Oncology, Brady Foundation
Department of Urology, Weill Medical College
of Cornell University; and Director, Lefrak
Institute of Robotic Surgery, New York
Presbyterian Hospital, New York, New York

VASSILIOS TZORTZIS, MD, PhD
Department of Urology, University of Thessaly,
School of Medicine, Larissa, Greece

OSAMU UKIMURA, MD
Associate Professor, Department of Urology,
Kyoto Prefectural University of Medicine,
Kyoto, Japan; and Professor, USC Institute
of Urology, Keck School of Medicine,
University of Southern California, Los Angeles,
California

GINO J. VRICELLA, MD
Resident Physician, Department of Urology,
University Hospitals Case Medical Center,
Cleveland, Ohio

JEFFERY C. WHEAT, MD
Resident Physician, Department of Urology,
University of Michigan Medical Center, Ann
Arbor, Michigan

WESLEY M. WHITE, MD
Section of Laparoscopic and Robotic Urologic
Surgery, Glickman Urological and Kidney
Institute, Cleveland Clinic, Cleveland, Ohio

HESSEL WIJKSTRA, MSc, PhD
Department of Urology, Academic Medical
Center, University of Amsterdam, Amsterdam,
The Netherlands

J. STUART WOLF, Jr., MD
David A. Bloom Professor of Urology,
Department of Urology, University of Michigan
Medical Center, Ann Arbor, Michigan

LAWRENCE L. YEUNG, MD
Urology Resident, Department of Urology,
University of Florida, Gainesville, Florida

Contents

> Computer-aided surgical navigation systems with fusion or overlaying capability, coupled with newer position tracking systems, can provide new opportunities to improve the precision of minimally invasive urology. Three-dimensional feedback of spatial position of surgical targets, and the predictive ability to guide laparoscopic dissection along the ideal surgical plane, with built-in safety checks and balances may help to lay the foundation for automated surgery in the future.

> Recently, advances in imaging technology have made possible the ability to image noninvasively specific molecular pathways in vivo that are involved in disease processes. Molecular imaging evaluates changes in cellular physiology and function rather than anatomy, which are likely to be earlier and more sensitive manifestations of disease. In addition, as newer drugs to treat disease become increasingly molecule specific, molecular imaging has become necessary to provide noninvasive determination of patients likely to benefit from treatment and early therapy response. This article reviews current and emerging molecular imaging technologies relevant to urologic surgery.

> Continuous innovations and clinical research in ultrasound (US) technology have upgraded the position of US in the imaging armamentarium of urologists. In particular, contrast-enhanced US and sonoelastography seem to be promising in the diagnosis of urologic cancers, implementation of ablative treatments, and monitoring of treatment response. This article focuses on the potential clinical applications of recent advances in US technology in oncologic urology.

> This article presents a fair and balanced review of natural orifice translumenal endoscopic surgery. The article chronicles the history and technical aspects of natural orifice translumenal endoscopic surgery with particular emphasis on its application in urology. It is hoped that this article serves as a straightforward and pragmatic reference for practicing and academic urologists.

Robotic technology is being increasingly used for a variety of surgical procedures. This article describes some novel flexible robotic platforms that may enhance the capabilities of flexible endoscopy and provides a rationale for robotic technology's further development and future use. It also reviews some recent experimental and clinical usages of flexible robotic technology to perform ureterorenoscopy and to provide treatment of stones.

Driven by patient preference and a more favorable oncologic prognosis at diagnosis, there has been a paradigm shift in the treatment of urologic cancers. Although the standard of care for most urologic malignancies continues to be surgical extirpation, ablation, in the form of needle-based or extracorporeal approaches, is quickly establishing itself as a viable primary treatment option. If there is anything to be learned from pioneering studies, it is that there must be strict adherence to inclusion criteria for patient enrollment and that there are real limitations with each approach. It is only with this awareness that we can achieve maximal benefit while limiting the number of unnecessary complications and poor oncologic outcomes.

Nanomedicine is a new distinct scientific discipline that explores applications of nanoscale materials for various biomedical applications. Translational nanomedicine is undergoing rapid transition from development and evaluation in laboratory animals to clinical practices. In the future, it is anticipated that nanotechnology can provide urologists a new point of view to understand the mechanism of disease, tools for early diagnosis of the disease, and effective modality for treatment. This article summarizes some of the emerging applications of nanomedicine in urology.

Since the Ruby laser was first developed in 1960 as the first successful optical laser, laser energy has continued to be developed and used in industry and medicine alike. Laser use in urology has been limited, however, largely until the last decade. The unique properties of laser energy have now led to its widespread use within urology, particularly in the treatment of benign prostatic hyperplasia, urolithiasis, stricture disease, and novel laparoscopic applications. This article details laser developments in each of these areas.

Tissue engineering efforts are currently being undertaken for every type of tissue and organ within the urinary system. Most of the effort expended to engineer genitourinary tissues has occurred within the past decade. Tissue engineering techniques require a cell culture facility designed for human application. Personnel who have mastered the techniques of cell harvest, culture, and expansion in addition to polymer design are essential for the successful application of this technology. Before these engineering techniques can be applied to humans, further studies need to be performed in many of the tissues described. Recent progress suggests that engineered urologic tissues and cell therapy may have clinical applicability.

Articles of Interest

Robotic surgical systems, such as the da Vinci Surgical System (Intuitive Surgical, Inc., Sunnyvale, California), have revolutionized laparoscopic surgery but are limited by large size, increased costs, and limitations in imaging. Miniature in vivo robots are being developed that are inserted entirely into the peritoneal cavity for laparoscopic and natural orifice transluminal endoscopic surgical (NOTES) procedures. In the future, miniature camera robots and microrobots should be able to provide a mobile viewing platform. This article discusses the current state of miniature robotics and novel robotic surgical platforms and the development of future robotic technology for general surgery and urology.

The use of bioadhesives, tissue sealants, and hemostatic agents has allowed for increased use of minimally invasive techniques for complex reconstructive urologic procedures. Hemostatic agents can facilitate clot formation through enzymatic reactions with host factors, mechanical compression, or a combination of the two. Tissue sealants and bioadhesives act through polymerization between themselves and adjacent tissues. This article reviews the unique features, mechanism of action, safety profile, and prototypical applications of the agents most commonly used in urologic surgery.

GOAL STATEMENT
The goal of *Urologic Clinics of North America* is to keep practicing urologists and urology residents up to date with current clinical practice in urology by providing timely articles reviewing the state of the art in patient care.

ACCREDITATION
The *Urologic Clinics of North America* is planned and implemented in accordance with the Essential Areas and Policies of the Accreditation Council for Continuing Medical Education (ACCME) through the joint sponsorship of the University of Virginia School of Medicine and Elsevier. The University of Virginia School of Medicine is accredited by the ACCME to provide continuing medical education for physicians.

The University of Virginia School of Medicine designates this educational activity for a maximum of 12 *AMA PRA Category 1 Credits*™ for each issue, 60 credits per year. Physicians should only claim credit commensurate with the extent of their participation in the activity.

The American Medical Association has determined that physicians not licensed in the US who participate in this CME activity are eligible for a maximum of 12 *AMA PRA Category 1 Credits*™ for each issue, 60 credits per year.

Credit can be earned by reading the text material, taking the CME examination online at: http://www.theclinics.com/home/cme, and completing the evaluation. After taking the test, you will be required to review any and all incorrect answers. Following completion of the test and evaluation, your credit will be awarded and you may print your certificate.

FACULTY DISCLOSURE/CONFLICT OF INTEREST
The University of Virginia School of Medicine, as an ACCME accredited provider, endorses and strives to comply with the Accreditation Council for Continuing Medical Education (ACCME) Standards of Commercial Support, Commonwealth of Virginia statutes, University of Virginia policies and procedures, and associated federal and private regulations and guidelines on the need for disclosure and monitoring of proprietary and financial interests that may affect the scientific integrity and balance of content delivered in continuing medical education activities under our auspices.

The University of Virginia School of Medicine requires that all CME activities accredited through this institution be developed independently and be scientifically rigorous, balanced and objective in the presentation/discussion of its content, theories and practices.

All authors/editors participating in an accredited CME activity are expected to disclose to the readers relevant financial relationships with commercial entities occurring within the past 12 months (such as grants or research support, employee, consultant, stock holder, member of speakers bureau, etc.). The University of Virginia School of Medicine will employ appropriate mechanisms to resolve potential conflicts of interest to maintain the standards of fair and balanced education to the reader. Questions about specific strategies can be directed to the Office of Continuing Medical Education, University of Virginia School of Medicine, Charlottesville, Virginia.

The faculty and staff of the University of Virginia Office of Continuing Medical Education have no financial affiliations to disclose.

Please note that the articles entitled "Advances in Bioadhesives, Tissue Sealants, and Hemostatic Agents," "Intraoperative Tissue Characterization and Imaging," "Technological Advances in Robotic-Assisted Laparoscopic Surgery," "Laparoscopic Single Site (Less) surgery in Urology," and "Miniature in Vivo Robotics and Novel Robotic Surgical Platforms" are not eligible for CME credit.

The authors/editors listed below have identified no professional or financial affiliations for themselves or their spouse/partner:
Monish Aron, MD; Theodore M. de Reijke, MD, PhD; Mark Joseph Doerr, MD; Michael S. Gee, MD, PhD; Matthew Gettman, MD; Troy R.J. Gianduzzo, MBBS, FRACS (Urol); Stavros Gravas, MD, PhD; Georges-Pascal Haber, MD; Mukesh G. Harisinghani, MD; Kerry K. Holland (Acquisitions Editor); Shihua Jin, MD; Jason Lee, MBBS, MClinEpid; Charalampos Mamoulakis, MD, MSc, PhD; Jorge Rioja, MD, PhD; William Steers, MD (Test Author); Shahin Tabatabaei, MD; Vassilios Tzortzis, MD, PhD; Osamu Ukimura, MD; Gino Joseph Vricella, MD; Wesley M. White, MD; and Hessel Wijkstra, MSc, PhD.

The authors/editors listed below identified the following professional or financial affiliations for themselves or their spouse/partner:
Anthony Atala, MD is a consultant for Tenigon, Inc., and Plureon, Inc.
Jeffrey A. Cadeddu, MD is an industry funded research/investigator for, serves on the Advisory Committee for, and owns a patent with Ethicon Endosurgery.
Jean J. de la Rosette, MD, PhD is a consultant for Galil Medical, Boston Scientific, and American Medical Systems.
Mihir M. Desai, MD (Guest Editor) is a consultant for Hansen Medical and Baxter, Inc., and owns stock in Hansen Medical.
Inderbir S. Gill, MD owns stock options in Hansen Medical.
Vinod Labhasetwar, PhD is an industry funded research/investigator for, patent holder with, and received a licensing fee for intellectual property from Telomolecular Inc.
Lee E. Ponsky, MD is an industry funded research/investigator for Accuray.

Disclosure of Discussion of Non-FDA Approved Uses for Pharmaceutical Products and/or Medical Devices.
The University of Virginia School of Medicine, as an ACCME provider, requires that all faculty presenters identify and disclose any off label uses for pharmaceutical and medical device products. The University of Virginia School of Medicine recommends that each physician fully review all the available data on new products or procedures prior to clinical use.

TO ENROLL
To enroll in the *Urologic Clinics of North America* Continuing Medical Education program, call customer service at 1-800-654-2452 or visit us online at: www.theclinics.com/home/cme. The CME program is available to subscribers for an additional fee of $195.00.

Urologic Clinics of North America

FORTHCOMING ISSUES

August 2009

Vasectomy and Vasectomy Reversal
Jay Sandlow, MD and Harris Nagler, MD,
Guest Editors

November 2009

**Benign Prostatic Hyperplasia
and Lower Urinary Tract Symptoms**
Jerry Blaivas, MD and Jeffrey Weiss, MD,
Guest Editors

RECENT ISSUES

February 2009

**The Socioeconomics of Health Care
and the Practice of Urology**
Kevin R. Loughlin, MD, MBA, *Guest Editor*

November 2008

**Contemporary Understanding and Management
of Renal Cortical Tumors**
Paul Russo, MD, FACS, *Guest Editor*

August 2008

Minimally Invasive Genitourinary Procedures
Howard N. Winfield, MD, *Guest Editor*

RELATED INTEREST

Medical Clinics of North America, September 2007 (Vol. 91, No. 5)
Nanomedicine
Chiming Wei, MD, PhD, FACC, FAHA, FAAN, *Guest Editor*

THE CLINICS ARE NOW AVAILABLE ONLINE!

Access your subscription at:
www.theclinics.com

Preface

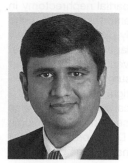

Mihir M. Desai, MD
Guest Editor

Technological advances have affected the scope and practice of medicine over centuries. However, the speed and magnitude of technological change over the past few decades are unparalleled in the history of medical science. Urology, long at the forefront of innovation, evaluation, and incorporation of technology, remains at the forefront in the twenty-first century. This issue of the *Urologic Clinics of North America*, comprising contributions by expert innovators, is devoted to important recent technological advances likely to influence urologic practice for years to come.

Radiological imaging has greatly affected the practice of medicine. Ongoing refinements in imaging technology with CT scans, MRI, and ultrasonography have certainly improved the process of diagnosing many disease conditions, leading to earlier detection and higher likelihood of cure. The next phase of innovations in imaging is in the arena of surgical navigation. These innovations, especially those related to laparoscopy and robotics, are likely to have a direct impact on surgical performance. Augmented reality, a recently introduced technology, allows real-time superimposition of preoperative imaging onto the surgical operative field. This will potentially allow surgeons to "see beyond" the immediate surgical field and therefore enhance the capabilities of the surgeon. Taking this concept a step further, "predictive navigation" may actually allow prediction of outcome of surgical dissection. That is, for example, it will predict whether or not

a specific dissection will achieve a negative margin. Another important area where imaging can aid intraoperative decision-making is that for tissue characterization. Initial studies with novel technologies, such as optical coherence tomography, confluorescent microscopy, and near-infrared spectroscopy, have been encouraging and may assist in intraoperative anatomic and pathological tissue characterization. Another exciting area of advance in imaging technology is the area of functional and molecular imaging. Molecular imaging takes advantage of the metabolic and functional characteristics of tissues and disease states and synchronizes them with anatomical imaging modalities. This may facilitate early diagnosis, improve accuracy of staging, and help targeted molecular therapy for various cancers. Ultrasonography has similarly evolved from an operator-dependant anatomic imaging modality to a sophisticated tool that can reliably assess vascularity and tissue characteristics. Ultrasonography forms the basis of many real-time tissue ablation techniques. Innovations are likely to expand the role of ultrasound technology in diagnosis and therapy of various urologic conditions.

Laparoscopy, increasingly in combination with robotics, now has an established role in the treatment of benign and malignant conditions across surgical disciplines. For many conditions, this has translated into lower morbidity, quicker recovery, and better cosmetic outcomes compared to open surgery with comparable

Five articles in this issue are not included in the CME post-test because they reference products by brand names. These articles are referenced as "Articles of Interest" and appear at the end of the issue. The five articles are: *Intraoperative Tissue Characterization and Imaging*; *Laparoendoscopic Single Site Surgery in Urology*; *Technological Advances in Robotic-Assisted Laparoscopic Surgery*; *Miniature In Vivo Robotics and Novel Robotic Surgical Platforms*; and *Advances in Bioadhesives, Tissue Sealants, and Hemostatic Agents*.

Urol Clin N Am 36 (2009) xiii–xiv
doi:10.1016/j.ucl.2009.03.001

efficacy. Various strategies have been employed to further minimize invasiveness and cosmetic sequelae of laparoscopic surgery. Natural orifice translumenal endoscopic surgery (NOTES) and laparoendoscopic single-site (LESS) surgery are novel approaches that share a common goal of making "scarless" surgery a reality. NOTES has generated considerable interest but has largely remained confined to the laboratory. Such issues as safety and reliability of closure of the intentional viscerotomy remain unanswered. Also, current instrumentation lacks the reliability, versatility, and robustness to perform complex intraperitoneal procedures. Most clinical NOTES procedures that have been reported are "hybrid" in that an additional transabdominal port is employed. LESS surgery, a term that has been recently introduced, encompasses a variety of laparoscopic surgical procedures performed using a single skin incision. Recent improvements in instrumentation and imaging have contributed to the rapid rise in LESS procedures across surgical specialties. The ability to conveniently conceal the single skin incision in the umbilicus makes it virtually "scar-free," thereby achieving a similar cosmetic outcome to NOTES. Further studies will determine the ultimate role of these minimally invasive techniques in the surgical armamentarium.

The use of robotics to perform laparoscopic procedures has risen exponentially over the past decade. It is estimated that in 2007 approximately 55,000 and in 2008 approximately 70,000 radical prostatectomies in the United States were performed with robotic assistance. With its role in the laparoscopic arena well established, novel surgical robotic platforms, such as flexible robotics and miniature in vivo robotics, are being developed for assisting NOTES, LESS, intraluminal endoscopy, and percutaneous image-guided interventions.

Another area where new technologies have made a significant impact on patient care is the field of solid organ ablation. Advances in ablative energy-form, image guidance, and delivery systems have all led to a rapid resurgence of tumor ablation as a potentially viable method of treating kidney and prostate cancers. Cryogenics, radiofrequency, high-intensity focused ultrasound are energy modalities already in clinical practice. Long-term follow-up data will determine the role of these promising technologies in the treatment of patients with renal and prostate cancer.

The last decade has also seen significant progress in the field of biological adhesives, sealants, and hemostats. These agents have already shown a benefit in such areas as partial nephrectomy in reducing postoperative hemorrhage and urine leak. These agents will likely play an increasingly important role in areas of laparoscopy, robotics, and percutaneous interventions by further enhancing the ability of the surgeon to achieve reliable hemostasis and watertight repair.

Other exciting technological advances have also occurred in the field of lasers, nanotechnology, and regenerative medicine. Developments in laser technology have affected many areas of urology, specifically stone disease and benign prostatic hyperplasia. More recently, investigators have explored the use of lasers to perform laparoscopic and robotic procedures. Early results have been encouraging. Nanomedicine, also an exciting area of research, uses nanoparticles for a wide variety of applications, including prevention, early diagnosis, treatment, and surveillance of various urologic conditions. Lastly, another exciting area of technologic marvel is that of regenerative medicine. Largely experimental, urologic applications of regenerative medicine have successfully created tissues to replace ureter, bladder, vagina, urethra, and phallic tissues. In its ultimate complexity, the creation of a complex functional organ system, such as the kidney, may also be within reach in the not-so-distant future.

Many of the presented technologic advances are in varying stages of development and, as such, are in their clinical infancy. The contributors, leaders in the field, have strived to present the current available evidence and an unbiased glimpse into the future. I would like to thank all the authors of this issue not just for their timely submission of manuscripts, but also, and more importantly, for their efforts in the quest to push the frontiers of what not long ago was considered impossible. All innovation we hope will ultimately result in the better care of our patients. I would also like to thank Kerry Holland and the editorial staff at Elsevier for their untiring efforts in creating this issue of the *Urologic Clinics of North America*.

Mihir M. Desai, MD
Stevan B. Streem Center for Endourology
Glickman Urological and Kidney Institute
Cleveland Clinic
9500 Euclid Avenue/Q10
Cleveland, OH 44195

E-mail address:
desaim1@ccf.org

Image-Fusion, Augmented Reality, and Predictive Surgical Navigation

Osamu Ukimura, MD[a,b,*], Inderbir S. Gill, MD[b]

KEYWORDS

- Computer-aided image-guided surgery
- Augmented reality • Prostate cancer
- Kidney cancer • Minimally invasive urology

Precise intraoperative decision-making requires extensive understanding of the three-dimensional topography of the surgical target, the three-dimensional course of the surrounding vasculature, and the proximity of vital anatomic structures in advance of embarking on the actual surgical procedure. Such information is typically obtained from evaluation of high-resolution radiographic images, such as CT or MRI; the surgeon's knowledge of the relevant surgical anatomy; and the surgeon's prior experience and expertise. The emergence of laparoscopic and robotic minimally invasive surgery has served to increase the surgeon's dependence on preoperative imaging. Although the magnification or three-dimensional picture capabilities of current endoscopes provides unparalleled visualization of the surgical field during laparoscopic and robot-assisted surgery, tactile feedback is somewhat diminished, increasing reliance on visual cues. As such, the novice surgeon's ability to be knowledgeable of anatomic structures beyond the endoscopic view may be somewhat decreased. Conventional intraoperative imaging for surgical navigation, such as two-dimensional real-time ultrasonography (US), has the considerable issue of being operator-dependent as regards expertise in performing the procedure, and in data interpretation.[1]

Intraoperative capability to visualize typically invisible surgical anatomy would be a considerable advance.

The recent revolution in high-speed computing, digital imaging software, and position-tracking technologies can provide new opportunities for real-time intraoperative surgical navigation. Fused-image or overlaid three-dimensional imaging for surgical navigation could be constructed from any imaging modality, such as preoperative CT, MRI, or positron emission tomography scanning, or intraoperative US, and serve to enhance the surgical capabilities of the surgeon.

"Virtual reality" implies surgical simulation of the three-dimensional world, for the purposes of educational training or preoperative surgical planning.[2] "Augmented reality" (AR) involves integrating radiologic images of anatomy with the real intraoperative view of the patient's anatomy to create computerized three-dimensional images of real surgical targets for the purpose of intraoperative decision-making.[3–6]

The authors initially reported the application of a US and CT-MRI fusion system to facilitate US-guided intervention.[7,8] They also first used AR technology in various urologic-oncologic laparoscopic procedures.[8,9] Their ongoing aims are to develop a predictive surgical navigation system

[a] Department of Urology, Kyoto Prefectural University of Medicine, Kawaramachi-Hirokoji, Kyoto 602-8566, Japan
[b] USC Institute of Urology, Keck School of Medicine, University of South California, 1975 Zonal Avenue, KAM 500, Los Angeles, CA 90089-9034, USA
* Corresponding author. Department of Urology, Kyoto Prefectural University of Medicine, Kawaramachi-Hirokoji, Kyoto 602-8566, Japan.
E-mail address: ukimura@koto.kpu-m.ac.jp (O. Ukimura).

Urol Clin N Am 36 (2009) 115–123
doi:10.1016/j.ucl.2009.02.012
0094-0143/09/$ – see front matter © 2009 Elsevier Inc. All rights reserved.

to guide the surgeon toward the ideal surgical direction or surgical plane before actually performing the surgical dissection to enhance intraoperative precision.

COMPUTER-AIDED IMAGE-GUIDED SURGERY

Every imaging modality has inherent advantages and disadvantages. Because most current imaging systems acquire and store data in a digital format they can be synchronized and fused using specialized software to create a system that combines advantages of two imaging modalities. Image-fusion systems provide a new opportunity to enhance the ability of an imaging modality by compensating for its shortcomings by fusing an additional imaging modality. Real-time virtual sonography (RVS) is the image-fusion system of real-time US with preoperative CT or MRI.[7,8] Herein, US provides real-time percutaneous or transrectal guidance; superimposition of preoperative CT or MRI images enhances the precision of the US-guided intervention. In RVS, images of the same section of the body are dynamically fused from its US plus its CT-MRI iterations, both images being synchronously shown in a side-by-side display. The unique advantages of each imaging modality are taken advantage of: the real-time images of US and the high-precision anatomic images of CT-MRI.

AR uses computerized digital imaging technology to project superimposed three-dimensional images onto the real-time endoscopic view. The authors used AR in a series of laparoscopic urologic surgical cases, mainly laparoscopic partial nephrectomy and laparoscopic radical prostatectomy.[8,9] During renal surgery, they primarily used preoperative CT data, whereas during prostate surgery they used preoperative MRI data and intraoperative transrectal US.

REAL-TIME VIRTUAL SONOGRAPHY

During percutaneous US-guided intervention, US allows real-time monitoring of the insertion of a needle into the target. The predicted puncture line is demonstrated on a display. For the novice practitioner, however, difficulty is often encountered during continuous visualization of the needle tip, the target organ, and adjacent anatomic structures, all of which have to be spatially located in the plane of the projected US beam. Difficulties include not only the technical visualization of the advancing needle, but also real-time interpretation of the US image.[1] The learning curve with US-guided interventions can often be significant. The reflected US echoes make it difficult to capture precise

images through stone, bone, gas, or air. Urologists typically prefer CT or MRI as the imaging modality of choice because of the higher resolution and availability of volume data acquisition. Taken together, the disadvantages of US-guided intervention include the relatively inferior image quality of US, especially for deep lesions located distant from the US probe, and operator dependence for technical aspects and interpretation.[1]

For energy-based needle ablation of renal tumor (cryoablation, radiofrequency ablation), reliable real-time image-guidance is necessary for (1) precise needle placement, (2) monitoring the entire extent of the ablative lesion, and (3) evaluation of ablation outcome. US can monitor ice-ball formation, yet visualization of the deep edge of the lesion is difficult, because US energy cannot penetrate through the body of the ice-ball. CT-guidance provides accurate images for cryoablation of renal tumors. Repeated CT-guided procedures confer the hazard of radiation-induced morbidity. Clearly, in children or young patients, US guidance is the safer choice.

Fundamentally, the RVS system constructs a tomogram from a previously acquired CT-MRI volume data-set and displays it in a synchronized manner along with the real-time US image. The physical position of the US transducer is tracked with an attached magnetic position sensor (**Fig. 1**).

The RVS system is comprised of (1) an US machine and display panel, (2) a computer workstation, (3) a magnetic field generator, and (4) an US probe with attached magnetic sensor. First, the Digital Imaging and Communication in Medicine formatted volume data of preoperative CT-MRI is obtained in the workstation of the RVS system before intervention. Second, this CT-MRI volume data is point-registered with the actual surgical target using fiducial or cross-section registration. Because a magnetic sensor is attached on the US probe in the RVS system, the angle and spatial position of the US probe is tracked in real-time, and the information is fed into the computer workstation. Movements of the magnetic sensor–attached US probe within the generated magnetic field around the body can be precisely tracked. The CT-MRI image can be automatically determined and reconstructed in real-time from the volume data, according to the real-time positional information of the US probe, which consists of both angle (to the x-, y-, or z-axis) and spatial position (x, y, z) of the US probe. The reconstructed "virtual" image of CT-MRI can be displayed in parallel with the US image for the same tomogram cut of the body in real-time (**Fig. 2**).

The most important advantage of the RVS is its presentation of enhanced high-resolution volume

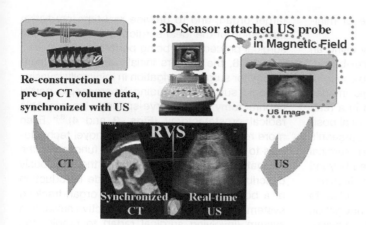

Fig. 1. Configuration of real-time virtual sonography. Synchronization of real-time ultrasound (US) tomography with preoperatively acquired CT/MRI tomography can be achieved by the high-speed computer-based workstation. Three-dimensional position and angle of US probe is identified by the signals from magnetic position sensor attached to the US probe within the magnetic field that is generated around the human body.

data. Any CT image (arterial phase, venous phase, delayed enhanced phase) or enhanced or functional MRI image can be selected from the preoperatively acquired volume data. Enhanced imaging, such as that provided by CT-MRI, can now be used for real-time navigation, while decreasing radiation exposure and costs.

The attractive feature of RVS is its side-by-side presentation of the real-time US and preoperative CT-MRI images (see **Fig. 2**). In monitoring the changing target lesion during ablative treatment, the display of the preoperative status, at the same tomogram level as the real-time US, can be important for confirming precision and safety of the ablation zone. Availability of only the real-time US image

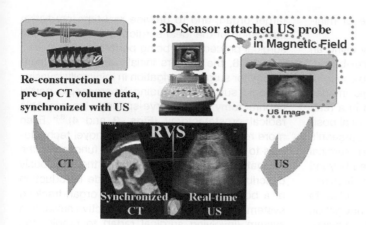

Fig. 2. Real-time virtual sonography image for percutaneous cryosurgery in a patient with a 1.8-cm upper pole renal tumor. The eleventh and twelfth rib bones create acoustic shadows on US images, especially during attempts to visualize an upper pole tumor. Real-time US can visualize the ice ball formation. Reconstructed synchronized CT helps visualize hidden anatomy beneath the ultrasound interface created by the eleventh and twelfth ribs.

after the formation of an ice-ball requires the surgeon to maintain a perfect mental picture of the spatial position of the pretreatment target lesion (whose shape may have become distorted by the ice-ball). Parallel displays of the initial and current status of the targeted tumor allow decision-making regarding the adequacy of the current treatment, and the possible necessity of an additional session to ablate completely the entire target.

For prostate applications, RVS is now also available for transrectal US-navigation fused with MRI. The high resolution of functional dynamic contrast-enhanced magnetic resonance imaging (DCE-MRI) could provide accurate diagnosis of prostate cancer in the future. Fusion of real-time images of needle ablation by transrectal RVS combined with high-resolution imaging of the prostate cancer nodule by functional DCE-MRI would enhance localization and targeted focal destruction. The authors' experience with RVS fusion of real-time transrectal US with high-resolution 3-T MRI volume data allows precise needle placement into the suspected lesion.

AUGMENTED REALITY IN UROLOGY

In minimally invasive laparoscopic or robotic surgery, the information about the targeted surgical anatomy is mainly visual-based, delivered by the magnified endoscopic view. As such, only the surface view of the surgical anatomy can be visualized; the opaque nature of organs and tissues precludes visualization of structures lying beneath the surface, or within the interior of organs. In surgical practice, much valuable information lies beyond what the surgeon can see directly. This includes various anatomic structures (vessels, nerves) often obscured by fat; small tumors; and cancers with varying depths of infiltration within or outside their native organs. Intraoperative, real-time information about these nuances facilitates expert performance of minimally invasive surgery.

Progress has been achieved recently using an AR visualization system.[3–6] This computer-based, image-assistance technology allows projection of preoperative or intraoperative radiologic images onto the displayed actual surgical field in a real-time manner. Importantly, three-dimensional positional correlation between the tip of the surgeon's surgical instruments and the targeted surgical anatomy, especially that which is located beyond what the surgeon can see directly, is now feasible.

This novel AR system has the potential to provide the surgeon with real-time navigation and predictive navigation. By "real-time" navigation the authors mean that the system can precisely provide the location of the surgeon's instrument tip vis-à-vis the targeted anatomy. By "predictive" navigation, the authors mean that the system has the potential to predict whether or not continuing in the current ongoing trajectory of surgical dissection will result in safe and accurate tumor excision, or in locating the desired anatomic structure. Currently, these systems are still in the prototype phase, and are not yet available for routine clinical use.

Over the last 10 years, AR navigation has been most commonly used in the field of neurosurgery. Surgery within the skull's stable bony frame has the advantage of minimal organ motion. This allows precise registration of the reconstructed three-dimensional surgical model onto the real surgical space.[3] Understandably, application of AR technology in abdominal surgery has been limited for various reasons including motion-deformation of abdominal soft and solid organs by insufflation, surgical manipulation, or ventilation.[4,5] In abdominal surgery, because the target organ is likely continuously to move or be displaced in comparison with the time of preoperative image acquisition, AR navigation is considerably more challenging to achieve. One way to overcome this problem is to use real-time image acquisition, such as by using intraoperative US.[4,6] In urologic surgery, however, not only US but also CT or MRI are used depending on the goal of each surgery. Additionally, even when using intraoperative images, repeated image acquisition is nevertheless necessary as the surgical procedure progresses, because the spatial position of the target organ changes compared with its position at the start of the surgery, when the previous image acquisition was performed. As such, significant efforts are underway to develop and introduce newer tracking systems to achieve dynamic real-time overlay of the three-dimensional surgical model according to the dynamic movement of the target organ, and to provide real-time predictive navigation of the ideal surgical plane even as the surgical procedure is being performed.[8,9]

In 2006, the authors initially applied AR technology for surgical navigation in minimally invasive urologic surgeries including laparoscopic partial nephrectomy and nerve-sparing laparoscopic radical prostatectomy (Figs. 3 and 4).[8,9] Even more recently, they are exploring novel technologies to improve the precision and function of the navigation system to overcome the previously described difficulties. These include introduction of a body-GPS system as a new organ-tracking system, and introduction of a predictive navigation system (involving surgical radar) to predict the ideal surgical plane before performing the actual surgical maneuver.[10,11]

Body-GPS and surgical radar are recent developments in surgical navigation. The authors' navigation software involves the concept of a color-coded zonal navigation system. The goal of procedures, such as laparoscopic partial nephrectomy and nerve-sparing laparoscopic radical prostatectomy, is to achieve better oncologic and better functional outcomes. With the color-coded zonal navigation system the authors seek to achieve those goals.

The spatial zone of the tumor or surgical target (eg, lymph node or a small renal tumor) is colored red; a 0- to 5-mm margin zone surrounding the tumor edge (target edge) is colored yellow; a 5- to 10-mm margin zone surrounding the yellow zone is colored green; and the greater than 10-mm margin zone is colored blue. For instance, during laparoscopic partial nephrectomy, this color-coded three-dimensional model is directly overlaid onto the small renal tumor. The surgeon's goal is to cut within the green zone (and never stray from it) to achieve a uniform, safe, 5-mm surgical margin (yellow zone) from the tumor (red zone), while simultaneously maximally preserving normal renal parenchyma (blue zone) (Figs. 4 and 5).

PREDICTIVE SURGICAL NAVIGATION SYSTEM: SURGICAL RADAR

Predictive navigation seeks to predict, in a dynamic, real-time manner, the ideal surgical plane, even as the surgical procedure unfolds. It alerts the surgeon by surgical radar, which is simultaneously shown in one corner of the surgical display, to predict or demonstrate the future anatomic end point of, for example, the surgical excision of a renal tumor, if the surgeon continues to cut along the current trajectory of the surgical scissors (Fig. 6).

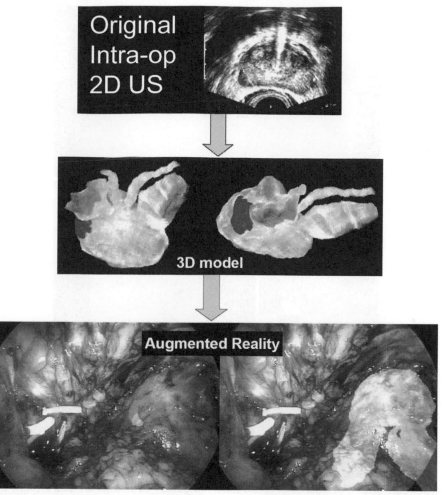

Fig. 3. Augmented reality navigation during laparoscopic radical prostatectomy. (*Upper*) Original intraoperatively acquired two-dimensional prostate transrectal US picture with traced hypoechoic lesion, already proved to be cancer on biopsy. (*Middle*) Reconstructed three-dimensional transrectal US surgical model of the prostate with biopsy-proved cancer area shown by blue. (*Bottom*) Augmented reality visualization using the three-dimensional transrectal US surgical model onto the real-time ongoing laparoscopic view; augmented reality demonstrates the precisely superimposed three-dimensional cancer area (*bottom left*, overlaid rainbow colored area) and three-dimensional prostate and seminal vesicles (*bottom right*, overlaid yellow area).

According to the previously mentioned color-coded zonal navigation system, the surgical target in the surgical radar is shown by a red zone, surrounded by yellow, green, and blue zones. The colored zones of the surgical radar with a 10-mm radius represent the presence of zones on the surface of the half-sphere up to a 10-mm distance from the tip of the surgeon's scissors. If the center of the 10-mm radius surgical radar display has turned red, it means that the tumor (red zone) is located 10 mm away from the scissors' tip along the current line of direction of the scissors. As such, if the surgeon continues to cut along the current trajectory for a depth of 10 mm, he or she runs the risk of cutting into the tumor.

Importantly, these colored zones are in real-time and dynamically changing like the radar in a weather forecast, according to the changing direction of the surgeon's scissors in real time. Taken together, the system has the potential to predict whether or not continuing in the current ongoing trajectory of surgical dissection results in safe and accurate excision of the tumor, or alternatively, in locating a desired anatomic structure (eg, renal artery), which may be hidden from view by the overlying renal hilar fat. This potentially allows the surgeon to make corrections in real-time of the ongoing surgical dissection toward the ideal direction, as guided by the surgical radar on the display monitor. Ultimately, surgical radar

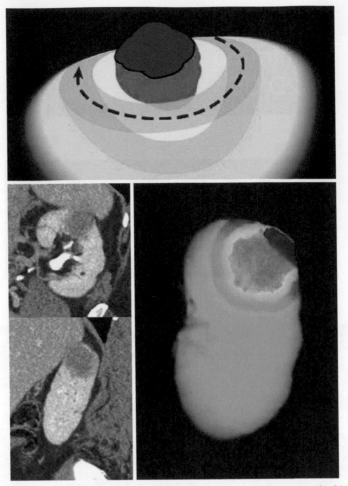

Fig. 4. Concept figure (*upper*) of "four-color coded zonal navigation" to indicate an ideal incision line within the green zone, to maintain safe surgical margin, and to maximize preservation of normal renal parenchyma. Example of the four-color coded surgical model of the intrarenal tumor (*bottom right*), which is reconstructed from original CT images (*bottom left*).

technology may find its application in robotic surgical systems.

INITIAL USE OF BODY-GPS FOR DYNAMIC REAL-TIME THREE-DIMENSIONAL NAVIGATION

Real-time tracking of organ motion, as occurs as the given surgical procedure progresses, is needed. The precision of overlaying a three-dimensional image onto the actual surgical view by the previously mentioned technology requires there be no organ motion or deformity between the time of acquisition of spatial co-ordinates and the time of superimposing the image.

Body-GPS technology has the potential to realize this goal. Because organ motion and organ deformity are unavoidable as the surgical procedure advances, real-time tracking of organ motion

is essential if real-time dynamic AR navigation is to be achieved.

A localization system provides real-time dynamic guidance to radiologic oncologists regarding the exact position and movement of the prostate during external-beam radiation treatment.[10] The system monitors prostate and tumor motion accurately, continuously, and in real-time.

The system consists of electromagnetic transponders that are percutaneously implanted in the prostate before the treatment. Each electromagnetic transponder is a small cylindrical-shaped device, approximately 8 mm in length and 2 mm in diameter; typically, three transponders are implanted. An electromagnetic console projects a magnetic field around the patient to receive the transmitted radiofrequency waves from the three implanted electromagnetic transponders, which transmit spatial-positioning

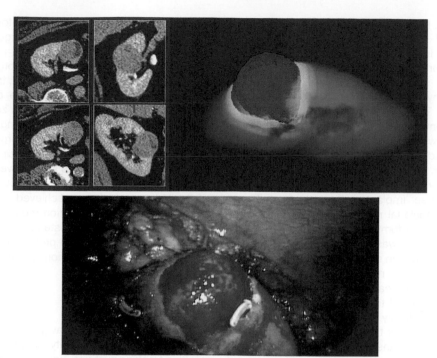

Fig. 5. Example of augmented reality navigation during laparoscopic partial nephrectomy. (*Upper left*) Original CT images. (*Upper right*) Four-color coded surgical model. (*Bottom*) Augmented reality image is superimposed onto the real-time surgical view.

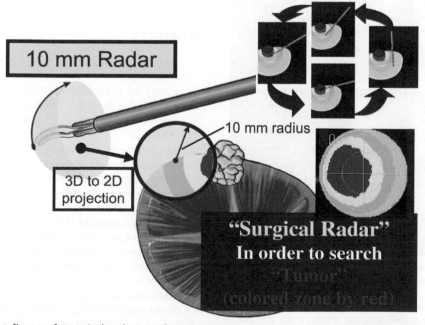

Fig. 6. Concept figure of "surgical radar" to demonstrate mapping of the four-color coded zones. When the surgeon changes the direction of the surgical instrument, the projected color mapping on a round of "surgical radar" changes according to the three-dimensional spatial positioning of the target zone (shown by red, surgical target, such as tumor), and surrounding zones (shown by yellow, 0–5-mm zone from the tumor; green, 5–10-mm zone from the tumor; blue, >10-mm zone from the tumor).

information. Real-time data on organ position can be tracked to localize the prostate precisely, thereby guiding radiation treatment.

The authors first evaluated this four-dimensional localization system during laparoscopic partial nephrectomy in an ex vivo bovine kidney model.[10,11] Three electromagnetic transponders were implanted onto the surface of an ex vivo calf kidney within a planned 5-mm surgical margin zone around a phantom tumor created with injected agar gel. A preoperative CT image was acquired, providing volume data of the tumor and the three implanted transponders. Then, a three-dimensional model for surgical planning of partial nephrectomy of the tumor, with a 5-mm surgical margin, was reconstructed using the predictive navigation software. Because the localization system can monitor the spatial co-ordinates (x, y, z) of each of the three implanted transponders in real-time, registration can be performed automatically by the computer software, with an error of less than 0.1 mm. The implanted electromagnetic transponders were successfully

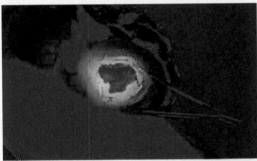
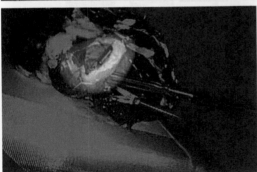

Fig. 7. Dynamic three-dimensional augmented reality navigation using body-GPS to achieve dynamic tracking of organ motion even during ongoing surgical procedure. (*Top*) Augmented reality to overlay the color-coded surgical model onto the tumor area. (*Bottom*) Dynamically tracked, overlaid three-dimensional surgical model onto the surgical target, according to the real-time positioning information provided by the implanted body-GPS sensors within the targeted area.

tracked by the system to provide information on the position and movement of the targeted organ, even as the partial nephrectomy progressed. Continuous, real-time monitoring of organ motion was provided by the system. As such, the surgeon could be alerted whenever the line of excision strayed outside the boundary (green zone) of the superimposed image, thereby enabling correction of the cutting line or plane as the surgical procedure progressed. **Fig. 7** shows the superimposed three-dimensional graphics images were dynamically overlaid in real-time onto the moving position of the kidney, which was achieved according to the data of the organ position monitored in real-time by the body-GPS system. The body-GPS system has the potential to provide an innovative solution for target localization and monitoring of mobile organs.

SUMMARY

Computer-aided surgical navigation systems with fusion or overlaying capability, coupled with newer position tracking systems, can provide new opportunities to improve the precision of minimally invasive urology. Three-dimensional feedback of spatial position of surgical targets, and the predictive ability to guide laparoscopic dissection along the ideal surgical plane, with built-in safety checks and balances may help to lay the foundation for automated surgery in the future.

REFERENCES

1. Ukimura O, Okihara K, Kamoi K, et al. Intraoperative ultrasonography in an era of minimally invasive urology. Int J Urol 2008;15:673–80.
2. Cameron BM, Robb RA. Virtual-reality-assisted interventional procedures. Clin Orthop Relat Res 2006; 442:63–73.
3. Iseki H, Masutani Y, Iwahara M, et al. Volumegraph (overlaid three-dimensional image-guided navigation): clinical application of augmented reality in neurosurgery. Stereotact Funct Neurosurg 1997; 68:18–24.
4. Sato Y, Nakamoto M, Tamaki Y, et al. Image guidance of breast cancer surgery using 3-D ultrasound images and augmented reality visualization. IEEE Trans Med Imaging 1998;17(5):681–93.
5. Marescaux J, Rubino F, Arenas M, et al. Augmented-reality-assisted laparoscopic adrenalectomy. Int J Radiat Oncol Biol Phys 2004;292:2214–5.
6. Nakamoto M, Nakada K, Sato Y, et al. Intraoperative magnetic tracker calibration using a magnetooptic hybrid tracker for 3-D ultrasound-based navigation in laparoscopic surgery. IEEE Trans Med Imaging 2008;27:255–70.

7. Ukimura O, Mitterberger M, Okihara K, et al. Real-time virtual ultrasonographic radiofrequency ablation of renal cell carcinoma. BJU Int 2008;101:707–11.

8. Ukimura O, Gill IS. Imaging-assisted endoscopic surgery: cleveland clinic experience. J Endourol 2008;22:803–10.

9. Ukimura O, Gill IS. Augmented reality for computer-assisted image-guided minimally invasive urology. Chapter 17. In: Ukimura O, Gill IS, editors. Contemporary interventional ultrasonography in urology. London: Springer; 2009. p. 179–84.

10. Kupelian P, Willoughby T, Mahadevan A, et al. Multi-institutional clinical experience with the Calypso system in localization and continuous, real-time monitoring of the prostate gland during external radiotherapy. Int J Radiat Oncol Biol Phys 2007;67:1088–98.

11. Ukimura O, Miki T, Nakamoto M, et al. Initial use of body-GPS for 4D Augmented reality navigation system. J Urol 2009;181(Suppl):790.

Molecular Imaging in Urologic Surgery

Michael S. Gee, MD, PhD, Mukesh G. Harisinghani, MD,
Shahin Tabatabaei, MD*

KEYWORDS

- Radiology • MRI • Optical imaging

Imaging plays an important role in the field of urologic surgery and is routinely used to diagnose genitourinary disease, stage urologic malignancies, and guide interventions. Multiple imaging modalities are currently used, including conventional radiography, x-ray fluoroscopy, ultrasound, CT, and MRI.[1] These imaging technologies all image structural anatomy by exposing the body to energy and resolving intrinsic contrast differences among tissues.[2] Recently, advances in imaging technology have made possible the ability to image noninvasively specific molecular pathways in vivo that are involved in disease processes.[3] Molecular imaging evaluates changes in cellular physiology and function rather than anatomy, which are likely to be earlier and more sensitive manifestations of disease. In addition, as newer drugs to treat disease become increasingly molecule specific, molecular imaging has become necessary to provide noninvasive determination of patients likely to benefit from treatment and early therapy response. This article reviews current and emerging molecular imaging technologies relevant to urologic surgery.

MOLECULAR IMAGING METHODS
Positron Emission Tomography

Positron emission tomography (PET) uses compounds labeled with positron-emitting radioisotopes as molecular probes.[4] The most commonly used clinical PET probe is the ^{18}F-labeled glucose analogue 2-^{18}F-2-deoxy-D-glucose (FDG). This probe is internalized into cells through glucose transporters and phosphorylated; however, the phosphorylated product does not undergo further processing and is retained within cells in proportion to their rate of glycolysis.

Many tumor cells are known to have increased glycolytic rates relative to normal cells even under aerobic conditions (known as the Warburg effect), which is thought to confer a selective advantage to transformed cells by allowing higher rates of proliferation and facilitating invasion and metastasis.[5] This association of increased glycolysis with malignancy forms the rationale for using FDG-PET as a method of detecting tumors. FDG-PET imaging of some urologic malignancies has been problematic. For example, FDG-PET has been shown to have lower sensitivity for prostate cancer detection compared with CT.[6,7] Additional studies have failed to demonstrate high accuracy rates of FDG-PET for distinguishing prostate cancer from benign prostate hypertrophy (BHP) or for detecting prostate cancer recurrence after surgery.[8,9] The relative indolence of prostate cancer, associated with low levels of tumor cell glycolysis, has been used to explain the poor detection rates with FDG-PET.[10] PET imaging with ^{11}C-choline, which accumulates in proliferating tumor cells undergoing increased cell membrane lipid synthesis, may prove to be superior to FDG-PET for detecting primary prostate malignancies and metastases.[11,12] FDG-PET imaging of renal cell carcinoma (RCC) and transitional cell carcinoma is limited by the renal excretion of tracer, which obscures detection of urinary tract tumors.[13] PET imaging with other metabolic tracers that do not undergo urinary excretion, such as ^{11}C-methionine, are being explored for detection of urinary tract malignancies.[14]

Lymphotropic Nanoparticle-Enhanced MRI

Lymphotropic superparamagnetic iron oxide particles (USPIO) consist of a monocrystalline

Massachusetts General Hospital, 55 Fruit Street, Boston, MA 02114, USA
* Corresponding author.
E-mail address: stabatabaei@partners.org (S. Tabatabaei).

Urol Clin N Am 36 (2009) 125–132
doi:10.1016/j.ucl.2009.02.007

superparamagnetic iron oxide core coated with dextrans to prolong circulation time. These particles, when injected intravenously, are taken up by lymphatic vessels and accumulate within lymph nodes, wherein they are internalized by macrophages. Normal uptake of USPIO in lymph nodes results in magnetic susceptibility effects of iron oxide manifesting as a decrease in signal intensity on T2* MRI.[15] In malignant lymph nodes, however, tumor cells displace normal sinus macrophages, leading to reduced USPIO uptake and maintenance of high signal on T2* MRI. Lymphotropic nanoparticle-enhanced MRI (LNMRI) provides a way to distinguish malignant versus benign lymph nodes during cancer staging, which is often difficult based on size criteria alone.

Magnetic Resonance Spectroscopy

Magnetic resonance spectroscopy (MRS) combines conventional MRI anatomic imaging with spectroscopic evaluation of cellular metabolites. In the prostate, the important metabolites are choline and citrate. Choline is an important component of cell membranes, integrated into the phospholipid bilayer. Prostate malignancy is hypothesized to lead to increased choline because of increased cell proliferation. Citrate is a component of the citric acid cycle that normally accumulates within the glandular ducts formed by prostate epithelial cells. Prostate malignancy is thought to lead to decreased choline levels by means of increased tumor metabolic activity and decreased glandular differentiation.[16] High-resolution, three-dimensional, quantitative proton spectroscopy can be performed using endorectal surface coils and volumetric spectroscopic sequences.

Optical Imaging

Optical imaging measures light photons of a given wavelength spectrum transmitted through tissues.[17] Optical techniques generate useful images from tissues by exploiting endogenous differences in tissue contrast or through the administration of optical probes designed to increase target tissue photon transmission. Optical coherence tomography (OCT) takes advantage of different light optical backscattering properties among cell layers to create real-time optical scattering images of tissue microarchitecture with a spatial resolution on the order of 10 μm.[18] Although originally conceived for ophthalmologic use because of limited tissue penetration (2–3 mm), the recent development of endoscopic OCT probes has made minimally invasive evaluation of microstructure in other epithelialized tissues possible.[19] Most exogenously administered

optical probes being considered for human molecular imaging applications are fluorescent probes consisting of a molecularly targeted agent conjugated with a fluorophore that absorbs and emits light within a defined spectral range. Fluorescent probes generate high contrast levels because of low background tissue autofluorescence but are often limited by poor transmission of emitted light through tissue, precluding imaging of deep structures.[20] Near-infrared fluorescence (NIRF) imaging uses fluorescent probes in the near-infrared range (640–900 nm) that can transmit light through tissues easily with minimal absorption by water and hemoglobin.[17] NIRF probes can be imaged up to 10 cm deep within the body and can be combined with tomographic imaging techniques to generate three-dimensional quantitative determination of probe distribution in vivo.[21] Additional advantages of NIRF optical imaging include lack of ionizing radiation exposure to patients and the ability to image multiple probes simultaneously.

Applications

Positron emission tomography of testicular germ cell tumors

A 1995 study examining FDG-PET imaging of 11 who had with testicular germ cell tumors (GCTs) demonstrated increased tracer uptake within the tumors and their metastases relative to fibrotic regions, normal tissues, and mature teratomas (**Fig. 1**).[22] A 1999 study comparing FDG and CT for initial staging in 37 patients who had testicular GCTs showed that FDG-PET was superior to CT for detection of lymphatic and distant metastases and correctly staged disease in 92% of cases compared with 68% for CT.[23] A 2004 study directly compared FDG-PET and CT for assessing viable residual tumor in 51 patients who had metastatic seminoma and were undergoing chemotherapy. Correlation with histology demonstrated FDG-PET to be superior to CT for detection of residual malignancy, with 100% specificity and 80% sensitivity compared with 70% and 74%, respectively, for CT.[24]

Lymphotropic Nanoparticle-Enhanced MRI for Lymph Node Metastasis

Prostate cancer

A study of 80 patients who had resectable prostate cancer (T1–T3) undergoing LNMRI with USPIO (Ferumoxtran-10) followed by histologic lymph node sampling demonstrated 91% sensitivity and 98% specificity for LNMRI on a node-by-node basis (**Fig. 2**).[25] The sensitivity of LNMRI for lymph node metastasis was statistically increased compared with conventional MRI. Within the

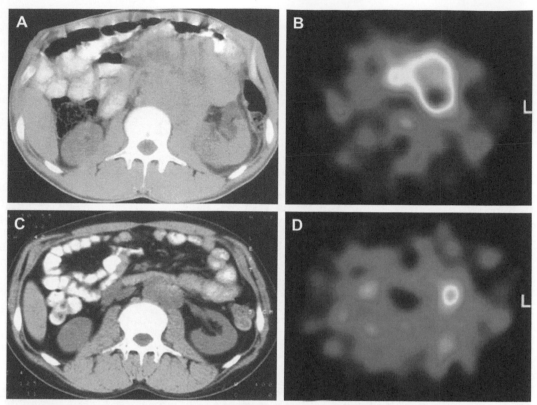

Fig. 1. FDG-PET of testicular germ cell tumors. Pretreatment (*A*) and posttreatment (*B*) CT scans of abdominal stage II seminoma show a marked reduction in tumor size after chemotherapy. The on-treatment FDG-PET scan (*D*) shows decreased tumor uptake compared with the pretreatment scan (*C*). (*From* Wilson CB, Young HE, Ott RJ, et al. Imaging metastatic testicular germ cell tumours with 18FDG positron emission tomography: prospects for detection and management. Eur J Nucl Med 1995;22:512; with permission).

subset of smaller lymph node metastases (5-10 mm in short-axis diameter) that would be considered normal on conventional CT or MRI, LNMRI demonstrated 96.4% sensitivity for metastasis. A 2008 study of 60 patients who had prostate cancer undergoing LNMRI also examined whether USPIO could detect the primary prostate malignancy. This study found a statistically significant association between the magnitude of the decrease in prostate gland T2* intensity after USPIO administration and the histologic tumor grade for intermediate- and high-grade prostate malignancies.[26] In this case, the USPIO are thought to be taken up by infiltrating macrophages within the prostate tumor and surrounding stroma.

Bladder cancer

Identification of lymphatic metastasis in patients who have muscle invasive bladder cancer is important to identify patients likely to require adjuvant chemotherapy. Accurate noninvasive determination of pelvic lymphatic metastasis before surgery would be a useful surgical guide for

resection of lymphatic metastases and would potentially help to reduce complications associated with extensive pelvic lymphadenectomy. A study of 58 patients who had bladder cancer undergoing LNMRI before surgical lymph node dissection demonstrated 96% sensitivity and 95% specificity compared with histology (n = 172 lymph nodes).[27] This study included 9 patients in whom LNMRI identified metastatic lymph nodes outside of the surgical dissection field.

Renal cell carcinoma

The presence of lymph node metastases in RCC is known to confer decreased life expectancy. The optimal extent of lymphadenectomy accompanying surgical nephrectomy remains a topic of active investigation,[28,29] however, particularly given the relatively low incidence of unsuspected lymphatic metastases[30] and the potential morbidity of lymph node dissection compared with nephrectomy alone. A 2008 study of nine patients with renal masses who underwent USPIO LNMRI before nephrectomy and lymph node

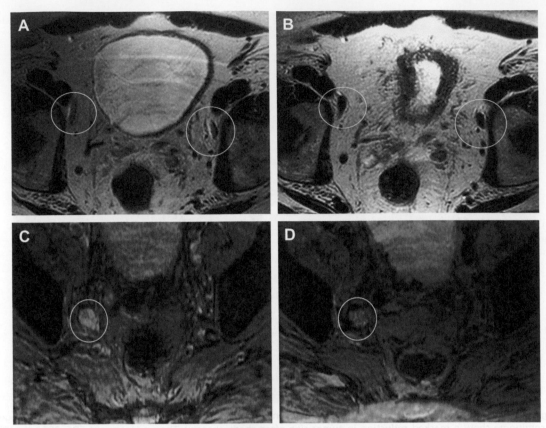

Fig. 2. LNMRI detection of prostate cancer metastasis. T2-weighted MRI of lymph nodes in patients who have prostate cancer are shown before (*A, C*) and after (*B, D*) administration of USPIO. The top row shows two benign lymph nodes (*circles*) that demonstrate avid contrast uptake (*B*). The bottom row shows a malignant lymph node that fails to take up contrast (*D*).

dissection showed that LNMRI demonstrated high sensitivity (100%) and specificity (95.7%) for detection of RCC lymphatic metastases.[31] This included accurate diagnosis of a benign enlarged lymph node in one patient that would have been considered metastatic on conventional CT or MRI based on size alone. The study also demonstrated a difference in USPIO-associated reduction in T2* signal intensity between benign oncocytomas and RCCs (77.8 versus 5 milliseconds), suggesting a possible additional role of USPIO for discriminating benign from malignant primary renal masses.

Magnetic resonance spectroscopy of prostate cancer

Prostate adenocarcinoma has been shown to demonstrate higher choline levels and lower citrate levels compared with benign prostatic hypertrophy and normal prostate peripheral zone tissue.[16,32] A 1996 study performed MRS on nine healthy volunteers, 5 patients who had BPH, and 85 patients who had biopsy-proved prostate cancer and BPH to determine whether MRS could discriminate prostate adenocarcinoma from normal prostate and BPH (**Fig. 3**).[32] MRS of prostate cancer demonstrated significantly lower mean citrate and higher mean choline levels compared with normal peripheral zone tissue in the same patient. A peak area ratio of [(choline + creatine)/citrate] was adopted to quantify the opposing changes in choline and citrate levels in prostate cancer into a single value. The peak area ratio was significantly elevated in prostate cancer compared with BPH or normal peripheral zone. Additionally, there was no overlap in peak area ratios between prostate cancer and BPH or normal in any of the patients imaged. These results suggest a role for MRS in detecting prostate cancer and evaluating its spatial distribution.

MRS has also been investigated as an imaging technique to determine prostate tumor volume more accurately before treatment, because tumor volume has been shown to be an independent predictor of disease recurrence after radical prostatectomy.[33] A 2002 study examined 37 patients

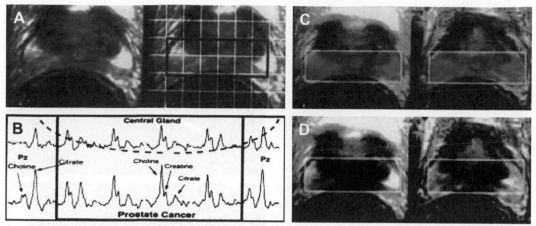

Fig. 3. MRS of prostate cancer. (*A*) MRI and MRS were performed at the level of the prostate base in a patient who had prostate cancer. (*B*) Multivoxel MRS demonstrates decreased citrate (*C*) and elevated choline (*D*) levels in the prostate regions corresponding to histologically proved prostate cancer. Pz, peripheral zone. (*From* Kurhanewicz J, Vigneron DB, Hricak H, et al. Three-dimensional H-1 MR spectroscopic imaging of the in situ human prostate with high (0.24-0.7-cm³) spatial resolution. Radiology 1996;198:801; with permission.)

who had prostate cancer and underwent MRI with MRS before radical prostatectomy.[34] Tumor volumes were measured by conventional MRI and MRS and then compared with histologic assessment. MRS proved to be superior to conventional MRI for estimating tumor volume for all tumors, in addition to tumors greater than 0.50 mL in volume, which are considered more clinically relevant.

Lymphotropic nanoparticle-enhanced MRI optical imaging of urolithiasis

A 2008 study tested the ability of an exogenous calcium-seeking NIRF optical probe to detect calcium stones in the kidney and ureter.[35] The probe consisted of a calcium-binding bisphosphonate conjugated with a near-infrared fluorochrome. The probe demonstrated avid binding to multiple types of calcium stones in vitro, in addition to in vivo binding to calcium stones surgically implanted into the renal pelvis of mice (**Fig. 4**). Stones as small as 1 mm in diameter could be detected by optical imaging. Future studies involving NIRF imaging systems incorporated into endoscopic devices would help to make this technology more clinically translatable.

Optical coherence tomography for bladder cancer staging

Determination of depth of bladder tumor invasion into the bladder wall is an important determinant of tumor staging and treatment. Currently, this is assessed by cystoscopic transurethral tumor resection, which is invasive and may be associated with tumor understaging in some cases.[36] A 2008 study used near-infrared OCT as

a cystoscopic adjunct to assess depth of bladder cancer invasion in 32 patients.[37] This study used a fiberoptic optical imaging probe that could be introduced into the working channel of a standard rigid cystoscope sheath. Taking advantage of the differing light backscattering pattern of different bladder tissue layers, OCT was able to distinguish the mucosa, lamina propria, and muscularis propria bladder layers (**Fig. 5**). Compared with histologic assessment of resected tumor, OCT detection of tumors confined to urothelial mucosa (Ta) demonstrated 90% specificity and 89% specificity, whereas OCT detection of muscle-invasive tumors (T2 or higher) demonstrated 100% sensitivity and 90% specificity. Additionally, based on morphologic features, OCT was able to differentiate malignant from benign bladder lesions with an 89% positive predictive value and 100% negative predictive value.

FUTURE APPLICATIONS

Molecular imaging is likely to be of increasing importance in the near future as treatments for urologic malignancies become more molecularly targeted. For example, multiple small-molecule tyrosine kinase inhibitors (eg, sunitinib, sorafenib) have recently been introduced into the clinic for treating metastatic RCC. An effective molecular imaging technique to assess the degree of molecular inhibition by these agents would be of tremendous benefit in this patient population as a screen for drug susceptibility, an aid in optimizing individual patient drug dosing, and an early marker of drug efficacy or refractoriness. These issues

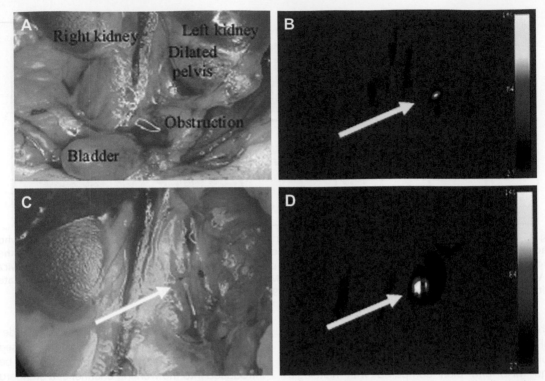

Fig. 4. NIRF optical imaging of urinary stones. A 1-mm calcium phosphate/struvite stone was surgically implanted into a mouse renal pelvis. The stone is not visible under bright light (*A*) but can be visualized by optical imaging after intravenous administration of a calcium-seeking NIRF probe (*arrow; B, D*). (*C*) Renal pelvis is subsequently opened surgically, revealing the presence of the stone (*arrow*). (*From* Figueiredo JL, Passerotti CC, Sponholtz T, et al. A novel method of imaging calcium urolithiasis using fluorescence. J Urol 2008;179:1612; with permission.)

are particularly important for molecular-based therapies that are often extremely costly and have their own set of toxicities.[38] In addition to RCC, there is preclinical evidence that molecular therapies targeting the fibroblast growth factor receptor 3 and platelet-derived growth factor receptor-β receptors demonstrate efficacy against bladder cancer.[39] Finally, recent technologic advances leading to the development of catheter-based multichannel molecular imaging devices create enormous potential for cystoscopy-based molecular imaging and interventions.[40]

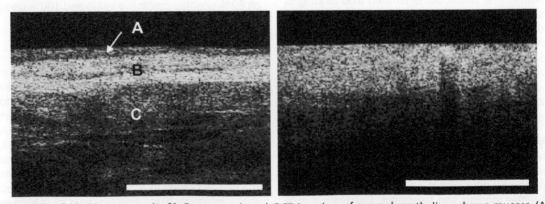

Fig. 5. OCT of bladder cancer. (*Left*) Cystoscopy-based OCT imaging of normal urothelium shows mucosa (A), lamina propria (B), and muscularis (C) layers. (*Right*) OCT imaging of muscle-invasive transitional cell carcinoma demonstrates loss of normal bladder wall layers. (*From* Lerner SP, Goh AC, Tresser NJ, et al. Optical coherence tomography as an adjunct to white light cystoscopy for intravesical real-time imaging and staging of bladder cancer. Urology 2008;72:134; with permission.)

REFERENCES

1. Nascimento RG, Coleman J, Solomon SB. Current and future imaging for urologic interventions. Curr Opin Urol 2008;18:116–21.
2. Weissleder R, Ntziachristos V. Shedding light onto live molecular targets. Nat Med 2003;9:123–8.
3. Weissleder R, Mahmood U. Molecular imaging. Radiology 2001;219:316–33.
4. Phelps ME. Inaugural article: positron emission tomography provides molecular imaging of biological processes. Proc Natl Acad Sci U S A 2000;97:9226–33.
5. Gatenby RA, Gillies RJ. Why do cancers have high aerobic glycolysis? Nat Rev Cancer 2004;4:891–9.
6. Salminen E, Hogg A, Binns D, et al. Investigations with FDG-PET scanning in prostate cancer show limited value for clinical practice. Acta Oncol 2002;41:425–9.
7. Sung J, Espiritu JI, Segall GM, et al. Fluorodeoxyglucose positron emission tomography studies in the diagnosis and staging of clinically advanced prostate cancer. BJU Int 2003;92:24–7.
8. Effert PJ, Bares R, Handt S, et al. Metabolic imaging of untreated prostate cancer by positron emission tomography with 18fluorine-labeled deoxyglucose. J Urol 1996;155:994–8.
9. Hofer C, Laubenbacher C, Block T, et al. Fluorine-18-fluorodeoxyglucose positron emission tomography is useless for the detection of local recurrence after radical prostatectomy. Eur Urol 1999;36:31–5.
10. Margolis DJ, Hoffman JM, Herfkens RJ, et al. Molecular imaging techniques in body imaging. Radiology 2007;245:333–56.
11. Kotzerke J, Prang J, Neumaier B, et al. Experience with carbon-11 choline positron emission tomography in prostate carcinoma. Eur J Nucl Med 2000;27:1415–9.
12. Yamaguchi T, Lee J, Uemura H, et al. Prostate cancer: a comparative study of 11C-choline PET and MR imaging combined with proton MR spectroscopy. Eur J Nucl Med Mol Imaging 2005;32:742–8.
13. Powles T, Murray I, Brock C, et al. Molecular positron emission tomography and PET/CT imaging in urological malignancies. Eur Urol 2007;51:1511–20 [discussion: 1520–11].
14. Ahlstrom H, Malmstrom PU, Letocha H, et al. Positron emission tomography in the diagnosis and staging of urinary bladder cancer. Acta Radiol 1996;37:180–5.
15. Weissleder R, Elizondo G, Wittenberg J, et al. Ultrasmall superparamagnetic iron oxide: characterization of a new class of contrast agents for MR imaging. Radiology 1990;175:489–93.
16. Kurhanewicz J, Vigneron DB, Nelson SJ, et al. Citrate as an in vivo marker to discriminate prostate cancer from benign prostatic hyperplasia and normal prostate peripheral zone: detection via localized proton spectroscopy. Urology 1995;45:459–66.
17. Bremer C, Ntziachristos V, Weissleder R. Optical-based molecular imaging: contrast agents and potential medical applications. Eur Radiol 2003;13:231–43.
18. Huang D, Swanson EA, Lin CP, et al. Optical coherence tomography. Science 1991;254:1178–81.
19. Pan Y, Lavelle JP, Bastacky SI, et al. Detection of tumorigenesis in rat bladders with optical coherence tomography. Med Phys 2001;28:2432–40.
20. Jaffer FA, Weissleder R. Molecular imaging in the clinical arena. JAMA 2005;293:855–62.
21. Ntziachristos V, Bremer C, Weissleder R. Fluorescence imaging with near-infrared light: new technological advances that enable in vivo molecular imaging. Eur Radiol 2003;13:195–208.
22. Wilson CB, Young HE, Ott RJ, et al. Imaging metastatic testicular germ cell tumours with 18FDG positron emission tomography: prospects for detection and management. Eur J Nucl Med 1995;22:508–13.
23. Albers P, Bender H, Yilmaz H, et al. Positron emission tomography in the clinical staging of patients with Stage I and II testicular germ cell tumors. Urology 1999;53:808–11.
24. De Santis M, Becherer A, Bokemeyer C, et al. 2-18fluoro-deoxy-D-glucose positron emission tomography is a reliable predictor for viable tumor in postchemotherapy seminoma: an update of the prospective multicentric SEMPET trial. J Clin Oncol 2004;22:1034–9.
25. Harisinghani MG, Barentsz J, Hahn PF, et al. Noninvasive detection of clinically occult lymph-node metastases in prostate cancer. N Engl J Med 2003;348:2491–9.
26. Li CS, Harisinghani MG, Lin WC, et al. Enhancement characteristics of ultrasmall superparamagnetic iron oxide particle within the prostate gland in patients with primary prostate cancer. J Comput Assist Tomogr 2008;32:523–8.
27. Deserno WM, Harisinghani MG, Taupitz M, et al. Urinary bladder cancer: preoperative nodal staging with ferumoxtran-10-enhanced MR imaging. Radiology 2004;233:449–56.
28. Freedland SJ, Dekernion JB. Role of lymphadenectomy for patients undergoing radical nephrectomy for renal cell carcinoma. Rev Urol 2003;5:191–5.
29. Pantuck AJ, Zisman A, Dorey F, et al. Renal cell carcinoma with retroperitoneal lymph nodes: role of lymph node dissection. J Urol 2003;169:2076–83.
30. Blom JH, van Poppel H, Marechal JM, et al. Radical nephrectomy with and without lymph node dissection: preliminary results of the EORTC randomized phase III protocol 30881. EORTC Genitourinary Group. Eur Urol 1999;36:570–5.

31. Guimaraes AR, Tabatabei S, Dahl D, et al. Pilot study evaluating use of lymphotrophic nanoparticle-enhanced magnetic resonance imaging for assessing lymph nodes in renal cell cancer. Urology 2008;71:708–12.

32. Kurhanewicz J, Vigneron DB, Hricak H, et al. Three-dimensional H-1 MR spectroscopic imaging of the in situ human prostate with high (0.24–0.7-cm^3) spatial resolution. Radiology 1996;198:795–805.

33. Stamey TA, McNeal JE, Yemoto CM, et al. Biological determinants of cancer progression in men with prostate cancer. JAMA 1999;281:1395–400.

34. Coakley FV, Kurhanewicz J, Lu Y, et al. Prostate cancer tumor volume: measurement with endorectal MR and MR spectroscopic imaging. Radiology 2002;223:91–7.

35. Figueiredo JL, Passerotti CC, Sponholtz T, et al. A novel method of imaging calcium urolithiasis using fluorescence. J Urol 2008;179:1610–4.

36. Shariat SF, Palapattu GS, Karakiewicz PI, et al. Discrepancy between clinical and pathologic stage: impact on prognosis after radical cystectomy. Eur Urol 2007;51:137–49 [discussion: 149–51].

37. Lerner SP, Goh AC, Tresser NJ, et al. Optical coherence tomography as an adjunct to white light cystoscopy for intravesical real-time imaging and staging of bladder cancer. Urology 2008;72: 133–7.

38. Johannsen M, Florcken A, Bex A, et al. Can tyrosine kinase inhibitors be discontinued in patients with metastatic renal cell carcinoma and a complete response to treatment? A multicentre, retrospective analysis. Eur Urol 2008 Oct 18. [Epub ahead of print].

39. Black PC, Dinney CP. Bladder cancer angiogenesis and metastasis—translation from murine model to clinical trial. Cancer Metastasis Rev 2007;26: 623–34.

40. Sheth RA, Upadhyay R, Weissleder R, et al. Real-time multichannel imaging framework for endoscopy, catheters, and fixed geometry intraoperative systems. Mol Imaging 2007;6:147–55.

Advances in Ultrasound Technology in Oncologic Urology

Stavros Gravas, MD, PhD[a],
Charalampos Mamoulakis, MD, MSc, PhD[b],
Jorge Rioja, MD, PhD[b], Vassilios Tzortzis, MD, PhD[a],
Theodor de Reijke, MD, PhD[b],
Hessel Wijkstra, MSc, PhD[b], Jean de la Rosette, MD, PhD[b],*

KEYWORDS
- Ultrasonography
- Contrast-enhanced ultrasound
- Elastography • Prostate • Kidney
- Bladder • Testis • Cancer

Ultrasonography (US) represents a key instrument in the diagnostic armamentarium of urologists because it is rapid, effective, noninvasive, radiation-free, and relatively inexpensive. During the past 15 years, continuous innovations in transducer engineering, electronics, computers, signal processing, and the development of contrast agents have resulted in advances in image resolution, three-dimensional (3D) and four-dimensional US, harmonic imaging, compound imaging, contrast-enhanced (CE) US, and sonoelastography.[1] In light of these developments, there is an increasing flow of data from studies investigating the role of US in the diagnosis, management, and follow-up of urologic patients. This article indicates the recent advances in US technology and focuses on their potential clinical applications in oncologic urology.

ADVANCES IN THE DIAGNOSIS OF PROSTATE CANCER
Three-Dimensional Imaging

3D technology offers several advantages over two-dimensional (2D) transrectal ultrasound (TRUS) imaging of the prostate, such as improving diagnosis of prostate cancer (PCa), assessment of brachytherapy seed placement or treatment mapping, cryoablation guidance, accurate diagnosis of extraprostatic tumor extension, and staging.[2–4]

Prostate HistoScanning is a novel computer-aided ultrasonographic technology based on tissue characterization algorithms. The characterization algorithms exploit the physical changes to sound waves that result from the interaction of the US beam and the cancer tissue (energy loss, erratic spatial energy distribution, and increased entropy). These can be applied in discrete regions of interest in the prostate. Thus, the presence of PCa can be ascertained within minute discrete tissue volumes. Prostate HistoScanning enables determination of PCa location and volume (**Fig. 1**). It has been reported that foci 0.50 mL or greater can accurately be detected, and this technology has been proposed as a potential triage test for men deemed to be at risk for PCa who wish to avoid biopsy.[5]

Elasticity Imaging

The use of US-based elasticity imaging for the detection of PCa relies on the fact that these tumors can be detected because they are firmer than the surrounding normal parenchyma (**Fig. 2**A). The results of several recent studies

[a] Department of Urology, University of Thessaly, School of Medicine, Feidiou 6-8, 412 21 Larissa, Greece
[b] Department of Urology, Academic Medical Center, University of Amsterdam, PO Box 22660, Meibergdreef 9, 1105 AZ Amsterdam, The Netherlands
* Corresponding author.
E-mail address: j.j.delarosette@amc.uva.nl (J. de la Rosette).

Urol Clin N Am 36 (2009) 133–145
doi:10.1016/j.ucl.2009.02.006

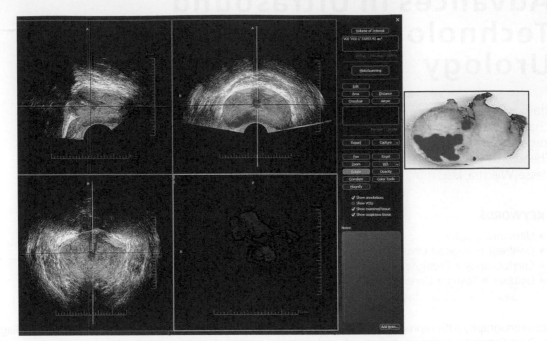

Fig. 1. Example of Prostate HistoScanning technology. (*Left*) 3D-US imaging with calculated probability for prostate cancer (in red). (*Right*) Histologic specimen. (*Courtesy of* Advanced Medical Diagnostics SA, Waterloo, Belgium; with permission.)

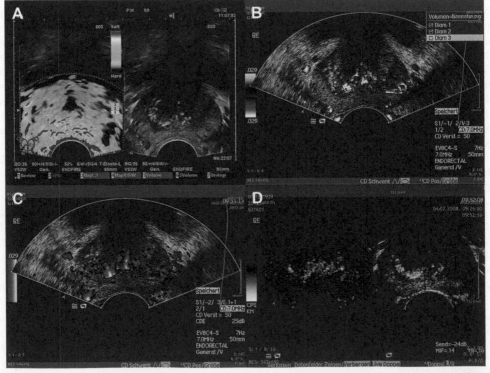

Fig. 2. Detection of a tumor located at the peripheral zone of the left prostate lobe by TRUS using different technologies in the same patient. Elastography (*A*), color Doppler (*B*), power Doppler (*C*), and contrast enhancement (cadence contrast-pulse sequence technology) (*D*). (*Courtesy of* F. Frauscher, MD, Innsbruck, Austria.)

are promising.[6–17] These studies can be schematically divided into two conceptually overlapping categories. The first category is studies based on images (no targeted biopsies obtained) to evaluate the technique as a diagnostic tool for PCa detection.[7–11,14,15,17] Most of these studies showed that elastography improved the detection rate of PCa, and the detection increased with higher Gleason scores. Detailed results are displayed in **Table 1**. The second category is studies based on elastography-targeted biopsy results to evaluate the method as a tool to support or replace TRUS-guided systematic random biopsy.[6,12,13,16]

Table 1
Evaluation of elasticity imaging role in the detection of prostate cancer

Reference	Patients (PCa)	Reference Standard	E Compared with	Main Study Results
Taylor et al, 2005[7,a]	19	RPS	3D-US	3D-E has a better diagnostic performance for PCa tumors ≥ 1 cm^3
Miyanaga et al, 2006[8]	29[b]	Biopsy	TRUS/DRE	Detection rates: E (93%),[c] TRUS 55%, DRE (59%) Two patients missed had well-differentiated PCa
	11[d]			Detection rates: E (55%), TRUS (55%), DRE (64%) in previously treated patients
Pallwein et al, 2007[9]	15	RPS	—	92% diagnostic accuracy, 80% overall sensitivity (100% at apex)
Tsutsumi et al, 2007[10]	51	RPS	TRUS	Detection rates: E (84%),[c] TRUS (31%); detection rate increases to 100% if modalities are combined Anterior tumors: excellent detection; for higher grade tumors, the detection rate is lower
Sumura et al, 2007[11]	17	RPS	TRUS/DRE CD/MRI	Detection rates: E (74.1%),[c] TRUS (48.1%), DRE (33.3%), CD (55.6%), MRI (47.4%) No difference in detection rates for anterior-posterior sides but higher for higher Gleason scores or tumor volumes
Pallwein et al, 2008[14]	492	Biopsy	—	87% sensitivity, 72% specificity (best at apex); good correlation with systematic biopsy results
Salomon et al, 2008[15]	109	RPS	—	75% sensitivity, 77% specificity, 76% accuracy; E findings correlate best at apex Higher detection rates for higher Gleason score (up to 93% for scores >7)
Eggert et al, 2008[17,e]	351	Biopsy	TRUS	E predicted histopathologic findings in only 44.5% of the cases; E does not improve detection rate

Abbreviations: CD, color Doppler; DRE, digital rectal examination; E, elastography; PCa, prostate cancer; RPS, radical prostatectomy specimens; TRUS, conventional transrectal ultrasound; US, gray-scale ultrasonography.
[a] Imaging performed in vitro.
[b] Previously untreated patients.
[c] Elastography superior to other modalities.
[d] Patients treated previously with hormone therapy. Elastography detection rate dropped, possibly attributable to softer rendered consistency of lesion by treatment.
[e] Randomized clinical trial in which both arms have been submitted to conventional TRUS-guided 10-core biopsy. One arm has additionally offered elastography before biopsy.

König and colleagues[6] evaluated 404 men with elastography in addition to a conventional TRUS-guided systematic sextant biopsy protocol. It was concluded that the sensitivity using this technique in conjunction with conventional diagnostic methods for guided biopsies is high (84.1% versus 64.2%). Elastography-targeted prostate biopsy was directly compared with systematic biopsy guided by conventional gray-scale TRUS in 230 screening volunteers.[12] The detection rate of patients who had PCa did not differ significantly between targeted and systematic biopsies (30% versus 25%, respectively). Detection rates per core differed significantly (targeted versus systematic: 12.7% versus 5.6%), however. A patient who has PCa was found to have a 2.9-fold higher probability of being detected by targeted compared with systematic biopsy.[12]

To compare the detection rate of PCa and the distribution of Gleason scores, targeted biopsies based on conventional TRUS, color Doppler (CD) US, and elastography were obtained, along with systematic sextant biopsies, in 137 patients.[13] The detection rate was higher for targeted than systematic cores, and positive results on CD-US and elastography were strongly associated with high-grade and moderate- to high-grade cancers, respectively. It was concluded that although CD-US and elastography may enhance PCa detection, a targeted biopsy protocol alone is not sufficient to replace the conventional sextant biopsy protocol.[13]

Kamoi and colleagues[16] compared the performance of elastography with conventional TRUS and power Doppler (PD) US in PCa detection by evaluating a clinical population of 107 men. TRUS sensitivity was significantly lower (50%) than that of PD-US (70%) or elastography (68%), whereas the accuracy was comparable among these modalities, ranging from 72% (TRUS) to 76% (elastography). Core analysis revealed a significantly lower detection rate for systematic biopsies compared with the combination of PD-US-elastography, however. It was concluded that elastography may complement conventional US to minimize the number of cancers missed.[16]

In conclusion, based on the available results, it seems that transrectal elasticity imaging allows for targeted prostate biopsies and may reduce the number of needed cores to detect cancer. Nevertheless, further clinical trials are still necessary to define the advantages and the exact role of this relatively novel technique better in the diagnosis of PCa.[18]

Contrast-Enhanced Ultrasonography

Microbubble-based contrast agents visualized with novel "contrast-specific" imaging modes represent a revolution in ultrasound. Contrast agents may facilitate the detection of PCa (**Fig. 3**), providing additional information on tumor size or aggressiveness, in addition to the monitoring of antiangiogenic treatment results, because of the increased vascularization of PCa, which can be visualized with CE-US.[19] An example of the depiction of a prostate tumor with the use CD-US, PD-US, and cadence contrast-pulse sequence (CPS) in the same patient is presented in **Fig. 2**B through D, respectively.

To determine the role of CE-US in PCa detection, localization, and treatment follow-up, a multicenter research coordination project has been conducted in four European countries during the period 2002 through 2006 (CONTRAST, QLRT-2001-2174). Recently, the results based on 3746 patients have been reported in comparison to published data outside this research group.[20] The individual studies of the project used various contrast agents imaged by CD-US,[21–26] 3D-PD-US,[27–30] and novel nonlinear imaging techniques (CPS).[31]

The correlation of histologic findings in radical prostatectomy specimens with preoperative CE-US images regarding tumor localization is promising. It seems that technical improvements have increased sensitivity for the detection of perfusion patterns. Lesions with increased microvascular density may be visualized with 3D-CE-PD-US[29] and CE-CD-US.[32] It has been reported that 3D-CE-PD-US is a superior diagnostic tool compared with digital rectal examination, prostate-specific antigen (PSA), and gray-scale US or PD-US and that the most suitable diagnostic predictor for PCa is the combination of 3D-CE-PD-US and PSA.[27] Despite improving sensitivity for PCa detection, CE-US may also demonstrate focal enhancement in areas of benign hyperplasia.[33] Nevertheless, accurate detection of localized tumors with 3D-CE-PD-US has been reported in up to 78% of patients.[30,34] In a study including 70 patients evaluated with the same technique, diagnosis by imaging alone has been improved from 61% with standard investigations to an average of 86% of tumors, with detection of foci 5 mm or greater in 68% to 79%.[35] In another small series, all T3 tumors could be identified using microvascular imaging.[20]

The clinical value of these initial results should be tested in a diagnostic setting. The effect of CE-US on the prostate biopsy protocols regarding the detection rate has been extensively investigated. The combined European research project demonstrated a clear association between prostate contrast enhancement and diagnosis of clinically significant PCa. The sensitivity is increased with the use of CE-US targeted biopsies; fewer

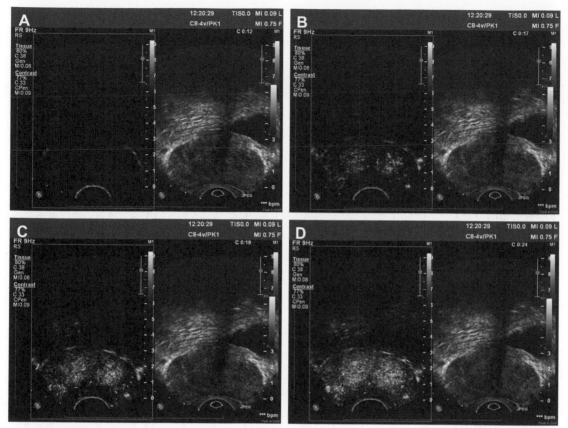

Fig. 3. CE-US of the prostate: contrast-only (*left*) and tissue-only (*right*) images are presented. (*A*) Enhancement is shown as a function of time. There is still no contrast in the prostate 12 seconds after the injection. (*B*) First (early) enhancement 17 seconds after the injection. Enhancement 19 seconds after the injection (*C*) and 23 seconds after the injection (*D*). (*C, D*) Suspicious lesion is seen on the right lobe at the peripheral zone.

biopsies are needed to obtain the same detection rate, and the tumors detected have a higher Gleason score than those detected by random biopsies.[20]

These findings are in agreement with the results from studies outside the European research project. Using various CE-US methods, including novel nonlinear imaging techniques (intermittent harmonic imaging, flash replenishment, and CPS), these studies directly compared gray-scale TRUS-guided systems with CE-US–targeted biopsy protocols (**Table 2**)[36–39] or investigated the contribution of CE-US on the systematic biopsy protocols[40–43] and its value in predicting the nature of hypoechoic lesions.[44–46]

Currently, CE-US enables visualization of PCa, and targeted biopsies applied on a random protocol do increase the detection rate. Sensitivity and specificity are still not sufficient to avoid systematic random biopsies, however. Therefore, the application of CE-US in routine clinical practice has not yet been established.

ADVANCES IN TREATMENT AND FOLLOW-UP OF PROSTATE CANCER

Apart from a possible role in the diagnosis of PCa, elasticity imaging techniques may monitor high-intensity focused ultrasound (HIFU) results in PCa, because HIFU-ablated lesions are stiffer than the surrounding normal untreated tissue. Promising results have recently been published, but further clinical trials are needed before this application can be considered established.[47,48]

CE-US might also enable visualization of the effects of minimal invasive or medical treatments that influence the perfusion of the organ (eg, HIFU/cryoablation, hormone therapy) and identify early PCa relapses indicated by the absence of blood signal.[49]

In patients undergoing HIFU before radical prostatectomy, it has been shown that the absence of blood flow indicated by 3D-CE-PD-US reflects ablated lesions and that volume measurements of these areas can quantify the amount of the

Table 2
Diagnostic performance of contrast-enhanced targeted compared with systematic gray-scale ultrasound-guided biopsies of the prostate

Reference	Patient Analysis PCa (%)				TB Versus SB P Value	Biopsy Core Analysis		PCa (%)			TB Versus SB		CE-US Imaging Technique
	Total	TB	SB	TB + SB		Total	TB	Total	TB	SB	OR (95% CI)	P Value	
European research coordination project													
Frauscher et al, 2002[21]	230	24.4	22.6	30.0	ns	3439	1139	7.0	10.4	5.3	2.6 (1.9–3.5)	<0.001	CD
Pelzer et al, 2005[23]	380	27.4	27.6	37.6	ns	5700	1900	8.6	32.6[a]	17.9[a]	3.1 (na)	<0.01	CD
Mitterberger et al, 2007[24,b]	690	26.1	24.1	32.0	ns	10,317	3417	7.6	11.1	5.8	na	<0.001	CD
Mitterberger et al, 2007[25,c]	100	32.0	26.0	29.0	0.04	750	250	9.7	15.6	6.8	—	<0.001	CD
Mitterberger et al, 2008[26,d]	36	33.3	16.7	33.3	0.04	540	180	12.2	17.0	10.0	2 (na)	0.027	CD
Pallwein et al, 2008[31]	20	40.0	25.0	40.0	ns	na	na	na	na	na	na	na	CPS
Frauscher et al, 2001[36]	84	27.4	20.2	28.6	0.034	1249	409	7.7	13.4	4.9	4.3 (2.6–7.1)	<0.001	CD
Halpern et al, 2005[37,e]	301	27.6	30.9	34.6	ns	2939	1133	363	15.4	10.4	2.0 (na)	<0.001	CD/PD/CHI/IHI
Linden et al, 2007[38]	60	21.7	26.7	30	ns	825	225	9.6	12.9	8.3	2.0 (na)	0.034	MFI
Colleselli et al, 2007[39]	345	77.4	73.0	na	ns[f]	5175	1725	—	—	—	—	—	CD

Abbreviations: CHI, continues harmonic imaging; CI, confidence interval; IHI, intermittent harmonic imaging; MFI, MicroFlow imaging (flash replenishment method); na, not available; ns, not significant; OR, odds ratio; SB, systematic biopsy; TB, targeted biopsy.

a Detection rate based on number of positive cores per total number of cores in the 143 men with PCa detected by the combined approach.
b Impact on Gleason score was studied: TB detected significantly higher Gleason scores compared with SB and may allow for identification of more aggressive tumors.
c Only randomized clinical trial to date. Two arms of 50 men underwent systematic or CE-targeted biopsies of the prostate.
d Short-term (14 days) application of dutasteride may be promising to improve cancer detection by CE- targeted US-guided biopsies because of blood flow reduction in benign prostatic tissue.
e IHI provides a statistically significant advantage over gray-scale and Doppler imaging but not over CHI. It significantly improves the characterization of tissue as benign versus malignant and may therefore improve PCa detection, but the technique is not sufficient to differentiate benign from malignant tissue definitely without biopsy confirmation.
f Statistically significant difference in PCa detection rate in favor of CE-US was detected only in small prostate glands (69% versus 88.1% and 70.4% versus 80.8% for prostate volumes of <20 mL and 20–30 mL, respectively).

affected tissue.[28] A study investigating the prediction of HIFU-induced destruction uniformity has shown that pretreatment evaluation cannot identify the nonresponders beforehand, however.[50] Thirty-five patients who had PCa underwent pre- and postcontrast CD-US of the prostate before HIFU treatment. Tissue destruction seen in post-treatment random biopsies did not correlate with the preoperative TRUS findings.[50]

Another potential application of CE-US is to monitor hormonal treatment in PCa. Vascular enhancement of the carcinoma, detected by CD-US and PD-US after the administration of a contrast agent, has been reported to decline with hormonal therapy similar to PSA levels.[22]

ADVANCES IN DIAGNOSIS OF RENAL TUMORS

US contrast agents can play an important role in differentiating solid lesions (**Fig. 4**) and in the characterization of complex cystic masses (**Table 3**). Tamai and colleagues[51] evaluated the usefulness of CE-US in the diagnosis of solid renal tumors in comparison to CT. They found that CE-US was more sensitive for detecting slight tumor blood flow and was helpful in diagnosing malignant hypovascular renal tumors. Recently, CE-CD imaging has been shown to achieve better results than unenhanced CD imaging for detecting tumor vascularity and discriminating benign and malignant small renal masses.[52] Ascenti and colleagues[53] compared CE-US with triple-phase helical CT scanning in the classification of complex renal cysts using the Bosniak system and found complete concordance in the differentiation of surgical and nonsurgical complex cysts, with a high interobserver agreement. In a similar study comparing CE-US with CT, Park and colleagues[54] found that CE-US might better visualize septa number, septa or wall thickness, solid

components, and the enhancement of some renal cystic masses than CT, resulting in upgrading of the Bosniak classification and a change in the patient's treatment plan. Quaia and colleagues[55] used an independent diagnostic classification system for CE-US based on the enhancement patterns involving or not involving the peripheral wall, intracystic septa, and mural or septal nodules. The overall accuracy of CE-US was better than that of unenhanced sonography and CT in the diagnosis of malignancy in complex cystic renal masses.

Recently, CPS imaging that is based on the characteristics of nonlinear bubble behavior has been introduced in the diagnosis of renal masses. This technique constructs images by transmitting a series of pulses with different amplitudes and phases and enables distinction between the nonlinear signals reflected by the contrast agent and the linear responses of the tissue. This makes simultaneous viewing of tissue-only and contrast-only images possible. A pilot study investigated the characteristics of perfusion imaging of renal tumors with CPS and compared them with clinical diagnosis and histologic findings when available.[56] It was concluded that CPS may have a future role in determining perfusion patterns in kidney tumors. Pallwein and colleagues[57] evaluated CE-US using CPS technology for the diagnosis of small renal masses (<4 cm) and found that CE-US using CPS had a similar diagnostic accuracy as multidetector CT scanning in renal masses between 2 and 4 cm, whereas in lesions smaller than 2 cm, CE-US was even superior.

The use of elastography in the imaging of renal masses has been applied in vivo recently. Fahey and colleagues[58] investigated the use of acoustic radiation force impulse (ARFI) imaging for real-time visualization of abdominal malignancies, including renal masses. These first human images of abdominal malignancies acquired in vivo using

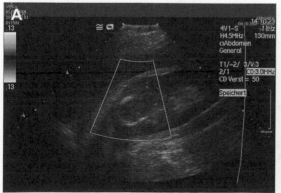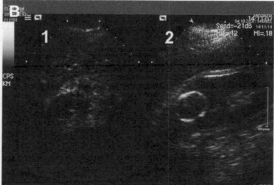

Fig. 4. Case of papillary renal cell carcinoma is presented. CD-US is negative (*A*), but CE-US shows contrast uptake within the tumor (*B*). (*Courtesy of* F. Frauscher, MD, Innsbruck, Austria.)

Table 3
Studies evaluating the role of ultrasound contrast agents in differentiating solid and complex cystic masses of the kidney

Reference	Patients	Lesions	Reference Standard	Histology Type		Diagnostic Modalities Compared	Main Results
				Malignant	Benign		
Tamai et al, 2005[51]	29	Solid masses	Resection of tumors	26	3	CE-US CCT	PPV in diagnosis of malignant tumors: CE-US (100%), CT (82.8%)
Park et al, 2007[54]	31	Cystic masses	Nephrectomies or biopsy	28	3	CE-US CT	Diagnostic accuracy for malignant tumor: CE-US (94%), CT (74%)
Pallwein et al, 2007[52]	51	Solid masses	Nephrectomies	35	16	ECDI UCDI	Sensitivity for malignancy: ECDI (83%), UCDI (46%) PPV: ECDI (81%), UCDI (70%), Specificity of both modalities (56%)
Quaia et al, 2008[55]	40	Cystic masses	Resection or follow-up imaging	21	19	CE-US UUS	Overall diagnostic accuracy[a]: CE-US (83%, 83%, 80%) UUS (30%, 30%, 30%), HCT (75%, 63%, 70%)

Abbreviations: CCT, contrast computed tomography; CDI, color Doppler imaging; ECDI, enhanced color Doppler imaging; HCT, helical computed tomography; UCDI, unenhanced color Doppler imaging; UUS, unenhanced ultrasonography; PPV, positive predictive value; UCDI, unenhanced color Doppler imaging; UUS, unenhanced ultrasonography.
[a] Three readers.

the ARFI method, or any other elasticity imaging technique, established the feasibility of visualizing liver and kidney malignancies and suggested that the ARFI method can provide improvements in boundary definition and contrast of tissue masses relative to the use of US alone.

ADVANCES IN TREATMENT OF RENAL TUMORS

Percutaneous ablative techniques for the treatment of renal cell carcinoma have been developed requiring an image-guided technique for the precise placement of the needles. Recently, the use of real-time virtual sonography (RVS) has been described. RVS is a novel technology that displays simultaneously the images of real-time US with the corresponding CT or MRI multiplanar views from a stored volume data set. Initial data showed that RVS seems to be a promising imaging method alternative to CT or MRI that provides excellent anatomic orientation and navigation for percutaneous radiofrequency ablation (RFA) of solid renal cell carcinomas with less radiation exposure.[59]

Pareek and colleagues[60] investigated the feasibility of elastography imaging during RFA in porcine kidneys by monitoring phase changes in the echo signals caused by variations in speed of sound and thermal expansion with temperature. A significant correlation between elastographic estimations of the area and volume of the thermal lesions and gross pathologic measurements was found. These results suggest that elastography may prove a reliable method for monitoring the zone of RFA of renal lesions, overcoming the inaccuracy of the current imaging modalities to provide real-time monitoring and resulting in improving the efficacy of RFA.[60]

ADVANCES IN FOLLOW-UP OF RENAL TUMORS

With the increasing use of ablation techniques for the management of small renal masses, urologists face the problem of optimal monitoring of the ablated tumors. Because success is defined as absence of contrast enhancement, US with the use of contrast agents may play a role in follow-up, resulting in reduction of radiation exposure, contrast toxicity, and costs after an ablative treatment. Indeed, CE-US has shown potential in monitoring RFA of tumors in animal models.[61] In addition, Wink and colleagues[62] demonstrated that CE-US based on CPS technology can be used to characterize perfusion defects at different times in the follow-up period after cryoablation (**Fig. 5**).

ADVANCES IN OTHER ORGANS
Bladder

Mitterberger and colleagues[63] compared 3D-US versus 2D-US of the bladder for the evaluation of patients who have hematuria. They found that 3D-US yielded an overall correct diagnosis in 86% of the cases, providing better diagnostic features than 2D-US, with 100% sensitivity for malignant bladder lesions and 71% sensitivity for benign bladder changes. In a similar study, Kocakoc and colleagues[64] evaluated the potential value of 3D-US and sonographic cystoscopy in the detection of bladder tumors. They found that 3D

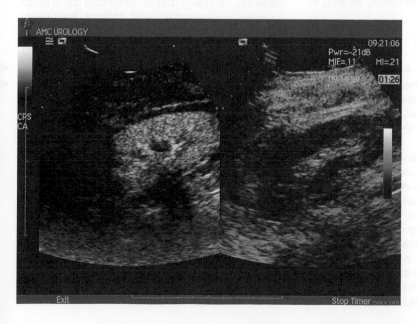

Fig. 5. CE-US 2 weeks after cryoablation of the kidney based on CPS technology (*left*) and conventional B-mode imaging (*right*). The perfusion defect after cryoablation of the renal tumor is more clearly depicted by CE-US.

virtual sonography had a sensitivity of 96.2%, specificity of 70.6%, positive predictive value of 93.9%, and negative predictive value of 80% for tumor detection. The combination of gray-scale sonography, multiplanar reconstruction, and 3D virtual sonography improved the diagnostic accuracy by increasing the sensitivity to 96.4%, specificity to 88.8%, positive predictive value to 97.6%, and negative predictive value to 84.2%.[64]

Testis

A minimally invasive technique for the treatment of testicular tumors in a solitary testis using HIFU therapy (eg, after surgical removal of the contralateral testis for a previous testicular tumor) has been described. Kratzik and colleagues[65] presented their long-term results of a phase II trial and reported that transcutaneous HIFU followed by prophylactic irradiation permits a minimally invasive, organ-preserving, curative treatment for tumors in a solitary testis.

The term *sonodynamic therapy* is often used for all non–thermal-related therapeutic US applications. In recent years, US-targeted microbubble destruction has evolved into a new tool for organ-specific gene and drug delivery. The incorporation, and subsequent destruction, of the bioactive substances of the microbubble shells in the target organ by US has been used to deliver plasmid DNA into cells.[66] The feasibility of delivering proteins to the extracellular tissue of testis has been evaluated by Bekeredjian and colleagues.[67] They found that US-targeted microbubble destruction is a feasible method for delivery of bioactive substances even in organs with moderate to low blood perfusion, as long as they are accessible to US.

FUTURE APPLICATIONS

More sophisticated potential applications of CE-US regarding diagnosis and treatment at a cellular level are emerging, such as molecular imaging and sonoporation, representing an exciting field of urologic research, and this is likely to be the next frontier that is reached.[19]

Molecular imaging views and quantifies early changes associated with diseases at a molecular level rather than the resulting morphologic changes. The superior sensitivity of "contrast-specific" imaging modes may render CE-US an ideal tool for molecular imaging of the vascular compartment. Efforts have recently been made in the design and preparation of specific ligands bound to the phospholipid-stabilized shell of the microbubbles. This should result in specific localization of the targeted bubbles on selected vascular receptors up-regulated in certain pathologic conditions, such as neoangiogenesis. They should then potentially serve as molecular targets for diagnosis or as therapeutic agents.

Sonoporation is a physical method that increases cell permeability with acoustic cavitation caused by US in the presence of contrast agents. One of the mechanisms is cavitation, which causes the implosion of microbubbles to generate microjets, which open transmembrane pores, allowing direct intracytoplasmic transfer of drugs or genetic material. Cell viability is preserved, because pore opening is reversible and transient with a duration of a few seconds.[68] Cell transfection is influenced by the properties of gas and the shell properties of the contrast agents.[69] Hard-shelled microbubbles (gas microcapsules) are promising candidates for US-mediated gene delivery.[70]

Recently, it has been shown that PCa cells can be transfected by means of microbubble-enhanced US with short antisense oligodeoxynucleotides that decrease the expression of the androgen receptor.[71] Intratumoral delivery of DNA-Optison, followed by therapeutic US, has been proposed as an effective nontoxic gene delivery method in PCa.[72] Delivery, for example, of angiogenic inhibitors by this method seems to be feasible.[73]

SUMMARY

Recent technologic developments in US seem to be promising and offer novel and great potential in numerous fields of management of the urologic patients, including better diagnosis of urologic cancers, implementation of ablative treatments, and improved monitoring of treatment response. Most of these techniques are still under investigation, depend on the operator, and require increased experience to guarantee the translation of imaging findings to clinical practice, however.

ACKNOWLEDGMENTS

The authors thank Advanced Medical Diagnostics SA, Waterloo, Belgium for supplying the images in **Fig. 1**. The authors thank Dr. F. Frauscher, Department of Radiology, Medical University Innsbruck, Innsbruck, Austria, for supplying the images in **Figs. 2** and **4**. C. Mamoulakis thanks the Alexander S. Onassis Public Benefit Foundation for a grant offered to attend a clinical fellowship program at the Academic Medical Center University Hospital, Department of Urology, University of Amsterdam, The Netherlands.

REFERENCES

1. Singer EA, Golijanin DJ, Davis RS, et al. What's new in urologic ultrasound? Urol Clin North Am 2006;33: 279–86.
2. Mehta SS, Azzouzi AR, Hamdy FC. Three dimensional ultrasound and prostate cancer. World J Urol 2004;22:339–45.
3. Mitterberger M, Pinggera GM, Pallwein L, et al. The value of three-dimensional transrectal ultrasonography in staging prostate cancer. BJU Int 2007; 100:47–50.
4. Zalesky M, Urban M, Smerhovský Z, et al. Value of power Doppler sonography with 3D reconstruction in preoperative diagnostics of extraprostatic tumor extension in clinically localized prostate cancer. Int J Urol 2008;15:68–75.
5. Braeckman J, Autier P, Garbar C, et al. Computer-aided ultrasonography (HistoScanning): a novel technology for locating and characterizing prostate cancer. BJU Int 2008;101:293–8.
6. König K, Scheipers U, Pesavento A, et al. Initial experiences with real-time elastography guided biopsies of the prostate. J Urol 2005;174:115–7.
7. Taylor LS, Rubens DJ, Porter BC, et al. Prostate cancer: three-dimensional sonoelastography for in vitro detection. Radiology 2005;237:981–5.
8. Miyanaga N, Akaza H, Yamakawa M, et al. Tissue elasticity imaging for diagnosis of prostate cancer: a preliminary report. Int J Urol 2006;13:1514–8.
9. Pallwein L, Mitterberger M, Struve P, et al. Real-time elastography for detecting prostate cancer: preliminary experience. BJU Int 2007;100:42–6.
10. Tsutsumi M, Miyagawa T, Matsumura T, et al. The impact of real-time tissue elasticity imaging (elastography) on the detection of prostate cancer: clinicopathological analysis. Int J Clin Oncol 2007;12:250–5.
11. Sumura M, Shigeno K, Hyuga T, et al. Initial evaluation of prostate cancer with real-time elastography based on step-section pathologic analysis after radical prostatectomy: a preliminary study. Int J Urol 2007;14:811–6.
12. Pallwein L, Mitterberger M, Struve P, et al. Comparison of sonoelastography guided biopsy with systematic biopsy: impact on prostate cancer detection. Eur Radiol 2007;17:2278–85.
13. Nelson ED, Slotoroff CB, Gomella LG, et al. Targeted biopsy of the prostate: the impact of color Doppler imaging and elastography on prostate cancer detection and Gleason score. Urology 2007;70:1136–40.
14. Pallwein L, Mitterberger M, Pinggera G, et al. Sonoelastography of the prostate: comparison with systematic biopsy findings in 492 patients. Eur J Radiol 2008;65:304–10.
15. Salomon G, Köllerman J, Thederan I, et al. Evaluation of prostate cancer detection with ultrasound real-time elastography: a comparison with step section pathological analysis after radical prostatectomy. Eur Urol 2008;54:1354–62.
16. Kamoi K, Okihara K, Ochiai A, et al. The utility of transrectal real-time elastography in the diagnosis of prostate cancer. Ultrasound Med Biol 2008;34: 1025–32.
17. Eggert T, Khaled W, Wenske S, et al. Impact of elastography in clinical diagnosis of prostate cancer: a comparison of cancer detection between B-mode sonography and elastography-guided 10-core biopsies. Urologe A 2008;47:1212–7.
18. Pallwein L, Aigner F, Faschingbauer R, et al. Prostate cancer diagnosis: value of real-time elastography. Abdom Imaging 2008;33:729–35.
19. Schneider M. Molecular imaging and ultrasound-assisted drug delivery. J Endourol 2008;22:795–802.
20. Wink M, Frauscher F, Cosgrove D, et al. Contrast-enhanced ultrasound and prostate cancer; a multi-centre European research coordination project. Eur Urol 2008;54:982–92.
21. Frauscher F, Klauser A, Volgger H, et al. Comparison of contrast enhanced color Doppler targeted biopsy with conventional systematic biopsy: impact on prostate cancer detection. J Urol 2002;167: 1648–52.
22. Eckersley RJ, Sedelaar JP, Blomley MJ, et al. Quantitative microbubble enhanced transrectal ultrasound as a tool for monitoring hormonal treatment of prostate carcinoma. Prostate 2002;51:256–67.
23. Pelzer A, Bektic J, Berger AP, et al. Prostate cancer detection in men with prostate specific antigen 4 to 10 ng/ml using a combined approach of contrast enhanced color Doppler targeted and systematic biopsy. J Urol 2005;173:1926–9.
24. Mitterberger M, Pinggera GM, Horninger W, et al. Comparison of contrast enhanced color Doppler targeted biopsy to conventional systematic biopsy: impact on Gleason score. J Urol 2007;178:464–8.
25. Mitterberger M, Horninger W, Pelzer A, et al. A prospective randomized trial comparing contrast-enhanced targeted versus systematic ultrasound guided biopsies: impact on prostate cancer detection. Prostate 2007;67:1537–42.
26. Mitterberger M, Pinggera G, Horninger W, et al. Dutasteride prior to contrast-enhanced colour Doppler ultrasound prostate biopsy increases prostate cancer detection. Eur Urol 2008;53:112–7.
27. Unal D, Sedelaar JP, Aarnink RG, et al. Three-dimensional contrast-enhanced power Doppler ultrasonography and conventional examination methods: the value of diagnostic predictors of prostate cancer. BJU Int 2000;86:58–64.
28. Sedelaar JP, Aarnink RG, van Leenders GJ, et al. The application of three-dimensional contrast-enhanced ultrasound to measure volume of affected tissue after HIFU treatment for localized prostate cancer. Eur Urol 2000;37:559–68.

29. Sedelaar JP, van Leenders GJ, Hulsbergen-van de Kaa CA, et al. Microvessel density: correlation between contrast ultrasonography and histology of prostate cancer. Eur Urol 2001;40:285–93.

30. Goossen TE, de la Rosette JJ, Hulsbergen-van de Kaa CA, et al. The value of dynamic contrast enhanced power Doppler ultrasound imaging in the localization of prostate cancer. Eur Urol 2003; 43:124–31.

31. Pallwein L, Mitterberger M, Pelzer A, et al. Ultrasound of prostate cancer: recent advances. Eur Radiol 2008;18:707–15.

32. Strohmeyer D, Frauscher F, Klauser A, et al. Contrast-enhanced transrectal color Doppler ultrasonography (TRCDUS) for assessment of angiogenesis in prostate cancer. Anticancer Res 2001;21: 2907–13.

33. Halpern EJ, McCue PA, Aksnes AK, et al. Contrast-enhanced US of the prostate with Sonazoid: comparison with whole-mount prostatectomy specimens in 12 patients. Radiology 2002;222: 361–6.

34. van Moerkerk H, Heijmink SW, Kaa CA, et al. Computerized three-dimensional localization of prostate cancer using contrast-enhanced power Doppler and clustering analysis. Eur Urol 2006;50: 762–8.

35. Sedelaar JP, van Leenders GJ, Goossen TE, et al. Value of contrast ultrasonography in the detection of significant prostate cancer: correlation with radical prostatectomy specimens. Prostate 2002; 53:246–53.

36. Frauscher F, Klauser A, Halpern EJ, et al. Detection of prostate cancer with a microbubble ultrasound contrast agent. Lancet 2001;357:1849–50.

37. Halpern EJ, Ramey JR, Strup SE, et al. Detection of prostate carcinoma with contrast-enhanced sonography using intermittent harmonic imaging. Cancer 2005;104:2373–83.

38. Linden RA, Trabulsi EJ, Forsberg F, et al. Contrast enhanced ultrasound flash replenishment method for directed prostate biopsies. J Urol 2007;178: 2354–8.

39. Colleselli D, Bektic J, Schaefer G, et al. The influence of prostate volume on prostate cancer detection using a combined approach of contrast-enhanced ultrasonography-targeted and systematic grey-scale biopsy. BJU Int 2007;100:1264–7.

40. Halpern EJ, Rosenberg M, Gomella LG. Prostate cancer: contrast-enhanced us for detection. Radiology 2001;219:219–25.

41. Halpern EJ, Frauscher F, Rosenberg M, et al. Directed biopsy during contrast-enhanced sonography of the prostate. Am J Roentgenol 2002;178: 915–9.

42. Roy C, Buy X, Lang H, et al. Contrast enhanced color Doppler endorectal sonography of prostate: efficiency for detecting peripheral zone tumors and role for biopsy procedure. J Urol 2003;170:69–72.

43. Taymoorian K, Thomas A, Slowinski T, et al. Transrectal broadband-Doppler sonography with intravenous contrast medium administration for prostate imaging and biopsy in men with an elevated PSA value and previous negative biopsies. Anticancer Res 2007;27:4315–20.

44. Tang J, Yang JC, Li Y, et al. Peripheral zone hypoechoic lesions of the prostate: evaluation with contrast-enhanced gray scale transrectal ultrasonography. J Ultrasound Med 2007;26:1671–9.

45. Tang J, Yang JC, Luo Y, et al. Enhancement characteristics of benign and malignant focal peripheral nodules in the peripheral zone of the prostate gland studied using contrast enhanced transrectal ultrasound. Clin Radiol 2008;63:1086–91.

46. Yang JC, Tang J, Li Y, et al. Contrast-enhanced transrectal ultrasound for assessing vascularization of hypoechoic BPH nodules in the transition and peripheral zones: comparison with pathological examination. Ultrasound Med Biol 2008;34:1758–64.

47. Souchon R, Rouvière O, Gelet A, et al. Visualisation of HIFU lesions using elastography of the human prostate in vivo: preliminary results. Ultrasound Med Biol 2003;29:1007–15.

48. Curiel L, Souchon R, Rouvière O, et al. Elastography for the follow-up of high-intensity focused ultrasound prostate cancer treatment: initial comparison with MRI. Ultrasound Med Biol 2005;31:1461–8.

49. Wondergem N, De La Rosette JJ. HIFU and cryoablation-non or minimal touch techniques for the treatment of prostate cancer. Is there a role for contrast enhanced ultrasound? Minim Invasive Ther Allied Technol 2007;16:22–30.

50. Rouvière O, Curiel L, Chapelon JY, et al. Can color Doppler predict the uniformity of HIFU-induced prostate tissue destruction? Prostate 2004;60: 289–97.

51. Tamai H, Tkigushi Y, Oka M, et al. Contrast-enhanced ultrasonography in the diagnosis of solid renal tumors. J Ultrasound Med 2005;24:1635–40.

52. Pallwein L, Mitterberger M, Aigner F, et al. Small renal masses: the value of contrast-enhanced colour Doppler imaging. BJU Int 2007;100:47–50.

53. Ascenti G, Mazzotti S, Zimbaro G, et al. Complex cystic renal masses: characterization with contrast-enhanced US. Radiology 2007;243:158–65.

54. Park BK, Kim B, Kim SH, et al. Assessment of cystic renal masses based on Bosniak classification: comparison of CT and contrast-enhanced US. Eur J Radiol 2007;61:310–4.

55. Quaia E, Bertolotto M, Cioffi V, et al. Comparison of contrast-enhanced sonography with unenhanced sonography and contrast-enhanced CT in the diagnosis of malignancy in complex cystic renal masses. Am J Roentgenol 2008;191:1239–49.

56. Wink MH, de la Rosette JJ, Laguna P, et al. Ultrasonography of renal masses using contrast pulse sequence imaging: a pilot study. J Endourol 2007; 21:466–72.

57. Pallwein L, Mitterberger M, Gradl J, et al. Diagnostic evaluation of small renal masses: value of contrast-enhanced US in comparison to multidetector CT. J Urol 2008;179(Suppl 4):331 [abstract 960].

58. Fahey BJ, Nelson RC, Bradway DP, et al. In vivo visualization of abdominal malignancies with acoustic radiation force elastography. Phys Med Biol 2008;53:279–93.

59. Ukimura O, Mitterberger M, Okihara K, et al. Real-time virtual ultrasonography radiofrequency ablation of renal cell carcinoma. BJU Int 2008;101:707–11.

60. Pareek G, Wilkinson ER, Bharat S, et al. Elastography measurements of in-vivo radiofrequency ablation lesions of the kidney. J Endourol 2006;20:959–64.

61. Slabaugh TK, Machaidze Z, Hennigar R, et al. Monitoring radiofrequency renal lesions in real time using contrast-enhanced ultrasonography: a porcine model. J Endourol 2005;19:579–83.

62. Wink MH, Laguna MP, Lagerveld BW, et al. Contrast-enhanced ultrasonography in the follow-up of cryoablation of renal tumors: a feasibility study. BJU Int 2007;99:1371–5.

63. Mitterberger M, Pinggera GM, Neuwirt H, et al. Three-dimensional ultrasonography of the urinary bladder: preliminary experience of assessment in patients with haematuria. BJU Int 2007;99:111–6.

64. Kocakoc E, Kiris A, Orhan I, et al. Detection of bladder tumors with 3-dimensional sonography and virtual sonographic cystoscopy. J Ultrasound Med 2008;27:45–53.

65. Kratzik C, Schatzl G, Lackner J, et al. Transcutaneous high-intensity focused ultrasonography can cure testicular cancer in solitary testis. Urology 2006;67:1269–73.

66. Bekeredjian R, Chen S, Frenkel P, et al. Ultrasound targeted microbubble destruction can repeatedly direct highly specific plasmid expression to the heart. Circulation 2003;108:1022–6.

67. Bekeredjian R, Kuecherer HF, Kroll RD, et al. Ultrasound-targeted microbubble destruction augments protein delivery into testes. Urology 2007;69:386–9.

68. Mehier-Humbert S, Bettinger T, Yan F, et al. Plasma membrane poration induced by ultrasound exposure: implication for drug delivery. J Control Release 2005;104:213–22.

69. Watanabe A, Otake R, Nozaki T, et al. Effects of microbubbles on ultrasound-mediated gene transfer in human prostate cancer PC3 cells: comparison among Levovist, YM454, and MRX-815H. Cancer Lett 2008;265:107–12.

70. Mehier-Humbert S, Yan F, Frinking P, et al. Ultrasound-mediated gene delivery: influence of contrast agent on transfection. Bioconjug Chem 2007;18: 652–62.

71. Haag P, Frauscher F, Gradl J, et al. Microbubble-enhanced ultrasound to deliver an antisense oligodeoxynucleotide targeting the human androgen receptor into prostate tumours. J Steroid Biochem Mol Biol 2006;102:103–13.

72. Duvshani-Eshet M, Machluf M. Efficient transfection of tumors facilitated by long-term therapeutic ultrasound in combination with contrast agent: from in vitro to in vivo setting. Cancer Gene Ther 2007;14: 306–15.

73. Duvshani-Eshet M, Benny O, Morgenstern A, et al. Therapeutic ultrasound facilitates antiangiogenic gene delivery and inhibits prostate tumor growth. Mol Cancer Ther 2007;6:2371–82.

Natural Orifice Translumenal Endoscopic Surgery

Wesley M. White, MD[a,*], Georges-Pascal Haber, MD[a],
Mark J. Doerr, MD[b], Matthew Gettman, MD[b]

KEYWORDS

- Laparoscopy • Robotics • Endoscopy • NOTES
- Minimally invasive surgery

Evolution is defined as a process of "change in a certain direction" or 'the process of working out or developing." Conversely, revolution is defined as "a fundamental change in the way of thinking about something...a change in paradigm" Whether natural orifice translumenal endoscopic surgery (NOTES) is best defined as evolutionary or revolutionary is debatable. On its most basic level, NOTES is simply a means of accessing the peritoneal cavity and organs by inserting a flexible endoscopic device through a natural orifice followed by incision through the lumenal wall. In reality, NOTES constitutes a fundamental change in how urologists think about and approach minimally invasive surgery. This conceptual transformation remains a complicated and tedious work in progress because the surgical skill set and dedicated instrumentation required to perform NOTES safely and reproducibly have yet fully to arrive. Regardless, the enthusiasm for NOTES among patients and industry is undeniable and urologists must be prepared to address questions from patients and colleagues regarding the role of NOTES in managing urologic diseases. This article provides a brief history of NOTES, summarizes the salient literature, offers a pragmatic overview of the technical aspects of NOTES, and addresses the inevitable concerns regarding this or any new revolutionary technique.

HISTORY OF NATURAL ORIFICE TRANSLUMENAL ENDOSCOPIC SURGERY

The concept of using a natural orifice for expedient surgical access or specimen extraction is extremely familiar to urologists and gastroenterologists. Indeed, transurethral and peroral diagnostic and therapeutic procedures represent the sine qua non of urology and gastroenterology, respectively. It holds that urologists and gastroenterologists stand at the forefront of NOTES research.

Before Kalloo and coworkers'[1] landmark description of transgastric peritoneoscopy, Breda and colleagues[2] reported removal of an intact tuberculous kidney through a posterior colpotomy to reduce morbidity and pain and improve cosmesis. Nearly a decade later, Gill and colleagues[3] at the Cleveland Clinic detailed the successful transvaginal extraction of intact laparoscopic radical nephrectomy specimens in 10 patients. Although both Gill and Breda performed hybrid procedures (standard laparoscopy was performed to complete the operation after which specimen extraction was performed through a natural orifice), the model of using a natural orifice to improve patient outcomes was established and arguably justified.

In 2002, Gettman and coworkers[4] published his experimental application of natural orifice nephrectomy in the porcine model. Using the transvaginal approach, six laparoscopic

a Section of Laparoscopic and Robotic Urologic Surgery, Glickman Urological and Kidney Institute, Cleveland Clinic, 9500 Euclid Avenue, Q-10, Cleveland, OH 44195, USA
b Department of Urology, Mayo Clinic, 200 First Street SW, Rochester, MN 55905, USA
* Corresponding author.
E-mail address: whitew@ccf.org (W.M. White).

Urol Clin N Am 36 (2009) 147–155
doi:10.1016/j.ucl.2009.02.014
0094-0143/ 09/$ – see front matter © 2009 Elsevier Inc. All rights reserved.

nephrectomies were performed, one of which was completed entirely through the vagina with the remaining five procedures performed with the assistance of a 5-mm laparoscope placed trans-abdominally ("hybrid" natural orifice surgery). Articulating laparoscopic instruments were used to ease technical constraints associated with in-line transvaginal placement. Operative time for the one pure transvaginal nephrectomy was 360 minutes. Mean operative time for the remaining hybrid procedures was 210 minutes. Mean blood loss was 30 mL excluding one catastrophic vascular injury that resulted in exsanguination and death. No additional perioperative complications were noted. The authors concluded that hybrid NOTES nephrectomy was feasible and reproducible in the porcine model but conceded that complete or pure transvaginal nephrectomy was, at that time, compromised by ill-adapted instrumentation and was not yet ready for human application.[4]

Building on the aforementioned studies, Kalloo and colleagues[1] successfully performed trans-gastric peritoneoscopy with or without liver biopsy in the porcine model in 2004. No immediate perioperative complications were noted and all survival animals thrived postoperatively. To address concerns of postgastrotomy bacterial contamination, postsacrifice peritoneal cultures were performed. Results were negative in most animals. The favorable results of this study generated considerable enthusiasm for NOTES and sparked a veritable litany of noncomparative diagnostic and therapeutic animal experiments including cholecystectomy, appendectomy, gastrojejunostomy, tubal ligation, and oophorectomy.[5–12]

Following this abundance of successful animal experiments, a consortium of gastroenterologists and general surgeons was convened to address frankly the benefits and limitations of NOTES. A white paper was generated during this meeting and the consortium was labeled the Natural Orifice Surgery Consortium for Assessment and Research (NOSCAR).[13] The consensus of this collaborative effort was that thoughtful and dedicated innovation is required to drive the field of NOTES forward, that NOTES research must be closely overseen by both local Institutional Review Boards and NOSCAR, and that technical limitations represented the most significant barrier to its safe application in humans.[13,14] In response to, and in accordance with, the recommendations of NOSCAR, additional animal experiments were performed transgastrically, transvaginally, and transvesically, and instrumentation and operating platforms were refined.[15–18]

The first human experience with NOTES was reported by Rao and Reddy in India during which transgastric appendectomy, tubal ligation, and cholecystectomy were performed. Although greater than 20 human NOTES procedures have been performed, this series has not yet been published. Although it remains difficult to accurately catalog all human NOTES procedures performed because of poor or ambiguous reporting, one can reliably state that transgastric, transvaginal, and transvesical peritoneoscopy, transgastric cholecystectomy, appendectomy, liver biopsy, and tubal ligation, and transvaginal appendectomy have all been successfully performed.[19–23]

Germane to urology, experience with NOTES has been relatively limited with the plurality of experiments confined to kidney surgery in the porcine model. Multiple centers have reported successful NOTES nephrectomy. In addition to Gettman's[4] aforementioned experience with transvaginal NOTES nephrectomy, Mathes and colleagues[24] reported transgastric and transvaginal nephrectomy in 2007. Using a dual-channel gastroscope, the left kidney was dissected and the renal hilum controlled with metallic clips. The kidney was morcellated and extracted. The animals were followed postoperatively with no clinical signs of abdominal infection at 19 days. Representative schematics and images of NOTES nephrectomy are found in **Figs. 1–5**.

Clayman and coworkers[25] at the University of California-Irvine presented and later published their experience with transvaginal NOTES nephrectomy in 2007. Using a specially designed operating platform, an acute experiment was performed in a female farm pig in which a 12-mm trocar was placed transabdominally through the midline with the operating platform placed trans-vaginally. Following dissection of the kidney through the transvaginal port, the renal hilum was controlled with an endovascular stapler deployed through the transabdominal trocar. The kidney was placed in an endoscopic retrieval bag and brought out through the vagina. This report received considerable commendation at the annual meeting of the American Urological Association and generated significant enthusiasm about the role of NOTES in urology.

In 2008, Crouzet and colleagues[26] reported bilateral transgastric and transvesical renal cryoablation in two female farm pigs (**Fig. 6**). The authors suggested that not only does NOTES and the use of flexible endoscopic instruments afford access to portions of the kidney that would otherwise be difficult to approach, but that cryoablation may also represent a natural transition into NOTES surgery because limited dissection and

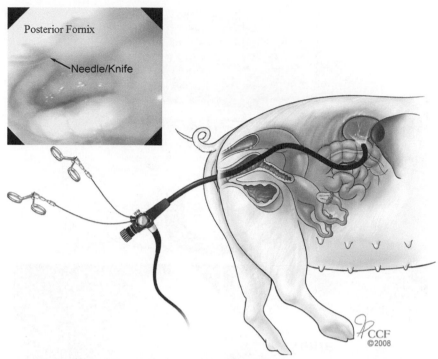

Fig. 1. Schematic representation of multichannel gastroscope inserted through a posterior colpotomy. The gastroscope is retroflexed to visualize the kidney. (*Courtesy of* the Cleveland Clinic Foundation, Cleveland, OH.)

reconstruction are needed. Indeed, the ability to perform difficult dissection or reconstruction during NOTES is viewed as a major impediment to its practical application.

In response to the poor instrumentation available to perform stapling, dissecting, and suturing during NOTES, Box and colleagues[27] reported their experience with combined transcolonic and

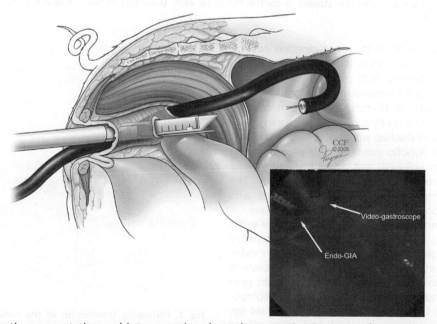

Fig. 2. Schematic representation and intraoperative photo demonstrating insertion of an endovascular stapler through the posterior colpotomy under direct vision. (*Courtesy of* the Cleveland Clinic Foundation, Cleveland, OH.)

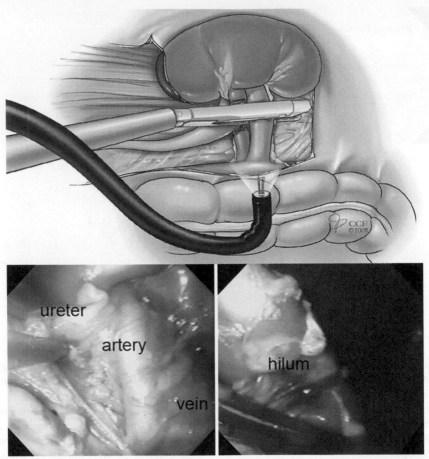

Fig. 3. Schematic representation and intraoperative photos demonstrating dissection of the renal hilum and deployment of an endovascular stapler to control the renal vein. (*Courtesy of* the Cleveland Clinic Foundation, Cleveland, OH.)

transvaginal, single-port, robot-assisted NOTES nephrectomy. An acute experiment was performed in a female farm pig in which a 12-mm trocar was placed transabdominally in the midline and two additional 12-mm ports were placed into the peritoneal cavity through the vagina and colon. The robot was docked with a port-in-port configuration. The robotic camera was placed in the midline with grasping and dissecting instruments placed through the colon and vagina. The nephrectomy was successfully performed with minimal blood loss and without complications.

Haber and colleagues[28] also applied the existing robotic platform during NOTES extirpative and reconstructive surgery in a porcine model. The authors successfully completed bilateral partial nephrectomy, bilateral dismembered pyeloplasty, and completion bilateral radical nephrectomy on 10 female farm pigs. In this hybrid set-up, the robotic camera and first arm were placed through the umbilicus, whereas the second arm was introduced through a posterior colpotomy

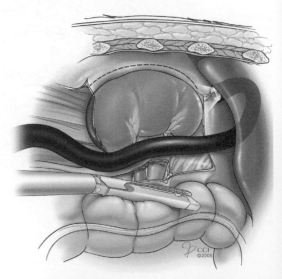

Fig. 4. Following transaction of the renal hilum, the lateral attachments of the kidney are dissected. (*Courtesy of* the Cleveland Clinic Foundation, Cleveland, OH.)

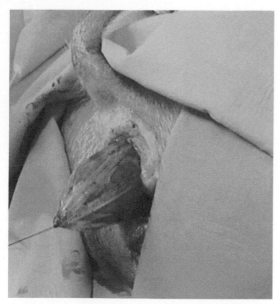

Fig. 5. Intraoperative photo demonstrating removal of an intact kidney through a posterior colpotomy in a porcine model.

(**Figs. 7** and **8**). Mean operative time was 154 minutes (range, 140–187 minutes). Mean estimated blood loss was 73 mL (range, 55–100 mL). No intraoperative complications were encountered and no technical constraints or robotic system failures occurred during either right- or left-sided procedures. The authors concluded that use of the robotic platform may overcome the learning curve and technical obstacles associated with NOTES.

In 2007, Gettman and Blute[21] successfully performed transvesical peritoneoscopy on a 56-year-old man before robotic prostatectomy.

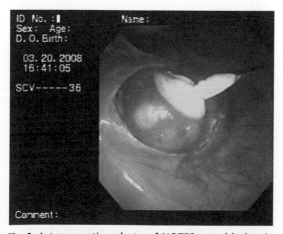

Fig. 6. Intraoperative photo of NOTES cryoablation in the porcine model. The evolving ice ball is easily visualized.

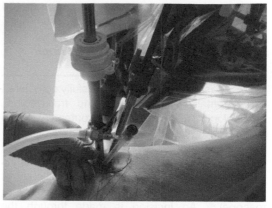

Fig. 7. Intraoperative photo of robotic NOTES procedure in a porcine model. The robotic camera holder and first arm are inserted transabdominally through a multichannel single port.

Under confirmatory standard laparoscopic guidance, an injection needle was used to perforate the bladder wall through which a flexible ureteroscope was passed. The peritoneal cavity was surveyed adequately and completely. The cystotomy was closed robotically before prostatectomy. No intraoperative or postoperative complications were reported.

In 2009, Kaouk and colleagues[29] at the Cleveland Clinic successfully performed the world's first transvaginal NOTES nephrectomy on a 57 year old female with a non-functioning right kidney. Following insufflation with a Veress needle, a camera was introduced into the abdominal cavity through a 5 mm umbilical port to allow vaginal access under direct vision. Using a standard Gel-Port® positioned through a 3 cm colpotomy, the kidney was dissected, the renal hilum exposed and controlled, and the kidney extracted exclusively through the vaginal incision. Operative time

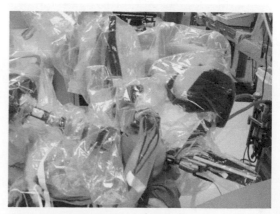

Fig. 8. Robotic NOTES set up. The second robotic arm is placed transvaginally.

was 307 minutes. Estimated blood loss was 100 mL. No intraoperative complications occurred.

Natural Orifice Translumenal Endoscopic Surgery Access

NOTES has thus far been successfully completed experimentally by the transgastric, transvaginal, transcolonic, and transvesical routes. Although strikingly singular organs, the logistics of trans-visceral surgery are universal. First, a natural orifice (mouth, anus, vagina, or urethra) is accessed with aid of a flexible multichannel videoscope (gastroscope, ureteroscope, or lapa-roscope).[30] An incision is made through the stomach, colon, vagina, or bladder using a needle knife and a wire is passed into the peritoneal cavity using a modified Seldinger technique (**Fig. 9**). A radially dilating balloon is variably used to enlarge the access tract (**Fig. 10**). A catheter, guide tube, or overtube is placed over the guidewire and insufflation is achieved with CO_2. A multichannel video-scope is then advanced further into the peritoneal cavity and the diagnostic or therapeutic procedure performed with flexible operating instruments (**Fig. 11**). The viscerotomy is closed at the termination of the procedure.[30] Although seemingly straight-forward, this step-wise approach to NOTES is overly simplistic and a dedicated evaluation of each access route and its comparative merits deserves mention.

Transgastric Natural Orifice Translumenal Endoscopic Surgery

Peroral access is obtained using a videogastro-scope. Typically, the incision in the stomach is made anteriorly to avoid vascular compromise or the spillage of enteric contents.[30] Alternatively,

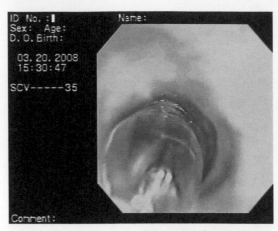

Fig. 10. Following incision of the stomach, a guidewire is passed into the peritoneal cavity followed by balloon dilation of the incision.

incisions have been made with the aid of ultra-sound guidance, transillumination, and even under direct laparoscopic visualization.[31–33] A guidewire is placed through the incision after which a dilating balloon or sphincterotome is used to dilate the tract.[32] Generally, a sphinctero-tome is faster than the dilating balloon and is preferred if repeated gastric crossing is required. Conversely, a dilating balloon preserves gastric muscle integrity and facilitates eventual gastric closure. This muscle preservation, however, can make repeated endoscopic passage tedious.[32] Pneumoperitoneum is achieved with CO_2 and the procedure performed using flexible endo-scopic instruments. Full-thickness gastrotomy closure is achieved using novel preplaced T-fasteners, a purse-string suture closure device, or with multiple clips.[10,26,34,35]

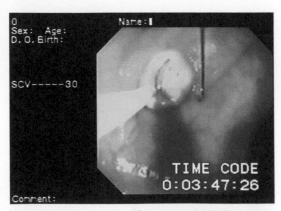

Fig. 9. Endoscopic view of transgastric NOTES procedure. The anterior aspect of the stomach is being incised with a needle-knife.

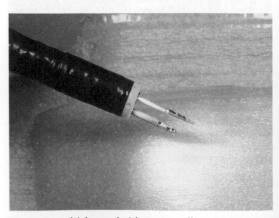

Fig. 11. A multichannel videoscope allows surgeons to deploy multiple instruments without obscuring the operative field.

Transvaginal Natural Orifice Translumenal Endoscopic Surgery

A needle knife is introduced in the posterior fornix of the vagina under direct vision. A guidewire is placed into the peritoneal cavity followed by balloon dilation and introduction of a videogastroscope. Following completion of the procedure, the colpotomy is closed in the usual fashion under direct vision.[36]

Transcolonic Natural Orifice Translumenal Endoscopic Surgery

Although some variation exists in the literature, most authors report deploying a purse-string suture around the planned incision site before perforation of the colon with a needle-knife.[37,38] No further dilation is generally needed because the colonotomies are easily widened.[5,37] A guide tube or catheter may be passed through the incision followed by passage of the videoscope. Visualization of the upper abdominal organs is considered superior with transcolonic access because retroflexion is obviated. Colotomy closure is very much a technical limitation at the present time, however, especially given the risk of peritoneal bacterial seeding with inadequate closure.[38,39] Despite using preplaced sutures, several authors have reported wound dehiscence and untoward complications secondary to use of novel closure devices.[5,39] These findings invoke very serious questions regarding the wisdom of transcolonic access. Certainly, secure and robust closure is of paramount concern during NOTES, regardless of the route of access. In several series, incomplete viscerotomy closure was strongly associated with significant infections and an unacceptably high mortality rate.[33,40] Most of these animal fatalities occurred following transcolonic access.[30] Undeniably, the consequences of complications associated with transcolonic access are more profound and morbid than those potentially associated with transvesical or transvaginal access and must be considered when applying NOTES in human trials.

Transvesical Natural Orifice Translumenal Endoscopic Surgery

A standard rigid or flexible cystoscope is passed into the bladder under direct vision.[41] The wall of the bladder is incised near the dome using a needle-knife. A guidewire and ureteral catheter are placed into the peritoneal cavity followed by dilation of the incision and placement of a transvesical overtube.[21] In most reported series, a flexible ureteroscope is passed into the peritoneal cavity as previously described by Gettman and Blute.[21] In Gettman's human study, the bladder was closed robotically during robotic prostatectomy. Lima and coworkers[41] reported significant contraction of the vesicotomy following withdrawal of the ureteroscope and left the hole unclosed without apparent sequelae. In a follow-up study, Lima and coworkers[42] reported use of a novel endoscopic closure to approximate the vesicotomy. In six female farm pigs, bladder perforations near the bladder dome were all successfully closed using an endoscopic suturing kit.

NATURAL ORIFICE TRANSLUMENAL ENDOSCOPIC SURGERY INSTRUMENTS AND TECHNICAL LIMITATIONS

Experience with standard laparoscopy has taught that safe and efficient minimally invasive surgery requires adequate visualization, maneuverability with triangulation, firm tissue grasping and manipulation, and precise dissection.[13] Beyond issues of access and secure closure, NOTES cannot be expected to flourish or survive if technical improvements are not realized. Myriad engineering barriers exist and purpose-built instruments must be developed.

Most successful NOTES procedures have been diagnostic (ie, peritoneoscopy) in nature. More complex procedures have required innovative but still suboptimal maneuvers to improve visualization including marked positional changes of the study subject, use of a minirobot to explore the peritoneal cavity, or with the aid of endoscopic ultrasonography.[30,31,43] Similarly, the ability to reliably grasp and manipulate tissue during dissection is woefully inadequate. There exists a distinct and pressing need for improved instrumentation and innovative approaches to tissue retraction and stabilization.

The previously cited operating platform is a purpose-built multilumen operating platform that has been used successfully to perform transvaginal NOTES nephrectomy.[25] The device is dynamic and accommodates flexible operating instruments through its four working channels. When the target tissue is reached, the platform can be locked rigidly into position to afford stable two-handed dissection. Although not yet applied in humans, this device represents the style of innovative engineering that will drive NOTES forward.

In response to issues of tissue retraction and improved visualization, Parks and colleagues[44] have reported use of a novel magnetic anchoring and guidance system that can be used to ease concerns related to fixed access, poor visibility, and operative field collapse secondary to adjacent organs. Zeltser and colleagues[45] have successfully performed laparoscopic nephrectomies in the porcine model using the magnetic anchoring and guidance system. Outcomes were favorable with minimal blood loss and no intraoperative complications. The authors concluded that the magnetic anchoring and guidance system may obviate many of the technical limitations associated with NOTES.

As mentioned, Haber and colleagues[28] at the Cleveland Clinic recently applied a robotic platform to complete complex hybrid NOTES renal surgery. According to the authors, the system's articulating instruments compensated for the absence of triangulation and made NOTES more accessible. Instrument conflict was still pronounced, however, and required significant compensation for the procedures to successfully be completed. This report underscores not only the importance of having an adaptable and stable operating platform during NOTES, but also the need for purpose-built instruments. The future of NOTES may very well reside in the development of a novel robotic platform that is designed to perform capably through a natural orifice.

SUMMARY

The promise of any new surgical technique requires a stringent and thorough inquisition of its comparative risks and benefits. When the field of laparoscopy was being conceptualized and applied nearly two decades ago, the benefits were immediate and tangible. Despite the complications associated with its initial use, laparoscopy was applauded by patients and surgeons for its substantial benefits of improved convalescence; less pain and morbidity; and, following the initial learning curve, equivalent or superior outcomes. Theoretically and optimally, NOTES should offer comparable efficacy to standard laparoscopic approaches with minimized patient discomfort and improved cosmesis. Although ostensibly noble goals, the magnitude of benefit associated with NOTES cannot possibly approach the quantum shift that accompanied the transition from open to laparoscopic surgery. The question becomes one of the use and role NOTES should play in the management of urologic diseases. The collective experience with NOTES has borne out several unifying issues, namely poor visibility and maneuverability and complications secondary to surgeon inexperience, technical constraints, or a combination thereof. Interestingly, these limitations also applied to the early experience with standard laparoscopy. Undeniably, many critical questions remain unanswered. The idea and promise of NOTES are revolutionary, but its maturation and widespread application will likely evolve slowly and with an uncertain fate.

REFERENCES

1. Kalloo AN, Singh VK, Jgannath SB, et al. Flexible transgastric peritoneoscopy: a novel approach to diagnostic and therapeutic interventions in the peritoneal cavity. Gastrointest Endosc 2004;60:114–7.
2. Breda G, Silvestre P, Giunta A, et al. Laparoscopic nephrectomy with vaginal delivery of the intact kidney. Eur Urol 1993;24:116–7.
3. Gill IS, Cherullo EE, Meraney AM, et al. Vaginal extraction of the intact specimen following laparoscopic radical nephrectomy. J Urol 2002;167:238–41.
4. Gettman MT, Lotan Y, Napper CA, et al. Transvaginal laparoscopic nephrectomy: development and feasibility in the porcine model. Urology 2002;59:446–50.
5. Pai RD, Fong DG, Bundga ME, et al. Transcolonic endoscopic cholecystectomy: a NOTES survival study in a porcine model. Gastrointest Endosc 2006;64:428–34.
6. Sumiyama K, Gostout CJ, Rajan E, et al. Pilot study of the porcine uterine horn as an in vivo appendicitis model for development of endoscopic transgastric appendectomy. Gastrointest Endosc 2006;64:808–12.
7. Bergstrom M, Ikeda K, Swain P, et al. Transgastric anastomosis by using flexible endoscopy in a porcine model. Gastrointest Endosc 2006;63:307–12.
8. Wagh MS, Merrifield BF, Thompson CC. Survival studies after endoscopic transgastric oophorectomy and tubectomy in a porcine model. Gastrointest Endosc 2006;63:473–8.
9. Wagh MS, Merrifield BF, Thompson CC, et al. Endoscopic transgastric abdominal exploration and organ resection: initial experience in a porcine model. Clin Gastroenterol Hepatol 2005;3:892–6.
10. Swanstrom LL, Kozarek R, Pasricha PJ, et al. Development of a new access device for transgastric surgery. J Gastrointest Surg 2005;9:1129–36.
11. Fritscher-Ravens A, Mosse CA, Mukherjee D, et al. Transluminal endosurgery: single lumen access anastomotic device for flexible endoscopy. Gastrointest Endosc 2003;58:585–91.
12. Kantsevoy SV, Jagannath SB, Niiyama H, et al. Endoscopic gastrojejunostomy with survival in a porcine model. Gastrointest Endosc 2005;62:287–92.
13. Rattner D, Kalloo A. ASGE/SAGES Working group on natural orifice translumenal endoscopic surgery 2005. Surg Endosc 2006;20:329–33.
14. Rattner D. Introduction to NOTES white paper. Surg Endosc 2006;20:185.
15. Kantsevoy SV, Jagannath SB, Niiyama H, et al. A novel safe approach to the peritoneal cavity for

per-oral transgastric endoscopic procedures. Gastrointest Endosc 2007;65:497–500.

16. Sumiyama K, Gostout CJ, Rajan E, et al. Submucosal endoscopy with mucosal flap safety valve. Gastrointest Endosc 2007;65:688–94.

17. Sumiyama K, Gostout CJ, Rajan E, et al. Transgastric cholecystectomy: transgastric accessibility to the gallbladder improved with the SEMF method and a novel multibending therapeutic endoscope. Gastrointest Endosc 2007;65:1028–34.

18. Onders R, Mcgee M, Marks J, et al. Diaphragm pacing with natural orifice transluminal endoscopic surgery: potential for difficult-to-wean intensive care unit patients. Surg Endosc 2007;3:475–9.

19. Hazey JW, Narula VK, Renton DB, et al. Natural-orifice transgastric endoscopic peritoneoscopy in humans: initial clinical trial. Surg Endosc 2008;22:16–20.

20. Tsin DA, Colombero LT, Lambeck J, et al. Minilaparoscopy-assisted natural orifice surgery. JSLS 2007; 11:24–9.

21. Gettman MT, Blute ML. Transvesical peritoneoscopy: initial clinical evaluation of the bladder as a portal for natural orifice translumenal endoscopic surgery. Mayo Clin Proc 2007;82:843–5.

22. Marks JM, Ponsky JL, Pearl JP, et al. PEG rescue: a practical NOTES technique. Surg Endosc 2007; 21:816–9.

23. Marescaux J, Dallemagne B, Perretta S, et al. Surgery without scars: report of transluminal cholecystectomy in a human being. Arch Surg 2007; 142:823–6.

24. Matthes D, Menke P, Koehler H, et al. Feasibility of endoscopic transgastric (ETGN) and transvaginal (ETVN) nephrectomy. Gastrointest Endosc 2007; 65:AB290.

25. Clayman RV, Box GN, Abraham JB, et al. Rapid communication: transvaginal single-port NOTES nephrectomy: initial laboratory experience. J Endourol 2007;21:640–4.

26. Crouzet S, Haber GP, Kamoi K, et al. Natural orifice translumenal endoscopic surgery (NOTES) renal cryoablation in a porcine model. BJU Int 2008;102: 1715–8.

27. Box GN, Lee HJ, Santos RJ, et al. Rapid communication: robot-assisted NOTES nephrectomy: initial report. J Endourol 2008;22:503–6.

28. Haber GP, Crouzet S, Kamoi K, et al. Robotic NOTES (natural orifice translumenal endoscopic surgery) in reconstructive urology: initial laboratory experience. Urology 2008;71:996–1000.

29. Kaouk JH, White WM, Goel RK, et al. NOTES transvaginal nephrectomy: first human experience. Urology 2009; in press.

30. Della Flora E, Wilson TG, Martin IJ, et al. A review of natural orifice translumenal endoscopic surgery (NOTES) for intra-abdominal surgery. Ann Surg 2008;247:583–602.

31. Fritscher-Ravens A, Mosse CA, Ikeda K, et al. Endoscopic transgastric lymphadenectomy by using EUS for selection and guidance. Gastrointest Endosc 2006;63:302–6.

32. Park PO, Bergstrom M, Ikeda K, et al. Experimental studies of transgastric gallbladder surgery: cholecystectomy and cholecystogastric anastomosis. Gastrointest Endosc 2005;61:601–6.

33. Merrifield BF, Wagh MS, Thompson CC. Peroral transgastric organ resection: a feasibility study in pigs. Gastrointest Endosc 2006;63:693–7.

34. Onders RP, McGee MF, Marks J, et al. Natural orifice transluminal endoscopic surgery (NOTES) as a diagnostic tool in the intensive care unit. Surg Endosc 2007;21:681–3.

35. Kratt T, Kuper M, Traub F, et al. Feasibility study for secure closure of natural orifice transluminal endoscopic surgery gastrotomies by using over-the-scope clips. Gastrointest Endosc 2008;68:993–6.

36. Swain P. Nephrectomy and natural orifice translumenal endosurgery (NOTES): transvaginal, transgastric, transrectal, and transvesical approaches. J Endourol 2008;22:811–7.

37. Wilhelm D, Meining A, von Delius S, et al. An innovative, safe and sterile sigmoid access (ISSA) for NOTES. Endoscopy 2007;39:401–6.

38. Fong DG, Pai RD, Thompson CC. Transcolonic endoscopic abdominal exploration: a NOTES survival study in a porcine model. Gastrointest Endosc 2007;65:312–8.

39. Pham BV, Raju GS, Ahmed I, et al. Immediate endoscopic closure of colon perforation by using a prototype endoscopic suturing device: feasibility and outcome in a porcine model. Gastrointest Endosc 2006;64:113–9.

40. Raju GS, Pham B, Xiao S-Y, et al. A pilot study of endoscopic closure of colonic perforations with endoclips in a swine model. Gastrointest Endosc 2005;62:791–5.

41. Lima E, Rolanda C, Pego JM, et al. Transvesical endoscopic peritoneoscopy: a novel 5 mm port for intra-abdominal scarless surgery. J Urol 2006;176: 802–5.

42. Lima E, Rolanda C, Osorio L, et al. Endoscopic closure of transmural bladder wall perforations. Eur Urol; 2008. Epub ahead of print.

43. Rentschler M, Dumpert J, Platt S, et al. Natural orifice surgery with an endoluminal mobile robot. Surg Endosc 2007;21:1212–5.

44. Parks S, Bergs R, Eberhart R, et al. Trocar-less instrumentation for laparoscopy: magnetic positioning of intra-abdominal camera and retractor. Ann Surg 2007;243:379–84.

45. Zeltser IS, Bergs R, Fernandez R, et al. Single trocar laparoscopic nephrectomy using magnetic anchoring and guidance system in the porcine model. J Urol 2007;21:2308–16.

Flexible Robotics

Monish Aron, MD, Mihir M. Desai, MD*

KEYWORDS

- Flexible robotics • Flexible robotic systems
- Robotic catheter • Steerable catheter

The initial foray into the use of robotics in urology began with transurethral resection of the prostate.[1,2] However, robotics in urology truly came into its own with the application of robotics to assist in laparoscopic surgery. The initial application of robotics in laparoscopy was the use of a voice-controlled robotic arm as a responsive and accurate camera holder (Aesop, Computer Motion).[3] This was followed by the development of more complex surgical robotic systems that operated on the master–slave principle (Zeus, Computer Motion; da Vinci, Intuitive Surgical). The development of the Zeus system was halted after Intuitive Surgical acquired Computer Motion in 2003.

The da Vinci system is a currently available, widely used surgical robotic system that features wristed instruments with increased degrees of freedom, three-dimensional visualization with depth perception, motion scaling, and elimination of tremor. Although the da Vinci system is a rigid, master–slave surgical manipulator designed and used for laparoscopic applications, recently several flexible robotic systems have been introduced primarily for intravascular catheter-based applications. In this article, the authors describe these novel flexible robotic platforms, review the initial experimental and clinical applications for flexible endoscopy, and postulate possible future roles for the platforms in performing single-port laparoscopic and natural orifice transluminal endoscopic surgery (NOTES).

THE NEED FOR FLEXIBLE ROBOTICS

With miniaturization and refinement in fiberoptic and endoscopic technology, endoscopic imaging of myriad bodily viscera through a multitude of natural orifices has become routine, and almost every body cavity is now accessible to some form of endoscopic inspection and manipulation. Despite significant progress, currently available endoscopic equipment continues to have limitations inherent to the manual control of endoscopes and their effectors. The ability to have fine control of the effector tip of flexible endoscopes and flexible catheters and to maintain these devices in a stable position in three-dimensional body cavities may be limited when using manual control. Using manual steering technologies for flexible endoscopes that provide navigation within a three-dimensional body cavity requires experience and expertise because moving the tip to a specific location requires a combined insert, roll, and articulation input that is complex and somewhat arbitrary. Additionally, the long duration of many procedures exposes the physician to considerable amounts of x-rays and the risk of nonergonomic strain. Despite these limitations when using manual endoscopes, the experienced endoscopist can perform a wide variety of diagnostic and therapeutic procedures.

Thus, there may be an advantage in developing a computer-controlled robotic platform that allows precise, controllable, complex, and reproducible maneuvers of flexible endoscopes inside hollow organs and three-dimensional anatomic spaces to further enhance the capabilities of manual endoscopy. Such a system should facilitate surgical manipulation within these complex spaces, thus transferring the advantages of a rigid robotic system into the endoscopic environment.

Two other philosophically similar but technically different, emerging areas have prompted renewed

Department of Urology, Stevan B. Streem Center for Endourology, Glickman Urological and Kidney Institute, Cleveland Clinic Foundation, 9500 Euclid Avenue/Q10, Cleveland, OH 44195, USA
* Corresponding author.
E-mail address: desaim1@ccf.org (M.M. Desai).

Urol Clin N Am 36 (2009) 157–162
doi:10.1016/j.ucl.2009.02.001

interest in flexible robotics. One such area is the use of NOTES, which involves traversing intact hollow viscera (eg, stomach, vagina, rectum, bladder) to access intra-abdominal organs for ablative or reconstructive surgery.[4] The instrumentation required to accomplish NOTES through various natural orifices is in evolution; clearly, additional work needs to be done. Safe, reliable, and reproducible techniques for foolproof visceral closure remain undefined. Whereas the tubular, hollow viscera are generally amenable to conventional endoscopy, NOTES will require far more complex movements in the peritoneal cavity, including complex retraction and suturing maneuvers. It is in this role that robotic platforms may provide an advantage in facilitating the performance of NOTES procedures.

The other emerging area is single-port laparoscopic surgery, or laparoendoscopic single-site surgery (LESS), which is a term recently coined to describe various techniques that are used to perform laparoscopic procedures through a single skin incision, which is often concealed within the umbilicus.[5–9] With currently available technology, the major limitations with LESS include the lack of triangulation of the closely situated instruments that are clustered together at the common entry point and the limited retraction and countertraction for heavy intra-abdominal tissues and organs. Although the current da Vinci system has been used for robot-assisted NOTES and LESS procedures,[10,11] challenges still remain from the clashing of the robotic arms and the instruments, which result in reduced range and precision of motion. Dedicated robotic platforms with a smaller profile or with steerable, flexible effector arms are likely to help circumvent these issues and make these procedures easier and more reproducible.

FLEXIBLE ROBOTIC SYSTEMS

Initially developed for cardiovascular applications, including endocardial ablation for arrythmia,[12] Hansen Medical, Inc. (Mountain View, CA) has adapted a flexible robotic catheter system to be used for performing ureterorenoscopy.[13] The robotic catheter consists of a remote master–slave control system (**Fig. 1**) consisting of: (1) a console for the surgeon, including an LCD display and a master input device (MID); (2) a steerable catheter system; (3) a remote catheter manipulator (RCM); and (4) an electronics rack. At the workstation, three adjacent LCD monitors display endoscopic, fluoroscopic, and other applicable procedure-specific imaging. The MID is a three-dimensional joystick that the surgeon uses to remotely manipulate the catheter tip, whose

movements mimic those of the surgeon's hand. The steerable catheter system (**Fig. 2**) has two components: an outer catheter sheath (14/12 Fr) that is manually inserted and an inner catheter guide (12/10 Fr) through which the steerable catheter is inserted and manipulated remotely. That the workstation can be positioned at a distance from the patient serves to limit radiation exposure to the surgeon.

Another commercially available flexible catheter manipulator system (NIOBE II, Stereotaxis, Inc.) uses a computer-controlled magnetic field for catheter steering. This system employs computer-controlled magnets placed on opposite sides of the patient, which create a magnetic field within which a catheter with a magnetic tip can be remotely steered with great accuracy. A motor is used to advance or retract the catheter, thus allowing for remote navigation. Manipulation of the catheter tip can be made in 1-mm increments with 1° of deflection. Recent improvements in the Stereotaxis system allow for integration with three-dimensional mapping software and image integration (eg, MRI) that can potentially decrease x-ray exposure to the patient by minimizing the need for real-time fluoroscopy. For cardiac ablative procedures, the external magnets are aligned with the patient's chest. Because a small magnet is embedded in the tip of the catheter, this system necessitates the use of specific, custom-designed catheters. When the outer magnets change their relative positions, the magnetic field is altered, thereby affecting tip deflection. The magnetic field sequences can be stored and played back to automate certain maneuvers. As with any remotely controlled system, the Stereotaxis system allows the physician to be protected from fluoroscopic radiation by being away from the operative field. The Stereotaxis system has been used predominantly for cardiac applications, and to the authors' knowledge has not been used for nonvascular endoscopic applications.[14–16]

Multiple remotely controlled flexible catheters, instruments, and scopes also have the potential to be combined inside a common channel. Separate devices could be positioned at independently desired locations to create necessary triangulation from a common entry point. The EndoVia System is one such system that incorporates independently controlled right- and left-hand effectors that are robotically controlled along with a flexible endoscope. Such a system, when refined further to achieve clinical applicability, has the potential to provide much greater control and capability for flexible endoscopy. In fact, preliminary experimental studies demonstrated that the ability of the EndoVia system to assist physicians in

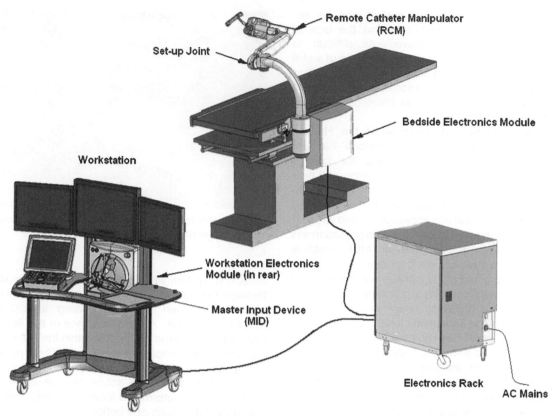

Fig. 1. Schematic system diagram of a robotic catheter control system. (*Courtesy of* Hansen Medical, Mountain View, CA. © 2009 Hansen Inc. Used with permission.)

performing complex tasks, such as suturing, that are not possible using current flexible endoscopes. These enhanced flexible robotic systems could also provide the necessary triangulation, degrees of freedom, and tensile strength so that physicians can perform complex intra-abdominal procedures within a compact yet robust platform for NOTES and LESS procedures. Whether the use of the electromechanical or magnetic systems, a combination of the two, or some other configuration not yet conceived will be the ultimate solution remains unknown and a subject of speculation.[17]

UROLOGIC APPLICATIONS

Flexible ureterorenoscopy has become increasingly popular for a wide variety of diagnostic and therapeutic applications. Existing flexible ureteroscopes, although commonly used in clinical practice, are fragile and their use involves a significant learning curve and the aid of a skilled assistant for advanced manipulations. In addition, positioning the tip of such ureteroscopes into a desired caliceal location is performed using a limited

mechanical lever and a combination of inserting and rolling movements. In a basic sense, the ureteroscope conforms passively to the ureteral contour, and the tip is maneuvered using a combination of active and passive deflection by maneuvering the proximal hand piece. These maneuvers provide less than ideal control and stability at the distal tip of the flexible ureteroscope. Although all

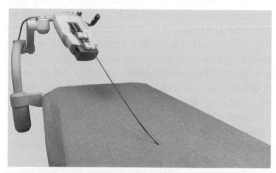

Fig. 2. Steerable guide catheter and sheath mounted on an RCM that is fixed to the side rail of the operating table. (*Courtesy of* Hansen Medical, Mountain View, CA. © 2009 Hansen Inc. Used with permission.)

locations in the collecting system can be accessed, breathing movements and the lack of stability make subtle movements difficult to control. Ureteroscopy is a good example of a skill set with many inherent limitations that the skilled endoscopist learns to overcome, and it has been an initial arena in which to investigate flexible robotics in urology.[17]

The software and hardware of the Hansen Medical Inc. remote flexible robotic catheter control system, initially designed for cardiac work, were modified for use in experimental flexible ureterorenoscopy. The steerable guide catheter, inside a steerable sheath, is inserted through an endoluminal access point, and its proximal end is attached to an RCM. The physician sits at a console equipped with an MID, which is essentially a three-dimensional joystick.

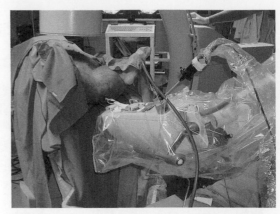

Fig. 3. Flexible robotic ureterorenoscopic examination in progress in the porcine model.

The sheath and guide catheter are manipulated using remotely controlled pull wires. These pull wires help the physician independently orient the tips of the guide and sheath for accessing various anatomic targets. The guide and sheath may be introduced and advanced in tandem along a guide wire. Articulation and precise control are provided by the manipulation of one or more of the following; the guide or sheath insertion axis, four independent pull-wire actuators in the guide, and two pull actuators in the sheath. The actuators can be pulled singly or in combination to produce various degrees of articulation in the guide catheter and to deflect the guide tip in any direction. The sheath works by the same principle but has two pull actuators. One is used for positive and negative sheath articulation in the distal tip toward one direction. The second pull actuator is used in conjunction with the first and limits the bending of the proximal portion of the sheath when the first actuator is activated.

The authors evaluated this system for use in flexible ureterorenoscopic examination of five female swine (**Fig. 3**).[18] The aim of the study was to manipulate a custom-built, passive, flexible fiberoptic ureteroscope that was inserted through the robotically controlled catheter system. The sheath and scope assembly was advanced manually up to the ureteropelvic junction (UPJ) using fluoroscopic control along a guide wire. When the catheter tip was positioned at the UPJ, the catheter sheath and guide were docked to the robotic manipulator arm. All subsequent maneuvers, including navigation in the collecting system, fragmentation of stones, and laser ablation of papilla were performed exclusively by using robotic assistance. Each minor calyx was individually examined (**Fig. 4**). Four-millimeter stones (three in each kidney) were inserted into the

collecting system in two animals (four kidneys) through the outer sheath of the system. These calculi were then pulverized using a 320-μ holmium laser fiber. A major advance of this flexible robotic system is its stability within the collecting system, as demonstrated by the ability to park the effector tip inside a given calyx for extended periods. In addition, the scope can be autoretracted to a predetermined location (in this case, the UPJ) at the touch of a button.

The robotic catheter system was introduced de novo into eight ureters; catheter introduction into two ureters required balloon dilation. The ureteroscope was successfully manipulated remotely in 83 (98%) of the 85 calyces. The time required to inspect all calyces within a given kidney decreased with experience, from 15 minutes in the first kidney to 49 seconds in the last (mean, 4.6 minutes). On

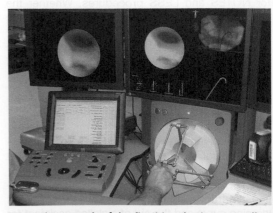

Fig. 4. The controls of the flexible robotic system allow the operator to perform detailed inspection of each calyx with remarkable stability while seated and at a distance from the C-arm radiation source.

a visual analog scale (from 1, worst, to 10, best), the reproducibility of calyceal access was rated at 8, and instrument tip stability was rated at 10. A renal pelvic perforation was the solitary complication. Histologic examination of the ureter showed changes consistent with acute dilation without areas of necrosis.

Based on lessons learned from this preclinical study and improvements made in the system, the authors performed the first clinical study in urology using a flexible robotic system for ureteroscopy. Robotic flexible ureteroscopic examinations using the Hansen Medical Inc. system were performed in 18 patients who had renal calculi. Inclusion criteria included having renal calculi from 5- to 15-mm in size. All procedures were done unilaterally, and patients who had coexisting ureteral calculi or obstruction, uncontrolled infection, renal insufficiency, or solitary kidney status were excluded from the study. Mean stone size was 11.9 mm. All patients were prestented for approximately 2 weeks. The robotic catheter system was introduced into the renal collecting system manually using fluoroscopic control along a guide wire. All intrarenal maneuvers, including stone relocation and fragmentation into 1- to 2-mm particles, were performed exclusively and remotely by the surgeon from the robotic console. All procedures were technically successful, and all calculi were fragmented to the surgeon's complete satisfaction, without need for conversion to manual ureteroscopy. Mean operative time was 91 minutes, including a robot docking time of 7 minutes; stone localization time was 9 minutes. The mean visual analog scale rating (from 1, worst, to 10, best) for ease of stone localization was 8.3, ease of maneuvering was 8.5, and ease of fragmentation was 9.2. Complete fragment clearance was achieved in 56% of patients at 2 months, based on CT examination, and in 89% of patients at 3 months, based on intravenous urographic examination. One patient required secondary ureteroscopy for a residual stone. Complications included pyelonephritis in two patients, pyrexia in one patient, and temporary positional limb paresis in one patient. There was negligible fluid absorption, based on calculated inflow and egress and on ethanol fluid absorption testing.[19]

The results of the initial clinical trial remain encouraging. Further refinements in robotic technology have the potential to provide additional benefits such as automated movements, surgical navigation, and incorporation and robotic control of endoscopic accessories by the surgeon at the console. Further studies will then determine the future place of flexible robotic technology in surgical endoscopy.

FUTURE DIRECTIONS

The role of flexible robotics in urology and other specialties is poised to expand for various intraluminal, transluminal, and laparoscopic applications. Existing flexible endoscopic equipment is designed to perform within a tubular, visceral lumen. Future robotic endoscopes, with an ability to create stable fixation points while maintaining precise tip maneuverability, might allow for an enhanced degree of precision that could facilitate the use of intraluminal therapeutic endoscopy and NOTES. Accessory instrumentation (eg, graspers, scissors, biopsy forceps, suction catheters) could be introduced and exchanged within working channels at the push of a button or even integrated within the flexible assembly.

A common finding in all NOTES studies has been the limitations of existing flexible videoendoscopes for use in complex surgical procedures inside the peritoneal cavity and for suture closure of a viscerotomy. In 2009, the clinical use of NOTES in urology remains a challenging endeavor when limited to the armamentarium of contemporary endoscopic equipment. Some groups are working on reducing these limitations by seeking mechanical solutions to improve the ability to suture and to triangulate operating instruments. It is here that flexible robotic technology could prove pivotal. Such technology could allow the endoscopic and laparoscopic surgeon to precisely position and maneuver a customized, robotically controlled, flexible video-endoscope. The working channels in this scope could carry independent, computer-controlled, robotic, flexible graspers; needle-drivers; monopolar and bipolar coagulators; and even ultrasonic scalpels, and suction and irrigation devices.

In contrast to the highly challenging NOTES procedures, LESS provides a more familiar, direct laparoscopic approach, albeit through a single incision. Given the equally scar-free and minimally morbid nature of NOTES and LESS, at this writing it seems that LESS offers superior clinical reliability, which is reflected in the wider clinical acceptance and repertoire of surgeons for LESS procedures. As such, the learning curve for LESS procedures is short, given adequate prior laparoscopic expertise by the surgeon. Having said that, current LESS procedures have several shortcomings that make them harder and riskier than conventional multiport laparoscopic surgery. The transition from conventional multiport laparoscopic surgery to single-port laparoscopic surgery (LESS) and then eventually to NOTES will to a large extent be facilitated by the use of dedicated robotic systems best suited individually for LESS and NOTES. These emerging areas of surgery most require and will benefit from advanced, robust, dependable, and versatile flexible robotic systems.

SUMMARY

The field of flexible robotics is nascent. However, it seems to be promising and may provide a natural progression from existing platforms for manual, flexible video-endoscopy. Improved precision, better ergonomics, and reduced occupational radiation exposure with the use of flexible robotic systems could lead to the incorporation of robotic technology across various disciplines that use flexible endoscopy for diagnosis and therapy. Refinements in software and hardware could potentially allow these systems to be used for NOTES or LESS in the future.

REFERENCES

1. Davies BL, Hibberd RD, Ng WS, et al. The development of a surgeon robot for prostatectomies. Proc Inst Mech Eng [H] 1991;205:35–8.
2. Harris SJ, Arambula-Cosio F, Mei Q, et al. The Probot—an active robot for prostate resection. Proc Inst Mech Eng [H] 1997;211:317–25.
3. Allaf ME, Jackman SV, Schulam PG, et al. Laparoscopic visual field. Voice vs foot pedal interfaces for control of the AESOP robot. Surg Endosc 1998; 12:1415–8.
4. Kaloo AN, Singh VK, Jagannath SB, et al. Flexible transgastric peritoneoscopy: a novel approach to diagnostic and therapeutic interventions in the peritoneal cavity. Gastrointest Endosc 2004;60:114–7.
5. Desai MM, Rao PP, Aron M, et al. Scarless single port transumbilical nephrectomy and pyeloplasty: first clinical report. BJU Int 2008;101:83–8.
6. Gill IS, Canes D, Aron M, et al. Single port transumbilical (E-NOTES) donor nephrectomy. J Urol 2008; 180:637–41.
7. Desai MM, Stein RJ, Rao P, et al. Embryonic natural orifice transumbilical endoscopic surgery (E-NOTES) for advanced reconstruction: initial experience. Urology 2009;73:182–7.
8. Kaouk JH, Haber GP, Goel RK, et al. Single-port laparoscopic surgery in urology: initial experience. Urology 2008;71:3–6.
9. Aron M, Canes D, Desai MM, et al. Transumbilical single-port laparoscopic partial nephrectomy. BJU Int 2009;103:516–21.
10. Haber GP, Crouzet S, Kamoi K, et al. Robotic NOTES (Natural Orifice Translumenal Endoscopic Surgery) in reconstructive urology: initial laboratory experience. Urology 2008;71:996–1000.
11. Kaouk JH, Goel RK, Haber GP, et al. Robotic single-port transumbilical surgery in humans: initial report. BJU Int 2009;103:366–9.
12. Saliba W, Cummings JE, Oh S, et al. Novel robotic catheter remote control system: feasibility and safety of transseptal puncture and endocardial catheter navigation. J Cardiovasc Electrophysiol 2006; 17(10):1102–5.
13. Aron M, Haber GP, Desai MM, et al. Flexible robotics: a new paradigm. Curr Opin Urol 2007; 17(3):151–5.
14. Pappone C, Vicedomini G, Manguso F, et al. Robotic magnetic navigation for atrial fibrillation ablation. J Am Coll Cardiol 2006;47(7):1390–400.
15. Di Biase L, Fahmy TS, Patel D, et al. Remote magnetic navigation: human experience in pulmonary vein ablation. J Am Coll Cardiol 2007;50(9): 868–74.
16. Pappone C, Augello G, Gugliotta F, et al. Robotic and magnetic navigation for atrial fibrillation ablation. How and why? Expert Rev Med Devices 2007;4(6):885–94.
17. Canes D, Desai MM, Aron M, et al. Transumbilical single-port surgery: evolution and current status. Eur Urol 2008;54(5):1020–9 [Epub 2008 Jul 14].
18. Desai MM, Aron M, Gill IS, et al. Flexible robotic retrograde renoscopy: description of novel robotic device and preliminary laboratory experience. Urology 2008;72:42–6.
19. Desai MM, Grover R, Aron M, et al. Remote robotic ureteroscopic laser lithotripsy for renal calculi: initial clinical experience with a novel flexible robotic system. J Urol 2008;179(4S):435 [Abstract # 1268].

Ablative Technologies for Urologic Cancers

Gino J. Vricella, MD[a], Lee E. Ponsky, MD[a],*,
Jeffrey A. Cadeddu, MD[b]

KEYWORDS

- Ablation • Cryotherapy • Percutaneous • Prostate cancer
- Radiofrequency • Radiosurgery • Renal tumors

KIDNEY

According to the American Cancer Society, an estimated 51,190 cases of newly diagnosed renal cancer occurred in 2007, more than double the reported incidence from just 3 years earlier.[1] This seemingly exponential increase in renal cancer incidence is attributable in large part to the increase in incidental detection of renal mass lesions by means of the widespread availability and use of cross-sectional abdominal imaging modalities (ie, CT, MRI).[2] This increased incidence has concurrently been met with a more favorable grade and stage migration for renal cell carcinoma (RCC). As a result, most small renal masses (SRMs), defined as less than 4.0 cm in diameter on cross-sectional imaging, manifest indolent biologic behavior with excellent prognosis.[3] Despite the benign nature of these SRMs, patients and surgeons alike favor treatment over observation, especially in patients with a long life expectancy.[4] It is in this clinical context that minimally invasive nephron-sparing surgery (MINSS) has been developed in an effort to preserve renal parenchyma and decrease morbidity while obtaining comparable oncologic results to established extirpative therapy. Ablative techniques for renal tumors include cryoablation, radiofrequency ablation (RFA), high-intensity focused ultrasound (HIFU), microwave therapy (MT), and radiosurgery.

Cryoablation

Percutaneous cryoablation (PCA) was first performed by Uchida and colleagues[5] in 1994 on canine kidneys. It was not until 1995 that Uchida's group described the initial application of PCA in two patients who had metastatic RCC, resulting in a decrease in their tumor size by 20% and 81%, respectively.[5] The practical limitations of cryotechnology at that time, namely, comparatively larger (6.8 mm) probes that used an exclusively liquid nitrogen medium, detracted from the interest and accessibility in applying this approach more broadly. The advent of smaller (2.4 mm) probes that use an argon gas medium, which allows for increased treatment precision by halting ice ball growth at the termination of the freeze, has allowed this technology to become more amenable to percutaneous applications. It is with these improvements and concurrent advances in real-time imaging modalities that we have seen a renewed interest in cryoablation as a formidable and more available treatment option for renal mass lesions.

Cryoablation is the best known and most well studied of all thermal ablative modalities. After renal mass biopsy, vacuum-insulated liquid nitrogen or argon-cooled probes are inserted directly into the renal lesions and an ice ball is rapidly generated around this core as these media are forced through a small aperture at the tip of the probe. The ensuing freeze-thaw cycles lead to complete and reproducible necrosis of renal parenchyma occurring at temperatures of −19.4°C or lower.[6] Rapid freezing causes cytotoxic intracellular and extracellular ice crystal formation leading to an increased extracellular osmotic concentration, which ultimately results in intracellular pH changes and protein denaturation

a Department of Urology, Center for Urologic Oncology and Minimally Invasive Therapies, University Hospitals Case Medical Center, 11100 Euclid Avenue, Cleveland, OH 44106, USA
b Clinical Center for Minimally Invasive Urologic Cancer Treatment, University of Texas Southwestern Medical Center, Dallas, TX, USA
* Corresponding author.
E-mail address: lee.ponsky@uhhospitals.org (L.E. Ponsky).

Urol Clin N Am 36 (2009) 163–178
doi:10.1016/j.ucl.2009.02.003

and extracellular mechanical disruption of the cell membrane.[7] Acute injury to the vasculature with resultant thrombosis and ischemia, particularly at the microcirculatory level, leads to delayed tissue necrosis over the ensuing hours to days after cryotherapy.[8] In addition to these mechanisms, apoptosis and freeze-induced immunologic sensitization are other means by which tumor cell destruction occurs.[9,10]

Chosy and colleagues[6] found that normal renal parenchyma needed exposure to a temperature at or lower than $-19.4°C$ for complete cell destruction. Given that cancer cells may need even lower temperatures for reliable cell death, most clinical protocols err on the side of caution and freeze to $-40°C$.[11] In experimental settings, these temperatures were reached only 3.1 mm inside the edge of the ice ball.[12] As a result, in clinical practice, the ice ball is usually extended 5 to 10 mm beyond the tumor margin. The end points of temperature and ice-ball monitoring can be determined by thermocouples at the tumor margin and real-time intraoperative ultrasound (US), CT, or MRI, respectively. In addition, most large clinical series use a double freeze-thaw cycle, which has demonstrated greater clinical efficacy when compared with a single cycle.[13]

Fortunately, not all renal structures are equally cryosensitive. This was demonstrated by Sung and colleagues,[14] who observed that in the absence of mechanical laceration with the cryoprobe, the collecting system heals in a watertight manner even when encompassed within the ice ball. Several researchers have duplicated these findings but have also discovered that hyperthermal ablation techniques (ie, RFA) were associated with an increased risk for urinary leak and fistula formation when compared with hypothermal cryoablation.[15] Proponents of RFA believe that the increased rate of urinary leak and fistula formation is secondary to the multiple tines used to measure impedance and monitor the ablation. Theoretically, the increased number of tines (up to 10) surrounding each electrode, as opposed to two to three cryoprobes, may make it easier to enter the collecting system, and ultimately damage it during ablation.

Currently, renal cryoablation is performed by one of two main minimally invasive approaches: laparoscopic cryoablation (LCA) and PCA. In LCA, the lesions can be approached in a transperitoneal or retroperitoneal fashion. In terms of facilitating exposure, tumors in an anterior or medial location are generally best approached in a transperitoneal manner, whereas posteriorly located tumors lend themselves to a retroperitoneal approach. LCA allows for direct intraoperative visualization, thereby permitting precise cryoprobe positioning and monitoring of ice-ball formation with the aid of a deflectable laparoscopic US transducer.[16] The US scan depicts the ice ball as hypoechoic with an advancing hyperechoic crescent with a posterior acoustic shadow. Once cryoablation has been accomplished and the probe has been withdrawn, hemostasis can be achieved by local compression with bioadhesive bolsters, argon beam coagulation, or a combination of both.

Laparoscopic Cryoablation

Davol and colleagues[17] reported their clinical experience with cryoablation, using an open technique in the first 24 patients and subsequently evolving their surgical method into LCA for the next 24 patients in their data set. The median tumor size in these 48 patients was 2.6 cm (range: 1.1–4.6 cm) with a median follow-up of 64 months (range: 36–110 months). The overall and cancer-specific survival rates were 89.5% and 100%, respectively. The disease-free survival rate after a single cryoablation procedure was 87.5%, which improved dramatically to 97.5% after a repeat procedure. There were no major adverse events and seven minor adverse events, which included four capsular fractures, 2 patients requiring postoperative packed red blood cell transfusions, and 1 patient who had postoperative ileus.

Schwartz and colleagues[18] presented their data using cryoablation, again, first with an open approach and subsequently with a laparoscopic approach. In the 85 consecutive patients who were treated at multiple centers, 70 procedures were performed in a laparoscopic fashion. The mean tumor size in this cohort was 2.6 cm (range: 1.2–4.7 cm), with a mean follow-up of 10 months (range: 3–36 months). The mean estimated blood loss (EBL) was 33 mL (range: <50–550 mL), with 2 patients requiring packed red blood cell transfusion. A total of seven laparoscopic cases were converted to an open procedure, two of which were considered technical failures. Abnormal postoperative enhancement occurred in 2 patients at 3 and 12 months. Radical nephrectomy in the first patient revealed no viable tumor, whereas needle biopsy in the second patient demonstrated RCC, which prompted nephrectomy.

Lawatsch and colleagues[19] reported on their experience with LCA of 81 tumors in 59 patients. The median tumor size in this group was 2.5 cm (range: 1.0–5.0 cm), with a median follow-up of 27 months. Mean pre- and postoperative creatinine levels were stable at 1.11 and 1.17 mg/dL, respectively. Two patients required open conversion, one of which required nephrectomy for bleeding. There were two recurrences identified by residual enhancement of the cryolesion on a contrast-enhanced CT scan. Both of these patients underwent salvage nephrectomy and had no evidence of disease (NED) at the time of publication.

Cestari and colleagues[20] presented data on 104 patients who underwent LCA with a mean tumor size of 2.2 cm (range: 0.7–6.0 cm). The mean operating time was 202 minutes (range: 90–320 min), with a mean EBL of 212 mL (range: 10–3200 mL). Thirty-six and 11 patients have had follow-up for 5 and 7 years, respectively. Delayed complications included one case of ureteropelvic junction (UPJ) obstruction requiring open pyeloplasty 8 months after surgery. One patient underwent open radical nephrectomy at 12 months for suspected tumor recurrence. Progressive reduction of the cryoablated lesions on MRI scans was demonstrated in all patients, with only a renal scar visible after 24 months of follow-up.

Aron and colleagues[21] recently reported an updated series from Gill and colleagues[22] on long-term (5-year minimum) outcomes after LCA in 82 patients who had sporadic single renal mass lesions. Mean tumor size was 2.3 cm (range: 0.9–5.0 cm), with a median follow-up of 83 months (range: 60–120 months). Follow-up consisted of MRI scans performed on postoperative day 1; at months 3, 6, and 12; and then annually thereafter. CT-guided biopsy of the cryolesion was performed 6 months after surgery and then repeated if MRI findings were abnormal. Of the 88 patients who underwent LCA and met the criterion of at least 5 years of follow-up, the mean operating time was just greater than 3 hours (range: 75–420 minutes), with a mean EBL of 106 mL (range: 10–800 mL). The 5-year actual overall, cancer-specific, and disease-free survival was 83%, 95%, and 78%, respectively, whereas the estimated Kaplan-Meier cancer-specific survival at 10 years was a promising 88%.

Modeled after the established principles of its open surgical counterpart, laparoscopic partial nephrectomy (LPN) has emerged as the main MINSS technique to address the SRM.[23] Although the cytocidal effect and durability of LCA seem promising, the fundamental difference between these two MINSS procedures is that whereas LCA leaves the ablated tumor in situ, LPN is extirpative. It is within this clinical context that Desai and colleagues[24] compared the perioperative and short-term outcomes of LPN (group 1, n = 153) versus LCA (group 2, n = 78) in patients who had small renal tumors (≤3 cm). LPN was associated with greater blood loss (211 vs 101 mL) and a higher incidence of delayed complications after discharge (16.3% vs 2.2%). Both groups were comparable with regard to operating time, intraoperative and postoperative complications, hospital stay, convalescence, and postoperative serum creatinine level. Local recurrence was detected over a mean follow-up of 5.8 months in group 1 (0.6%) and 24.6 months in group 2 (3%).

Expounding on Desai's work, Hruby and colleagues[25] compared 12 LPNs with 11 LCAs in the management of small tumors (≤3.2 cm) located in close proximity (≤5 mm) to the renal hilum. All 23 cases were successfully completed laparoscopically. The mean operating time for LPN and LCA was 2.8 hours and 2.3 hours, respectively. The mean EBL was 197 mL for LPN and 70 mL for LRC, whereas the mean hospital stay for the LPN and LCA groups was 3.9 days and 3.2 days, respectively. There were no apparent intraoperative complications in either group. Nine postoperative complications were seen in the LPN group (four of which were urine leaks), whereas the LCA group had no complications. No disease recurrence was seen in either group during the follow-up period of approximately 1 year.

Percutaneous Cryoablation

The percutaneous approach to cryoablation is even less invasive than LCA. In fact, several institutions have demonstrated that PCA can be successfully performed with just intravenous sedation and local anesthesia.[26] This last point is under debate, however, because others believe that general anesthesia optimizes patient tolerance and allows greater control of respiratory motion during probe placement.[27] In any case, PCA can be performed using real-time imaging modalities under US, CT, or MRI guidance. Although US is the most cost-effective and widely available of the imaging techniques, the attenuation of the ice ball limits cryoablation monitoring secondary to the posterior acoustic shadow. This factor precludes imaging deep to the superficial ice ball margin, which is an important consideration in terms of treatment efficacy and complications.[28,29] As a result, PCA is currently performed with the use of open-gantry MRI or CT scan guidance. The requisite for an open-access MRI unit or fluoroscopy-capable CT scanner for intraoperative monitoring could potentially limit this technique in terms of widespread availability.

Gupta and colleagues[26] reported on their clinical experience with CT-guided PCA in 27 renal tumors 5 cm or less in maximal diameter. The average tumor size was 2.5 cm (range: 1.0–5.0 cm), with

11 small (≤3 cm) and 5 large (>3 cm) tumors. The procedure was accomplished successfully in all patients using conscious sedation. Of the 20 treatments, there was only one complication (perinephric hematoma) requiring blood transfusion. Although mean follow-up imaging time was relatively short (5.9 months), 15 of 16 cryoablated lesions showed no residual enhancement. It should be noted that the single tumor that did show residual enhancement occurred in a patient who had a centrally located 4.6-cm tumor.

Silverman and colleagues[30] presented their initial experience using MRI-guided PCA in 23 patients. The 26 treated renal tumors had a mean diameter of 2.6 cm (range: 1.0–4.6 cm). Using general anesthesia, 24 of 26 tumors were successfully ablated, with a mean follow-up of 12 months (range: 3–43 months). In two cases, a small enhancing nodule located at the ablation zone margin proved to be recurrent tumor. The researchers noted that intraprocedure CT fluoroscopy seems promising in ablating renal tumors in one session.[30]

Sewell and Shingleton[31] reported on their updated clinical experience in 103 patients treated with MRI-guided PCA over a 5-year period. A total of 120 tumors were cryoablated in a broad range of 103 patients, including those with solitary kidneys, multiple or bilateral tumors, and renal insufficiency. Tumor size ranged from 1.1 to 7.5 cm, with a mean follow-up of 35 months (range: 4–99 months). Overall and disease-specific survival was 90.2% and 97%, respectively. Based on their results, 72 tumors were completely ablated with a single procedure, with 18 tumors requiring a second cryoablation procedure, 4 tumors requiring a third cryoablation procedure, and 11 tumors requiring a fourth cryoablation procedure. Ten patients had residual disease (or recurrence) at the time of death; however, only three of these cases were disease-related. Although these results are promising in terms of overall and disease-specific survival, they also underscore the importance of patient counseling on the possibility for additional procedures to treat renal tumors adequately and effectively using this MINSS therapeutic modality.

Atwell and colleagues[27] recently reported on their experience using CT-guided PCA in 110 patients. A total of 115 tumors with a mean tumor size of 3.3 cm (range: 1.5–7.3 cm) were treated. Of 90 renal mass biopsies performed, 52 (58%) showed RCC. All patients were admitted to the hospital after cryoablation, with most (87%) being discharged on postoperative day 1 (range: 1–12 days). There were seven major complications (6%) of 113 total procedures performed. Technical success was achieved in 97% of the treated tumors, with three failures occurring in centrally located tumors. Of these failures, 1 patient died while in hospice of nonrelated complex medical issues, 1 is being observed, and 1 has been lost to follow-up. There has been no local progression of 80 tumors (100% treatment success) followed for a mean of 13.3 months (range: 3–39 months). It should be noted that 25% of the tumors treated were 4.0 cm or larger, thereby making a case for technical feasibility in successfully ablating relatively larger tumors. The investigators also demonstrated that with the correct changes in patient positioning (eg, supine versus decubitus), and even fluid injection into the anterior pararenal space (ie, the creation of a "salinoma"), the overlying bowel can be displaced to treat anterior tumors successfully.

Complications of Cryoablation

The morbidity associated with cryoablation of renal tumors seems to be relatively low. With LCA, the most recent publication by Cestari and colleagues[20] reported only 3 major complications of 104 cases treated: one perinephric hematoma that required a blood transfusion, one abscess treated successfully with percutaneous drainage, and one UPJ obstruction that required open pyeloplasty. Although the results from this Italian group are promising, a recent study by Lehman and colleagues[32] reported that LCA of larger (≥3.0 cm) renal masses was associated with increased morbidity. This retrospective study of 44 procedures on 51 tumors stratified the subjects into two groups based on tumor size. Group 1 included 30 tumors in 23 patients with a maximum tumor diameter less than 3.0 cm (mean = 1.8 cm, range: 0.7–2.8 cm), and group 2 included 21 tumors in 21 patients with a maximum tumor diameter greater than or equal to 3.0 cm (mean = 4.0 cm, range: 3.0–7.5 cm). Although group 1 had no complications, group 2 had 13 (62%) complications, including two deaths. The most common complication was postoperative hemorrhage requiring blood transfusion (38%), with the two deaths secondary to aspiration pneumonia and myocardial infarction on postoperative days 16 and 37, respectively. With a mean follow-up of 9 months, there were no recurrences in group 1, whereas group 2 had one recurrence. The investigators concluded that although LCA was equally effective for larger renal masses (>3.0 cm) in terms of successful ablation, the laparoscopic approach to cryoablation should be performed only for lesions less than 3.0 cm because of the significantly higher complication rate.

One of the larger and more recent PCA studies by Atwell and colleagues[27] reported a complication rate of 6%, similar to the other PCA studies mentioned previously. The seven complications included worsening preexisting hypertension and pulmonary edema, delayed urosepsis, pulmonary embolus, hematuria requiring ureteral stent placement, and three patients who had retroperitoneal hematomas requiring angiography and red blood cell transfusion. The researchers mentioned the value of preablation selective angioembolization of renal tumors in decreasing the rate of major postoperative hematomas. Although the small number of tumors that were embolized before surgery precluded any meaningful statistical analysis, this does give some food for thought in terms of whether or not this optimizes patient safety by decreasing the number of major postoperative retroperitoneal hematomas and what effect this would have on renal function and the overall cost of the procedure.

In a multi-institutional retrospective series of 271 ablative cases, Johnson and colleagues[33] analyzed the complications of 139 cryoablation and 133 RFA procedures, of which 181 were performed percutaneously, with the remaining 90 procedures performed laparoscopically. A total of 20 complications (14.4%) occurred in the cryoablation series (4 after LCA and 16 after PCA). The cryoablative group reported 2 major complications: one significant postoperative hemorrhage requiring reoperation and blood transfusion after PCA and one open conversion attributable to the inability to access the tumor laparoscopically. Minor complications included 10 cases of flank pain and paresthesias at the operative site, two postoperative urinary tract infections, one small self-limited hematoma, one case of postoperative pneumonia, and one case of elevated serum creatinine. Most of these patients had a complete recovery. The researchers noted that more than half of the complications in this study occurred in the first third of the procedures performed, suggesting a learning curve associated with this new MINSS technique.

The theory that cryoinjury predisposes the kidney to further loss of renal function secondary to necrosis and scarring seems to be largely unfounded based on all clinical trials to date. Johnson and colleagues[33] showed promising results after cryoablation with only 1 of 139 patients sustaining a significant elevation in serum creatinine. In a retrospective review with a mean follow-up of 20.6 months, Carvalhal and colleagues[34] reported no significant differences in pre- and postoperative creatinine levels, blood pressure, or estimated creatinine clearance.

In a retrospective review, Finley and colleagues[35] compared the peri- and postoperative outcomes of PCA and LCA. A total of 37 patients underwent treatment for 43 renal masses; 24 tumors were approached laparoscopically (mean tumor size = 3.0 cm, range: 1.1–5.4 cm), whereas the remaining 19 tumors were treated with CT-guided PCA (mean tumor size = 2.7 cm, range: 1.7–4.7 cm). The transfusion rates in the PCA and LCA groups were 11.1% and 27.8%, respectively. Operative time was significantly longer in the LCA group (mean = 147 minutes, range: 89–209 minutes) than in the PCA group (mean = 250 minutes, range: 151–360 minutes). The overall complication rate was lower in the PCA group (22%) when compared with the LCA group (40%). Hospital stay was also significantly shorter in the PCA group than in the LCA group (1.3 versus 3.1 days; $P<.0001$). Among the patients who had biopsy-proved RCC, during a median follow-up of 11.4 and 13.4 months, the PCA and LCA groups had 100% cancer-specific survival and treatment failure rates of 5.3% and 4.2%, respectively. Given these findings, the investigators concluded that PCA seems to be superior to the laparoscopic approach to cryoablation for small renal tumors.

Radiofrequency Ablation

RFA acts through the conversion of radiofrequency waves into heat, resulting in thermal damage to tissue. A high-frequency monopolar alternating current flows from the needle electrode to the target tissue, resulting in ionic agitation and heat-producing molecular friction as an inverse function of the tissues' impedance (resistance to energy flow). Heat is not directly supplied by the probe itself.[36] RFA leads to cell death through instantaneous and irreversible protein denaturation, tissue cross-linking, and desiccation. The thermal effects of tissue desiccation and coagulative necrosis occur almost immediately when temperatures reach higher than 60°C.[37] Exposure to these high temperatures also has direct effects on cellular components, including cell membrane disintegration and cell nucleus unrest. In addition, RFA has a direct effect on tissue perfusion secondary to microvascular and arteriolar occlusion within the ablated zone, leading to ischemia of the treated tissue.[38]

Originally, RFA was applied in a "dry" fashion by an electrode causing rapid increases in temperature, with tissue desiccation and charring around the tip of the probe. Once tumors reach 4 cm and larger, however, this technique increases tissue impedance and results in an inefficient radiofrequency lesion. To circumvent this problem and make ablation more time-efficient, "wet" RFA was developed, in which saline is irrigated through the tissue to increase conductivity and help to dissipate energy, thereby resulting in a larger radiofrequency lesion.[39]

Because of the formation of microbubbles and the low intrinsic contrast between normal and ablated tissues, real-time imaging of the developing thermal lesion with intraoperative US, CT, or MRI has proved difficult.[40] The lesion created by the radiofrequency probe, however, is a function of its deployed diameter and minimum time activated; as a result, proponents of RFA argue that real-time monitoring of the ablation zone is not necessary, because activating the probe for longer periods does not change the lesion size. RFA is generally monitored by measuring impedance and temperature changes, with feedback provided from thermosensors integrated at the end of radiofrequency tines around the radiofrequency probes. Imaging immediately after the procedure can be difficult to interpret in terms of successful ablation because of peripheral inflammation; however, one study did demonstrate that MRI allowed differentiation of treated versus untreated renal parenchyma to within 2 mm when compared with pathologic examination.[41] Typically, the success of RFA is assessed by a contrast-enhanced CT scan or MRI 4 to 6 weeks after treatment by demonstrating a paucity of enhancement within the ablated tissue.

As with cryoablation, RFA can be used by means of an open, laparoscopic, or percutaneous approach, with the latter two techniques being the predominant ways in which radiofrequency waves are currently delivered. As with cryoablation, laparoscopic radiofrequency ablation (LRFA) has the advantage of tumor mobilization and placement of the probe under direct vision. This increased exposure and visualization of the kidney would theoretically allow for the avoidance of adjacent organ damage.

Early experience with LRFA was presented by Jacomides and colleagues[42] on 13 patients with a total of 17 renal tumors. In 5 patients, the tumor was subsequently excised completely, whereas in 7 patients, it was left in situ. Mean tumor size was 1.96 cm (range: 0.9–3.6 cm). Pathologic analysis revealed RCC in 10 patients, angiomyolipoma in 2 patients, and oncocytoma in 1 patient. None of the 8 patients who had RCC and at least 6 weeks of follow-up had any evidence of persistent tumor enhancement on surveillance CT scan. There was one focal positive margin in a patient who underwent RFA and excision of RCC, but the patient

has remained disease-free for 12 months after treatment.

The evolution of thinner diameter radiofrequency probes has rendered percutaneous radiofrequency ablation (PRFA) the most prevalent method currently for renal RFA, using CT or MRI guidance. Matsumoto and colleagues[43] reported on a series of 91 patients who had 109 small renal tumors; 63 were treated with PRFA, and the other 46 were treated with LRFA. The combined mean tumor size for the two groups was 2.4 cm (range: 0.8–4.7 cm), with a combined initial success rate of 98% (107 of 109 tumors). There was one local recurrence (1.7%) detected during a mean follow-up of 19.4 months (range: 12–33 months), with incomplete ablations and the local recurrence successfully treated with reablation. Paralleling the results from the CA literature, the percutaneous approach had a shorter mean operative time (105.8 versus 147.5 minutes) and lower mean EBL (4.2 versus 25.1 mL) than LRFA. Although the PRFA group reported no major complications, the LRFA group had three major complications, consisting of a UPJ injury that ultimately required nephrectomy, a urine leak, and a lower pole infarct.

Gervais and colleagues[44,45] reported on their clinical experience with CT- and MRI-guided PRFA for 100 renal masses in 85 patients over a period of more than 6 years. All the 68 peripheral exophytic lesions (52 of which were ≤3 cm) were ablated successfully after one treatment. This was in contrast to 78% (7 of 9 tumors) of central tumors and only 61% (11 of 18 tumors) of mixed-type tumors that had both central and exophytic components, which were completely ablated after one session. In addition, the researchers noted that small (<3 cm) peripheral lesions had a successful ablation rate of 100%, whereas larger tumors (>3 cm) and those that were centrally located had successful ablation rates of 92% and 25%, respectively. Results of the ad hoc analysis suggested that small size (P<.0001) and noncentral location (P<.005) proved to be independent predictors of complete necrosis after a single PRFA session.

Stern and colleagues[46] recently compared the intermediate-term outcomes of patients who had clinical T1a renal tumors treated with partial nephrectomy (open and laparoscopic) or RFA (laparoscopic and percutaneous). A total of 37 partial nephrectomies (30 open, 7 laparoscopic) were compared with 40 RFAs (14 laparoscopic, 26 percutaneous), with a mean tumor size of 2.41 cm and 2.43 cm, respectively. The mean (range) follow-ups for the RFA and partial nephrectomy groups were 30[18–42] and 47[7,24–92] months, respectively. There was one incomplete ablation and two recurrences in the RFA group, whereas the partial nephrectomy group had two recurrences (one local and one in the contralateral kidney). There were no disease-specific deaths in either group. The overall actuarial disease-free probability for the partial nephrectomy and RFA groups was 95.8% and 93.4%, respectively.

Levinson and colleagues[47] recently reported their long-term oncologic and overall outcomes of PRFA in 31 high-risk surgical patients who had solitary renal masses. Median tumor size was 2.0 cm (range: 1.0–4.0 cm), and patients had a mean follow-up of 60.5 months (range: 41–80 months). There was one primary treatment failure, which was successfully reablated, and three recurrences at 7, 13, and 39 months after PRFA. The recurrences were managed with repeat PRFA, PCA, and laparoscopic radical nephrectomy, respectively. The overall recurrence-free survival was 90.3%, with 100% metastasis-free and disease-specific survival. The difference between pretreatment and last known serum creatinine levels was 0.15 mg/dL ($P = .06$). The researchers concluded that in patients who have a limited life expectancy or are high-risk surgical candidates, RFA provides reasonable long-term oncologic control.

Complications of Radiofrequency Ablation

In the multi-institutional review by Johnson and colleagues,[33] of the 133 cases that underwent RFA, there were a total of 10 complications (7.6% complication rate) directly attributable to the procedure (3 major, 7 minor). The LRFA group had all 3 major complications, consisting of urine leak, UPJ obstruction, and ileus. The minor complications included four patients who had probe site pain or paresthesias, postoperative pneumonia, or self-limited liver-burn injury and one patient with an elevated serum creatinine level.

As with cryoablation, renal function after RFA is preserved in the most cases. In a study by Lucas and colleagues,[48] a total of 242 consecutive patients were treated for solitary renal masses 4 cm or less in diameter using RFA (86 patients), partial nephrectomy (85 patients), and nephrectomy (71 patients). Before surgery, stage 3 chronic kidney disease was identified in a total of 65 patients, including 26.7%, 27.1%, and 26.8% who underwent RFA, partial nephrectomy, and radical nephrectomy, respectively. After intervention, the 3-year freedom from a glomerular filtration rate decrease of less than 60 mL per minute per 1.73 m^2 for RFA, partial nephrectomy, and

radical nephrectomy was 95.2%, 70.7%, and 39.9%, respectively ($P<.001$). This article highlights the prevalence of impaired renal function in patients who have SRMs and the important consideration of long-term kidney function, particularly in those patients in whom renal function is already compromised.

Overall, the complications that were defined in the review by Johnson and colleagues[33] are similar to those reported by other smaller single-institution series. By far, the most common minor complication is pain and paresthesias at the percutaneous probe insertion site. In terms of major complications, most are secondary to thermal injury to the renal collecting system. Traver and colleagues[49] reported two cases of proximal ureteral strictures from a series of 73 tumors that were treated with PRFA. Single cases of ureteral stricture were also seen in the PRFA series of Matsumoto and colleagues,[43] Gervais and colleagues,[44] and Weiser and colleagues.[50] This last point further emphasizes the need to apply any thermal ablation technology in the vicinity of the proximal ureter or renal pelvis judiciously for the reasons discussed previously. In most of the reported clinical series, the preponderance of major complications secondary to cryoablation has to do with postoperative hemorrhage. The ability of RFA to avoid tract bleeding and tumor seeding by coagulating the puncture channel during probe withdrawal results in the decreased number of major bleeding complications associated with this procedure.

There are a few clinical studies in which renal tumors have been removed or biopsied after RFA that have called the success of this technology into question. In a recent study by Weight and colleagues,[51] they sought to correlate radiographic imaging with histopathologic examination after LCA and PRFA. There were a total of 109 lesions treated with PRFA, whereas 192 lesions were treated with LCA. Radiographic success at 6 months was 85% and 90% for PRFA and LCA, respectively. At 6 months, almost half of the lesions were biopsied and success in the PRFA cohort dropped to 64.8%, whereas success in the LCA group remained fairly high at 93.8%. Perhaps most alarming was that 6 (46.2%) of 13 patients in the PRFA group with a positive biopsy demonstrated no enhancement on posttreatment MRI or CT scans. In the patients treated with LCA, 100% of the positive biopsies revealed posttreatment enhancement on imaging just before biopsy. The investigators concluded that because of the poor correlation between postoperative imaging and biopsy to define success after RFA, all patients undergoing RFA should have a postoperative biopsy to rule out residual cancer cells left behind after ablation.

Standard histologic staining using hematoxylin and eosin (H&E) may be somewhat misleading, however, immediately after RFA.[52] Rather, staining with NADH diaphorase has been postulated to be a more accurate assessment of cell viability, because the activity of this ubiquitous cellular enzyme has been shown to cease several hours after cell death.[53] Essentially, the temperatures used during RFA are high enough to cause cell death and not necessarily acute architectural damage throughout the ablated lesion. Marcovich and colleagues[52] demonstrated this point by staining resected porcine renal tumors that had first been treated with RFA with H&E and NADH diaphorase. What they found was that although RFA produced discernable histologic changes on H&E, these were variable and patchy and alternated with areas in which the architecture had been well preserved. When these corresponding areas were then stained with NADH diaphorase, there was a complete absence of staining, indicating that cell death had taken place.

Taking these data into account, Michaels and colleagues[54] treated 20 tumors in 15 patients using a temperature-based electrode immediately before open partial nephrectomy. Although gross visualization indicated that all tumors were completely treated, 4 of 5 tumors stained with NADH diaphorase suggested residual activity. Matlaga and colleagues[55] also evaluated tumor cell destruction after RFA using histologic analysis. Ten patients underwent impedance-based US-guided RFA immediately before partial or radical nephrectomy. Overall, 8 of 10 tumors demonstrated no NADH activity within the tumor or surrounding rim of renal parenchyma. Of the 2 tumors that stained positively for NADH diaphorase, the first did not achieve an adequate increase in temperature (41°C), whereas the other was 8.0 cm in maximal diameter. The first failure was attributed to heat sink phenomena, whereas the second was not expected to be successful based on the size of the tumor.

The failures of renal RFA in these studies have largely been attributed to flaws in surgical and staining technique and immature technology used at that time. Among the reasons cited to explain the ablative failures are inappropriate use of NADH diaphorase staining, real-time US to monitor the ablation zone, impedance-based electrodes prematurely ceasing tissue ablation, short ablation times, and inadequate wattage. Recently, Stern and colleagues[56] reassuringly performed post-RFA biopsies on 20 lesions at a mean follow-up of 26.9 months (range: 13.1–58 months).

All biopsies were performed on patients who clinically had NED (absence of lesion growth or contrast enhancement by CT) 1 year or more after RFA. Preablation biopsies confirmed that 17 of 20 tumors were RCC, whereas the remaining 3 tumors were oncocytomas. At the time of repeat biopsy, all 20 specimens showed unequivocal cell death with no evidence of cellular viability.

Microwave Ablation

Microwave ablation (MWA) involves the insertion of flexible antennae placed directly into target tissue and channels microwave energy to create a rapidly alternating electromagnetic field. In turn, this leads to the oscillation of ions, with a subsequent increase in kinetic energy that is converted to heat and ultimately results in coagulative necrosis.[57] Most of the published literature on MT describes its use in achieving hemostasis at partial nephrectomy without the need to clamp hilar vessels. Until recently, no clinical experience had been reported regarding its use in renal tumor ablation as a curative approach. Liang and colleagues[58] recently evaluated the feasibility, safety, and efficacy of US-guided percutaneous MWA for small (<4.0 cm) RCCs. A total of 12 patients who had pathologically proved RCC on preoperative biopsy underwent US-guided percutaneous MWA. Mean tumor size was 2.5 cm (range: 1.3–3.8 cm), with 10 tumors being exophytic and the other 2 being intraparenchymal. Immediate treatment efficacy was assessed using thermocouples to monitor temperature in real time during ablation and 24 hours after ablation with contrast-enhanced US. Short-term efficacy was then assessed by a contrast-enhanced CT scan or US at 1, 3, and 6 months and every 6 months thereafter. All tumors were successfully ablated in one session, and there were no reported complications. No residual tumor recurrence was observed at a median follow-up of 11 months (range: 4–20 months). The researchers discuss some potential advantages of MWA, which include a broad zone of active heating and the fact that its transmission through tissue is not limited by desiccation and charring. MT is also less affected by the perfusion-mediated heat sink effect. Although the study is promising in terms of ablation success rate, complication rate, and short-term efficacy, it does have some limitations that must be addressed in subsequent series. The inclusion criteria were quite strict in terms of tumor size (<4.0 cm) and location (tumors near the hilum or adjacent to important structures, such as bowel or ureter, were excluded), and the relatively small sample size makes it somewhat difficult to interpret the results.

High-Intensity Focused Ultrasound

In HIFU, an US wave is propagated through biologic tissues, whereby it is progressively absorbed. This energy is converted into heat, leading to protein denaturation, coagulative necrosis, and subsequent cell death. The transducer is used for delivery and monitoring of the ablative therapy. The most vital aspect of this technology (which allows it to be applied in an extracorporeal fashion) is that the energy generated by means of the ultrasonic waves drops sharply outside of the focal zone, such that nearby tissues remain largely unchanged. This seemingly narrow range of focus also proves to be HIFU's main limitation in terms of lesion localization and targeting, especially when applied to renal tumors.

This last point was demonstrated by Marberger and colleagues,[59] who looked at 18 kidney tumors treated with HIFU. All tumors were subsequently removed, and histologic analysis found incomplete ablation in every case. The disappointing results were largely attributable to the difficulty in tissue targeting secondary to respiratory movement, intervening structures of the abdominal wall and ribs, and acoustic characteristics of the tumors themselves. In another study, Hacker and colleagues[60] applied HIFU to the healthy tissue of 24 kidneys monitored by US. For an in vivo study, 14 kidneys were removed immediately after ablation, with the other 10 kidneys removed after 1, 7, and 10 days of therapy. Side effects included grade 3 skin burns in two of the patients. In one case, there was a thermal lesion of the small intestine, which the investigators attributed to poor focusing. HIFU effects in the focal zone immediately after application were interstitial hemorrhage, fiber rupture, shrinking of collagen fibers, and coagulative necrosis. These effects occurred sporadically, and their number and size did not correlate with the number of HIFU pulses that were applied to the target tissue. After 7 and 10 days, there was a well-demarcated area of coagulative necrosis in vivo. Based on the cumulative clinical experiences of these and other researchers, it would seem that continued refinements in HIFU are essential to establish this ablative technology as a noninvasive treatment option for renal masses.

Radiosurgery

In contrast to the thermal ablation techniques discussed heretofore, radiation destroys dividing tumor cells by mitosis-linked apoptosis. At higher doses, radiation results in complete ablation of tissue, and thus provides the basis for solid mass ablation. The caveat to radiation's use for ablation was the unacceptable collateral damage that occurred to normal tissue at the treatment margins. In contrast to traditional external beam radiation, however, radiosurgical therapy is delivered using a frameless image-guided device that utilizes a linear accelerator mounted on a robotic arm and divides the high-dose radiation into more than 1000 beams. Therefore, the individual dose of each beam is relatively benign to skin and adjacent tissue, whereas at the focal point of the beams, the dose is additive and the desired ablative dose is attained.

As described previously, one of the major limitations to extracorporeal solid organ ablation of renal tumors is the inherent back-and-forth movement of the kidney associated with the respiratory cycle. This limitation is circumvented by a highly advanced radiosurgical image guidance system that allows the radiation beam to follow and "correct" for a moving target in real time. A unique tracking and compensation system uses external "fiducial" markers in conjunction with diagnostic radiographic images to guide the robotic arm so that the beam remains aligned with its target. With the aid of this technology, renal tumor motion can be tracked in three-dimensional (3D) space, allowing for exceptionally precise treatment (within 0.3 mm).

Still in its relative infancy, radiosurgical ablation is devoid of any long-term studies; however, short-term analysis has been promising. In 2003, Ponsky and colleagues[61] were the first to report their initial evaluation with stereotactic radiosurgery technology in eight swine. In each pig, bilateral kidneys were treated at predetermined sites (each approximately 2 cm in diameter) using a single dose of 24 to 40 Gy followed by organ harvest and histologic examination 4 to 8 weeks later. All targeted sites revealed complete tissue ablation surrounded by a small zone of partial fibrosis. Perhaps just as important, the remainder of the surrounding renal parenchyma was completely unharmed, and gross inspection at the time of kidney procurement failed to reveal any evidence of radiation injury to the body wall or surrounding organs. After this initial study, a clinical protocol was designed to address the safety of renal radiosurgery in humans. Ponsky and colleagues[62] treated three patients with a mean tumor size of 2.03 cm using 16 Gy divided into four fractions over 2 consecutive days. All patients had a CT scan 8 weeks after radiosurgery and subsequently underwent a partial nephrectomy for their renal mass. Histopathologic examination of the excised specimens demonstrated a cavity without evidence of viable tumor in one patient, whereas the remaining two showed evidence of residual RCC. This trial confirmed the safety of renal radiosurgery, because there were no acute or chronic toxicities using this low dose with a follow-up time of longer than 1 year. With a clinical protocol in place for gradual dose escalation, results are forthcoming with regard to clinical efficacy.

Promising work with radiosurgical technology has also been reported by Hong and colleagues.[63] Their initial evaluation included 14 patients with a mean tumor diameter of 4.1 cm treated with 21 Gy divided into three fractions. Patients were then imaged every 3 months with serial CT scans. Tumor volume decreased by a mean of 44%, with no signs of disease progression at 12 months of follow-up. Given that multiple radiosurgical units are currently in operation at radiation oncology centers worldwide, further experimental and clinical data should continue to become available for this promising ablative technology.

PROSTATE

Prostate cancer is the most frequently diagnosed cause and the second leading cause of death attributable to cancer among men in the United States. An estimated 186,320 cases of newly diagnosed prostate cancer have been predicted to occur in 2008 in the United States, with more than 28,000 of these men succumbing to the disease.[1] Over the past 25 years, the 5-year survival rate for all stages combined has increased from 69% to greater than 98%. According to the most recent data, relative 10- and 15-year survival is 91% and 76%, respectively.[1] The dramatic improvements in survival, particularly at 5 years, are attributable to earlier diagnosis and improvements in therapy. Widespread screening with serum prostate-specific antigen (PSA) and digital rectal examination (DRE) has allowed for earlier detection, with most cases being detected in a clinically localized stage. Because of this, along with the improved efficacy in treatment modalities, only approximately 15% of men diagnosed with prostate cancer ultimately die as a result of the disease.

The good and bad news about prostate cancer are one in the same: there are a variety of different treatment options for patients to choose from, and the advent of extracorporeal and needle-ablative technologies certainly does not make this choice any easier. Couple this with prostate cancer's protracted natural history, and it is easy to see how hard it becomes to develop a consensus for its optimal management. Given the fact that most men who are currently diagnosed ultimately have their disease eradicated by one of the many different treatment options available, the real focus of curative therapy has been on quality of life after treatment. It is in this clinical context that minimally invasive treatment options for prostate cancer, such as radiosurgery, HIFU, and cryosurgery, have come to the forefront of prostate cancer management in an effort to maintain sound oncologic outcomes while minimizing the well-known complications of extirpative therapy.

Stereotactic Hypofractionated Radiosurgery of the Prostate

As eluded to previously, eradication of tumor by radiation is believed to depend on dose; however, the dose beyond which no additional benefit is likely largely remains unknown. Newer radiation technologies, such as 3D conformal radiation therapy (CRT), intensity-modulated radiation therapy (IMRT), and now hypofractionated radiosurgery, have several interrelated goals. The ultimate in radiation therapy would provide for precise tumor targeting and safe delivery of higher doses of radiation while reducing the amount of normal tissue toxicity associated with these higher doses of radiation.

Hypofractionation refers to the use of larger than conventional dose-per-fraction sizes of radiation. Several investigators have recently argued that the α/β ratio for prostate cancer is much lower than previously thought, which implies a high sensitivity to dose-per-fraction size.[64,65] If this is true, a hypofractionated regimen would yield high tumor control rates while maintaining an equivalent dose to normal tissues (ie, bladder, rectum) for late toxicity and would reduce the acute toxicity seen with modern 3D-CRT. In addition, a shortened course of radiotherapy would be a much more appealing option than conventional radiotherapy in terms of logistics (1-week versus 6- to 9-week course of daily treatment) and cost differential.

The demands for high precision of delivery of large-dose fractions require a system that is capable of overcoming daily target position variations and potential organ motion to a high degree of precision while delivering CRT. The CyberKnife is a 6-MV linear accelerator mounted on a computer-controlled robotic arm. Real-time correction attributable to target organ daily position changes or motion during radiation delivery is accomplished by means of an orthogonal pair of digital radiographic imaging devices monitoring the position of fiducial markers placed within the target organ. These fiducial markers consist of three gold "seeds" placed within the apex, base, and midgland of the prostate (this is done by transrectal ultrasound [TRUS] guidance). Because the planning CT scan is obtained with these seeds in place, it is the relative position of the seeds with respect to the contoured organ that serves as the reference point. This allows radiation delivery with a precision of less than 0.5 mm and a tracking error of less than 1 mm.[66]

Results are limited, because few centers in the United States have adopted this technology (originally described for use on intracranial tumors) to treat carcinoma of the prostate. In a recent phase I/II trial, 40 patients were prospectively enrolled to evaluate the feasibility and toxicity of stereotactic hypofractionated radiotherapy to the prostate for localized low-risk prostate cancer. The median time to follow-up was 41 months, with 5 patients dying of non–prostate-related illnesses. Acute and late genitourinary (GU) and gastrointestinal (GI) toxicities were evaluated, and PSA values and self-reported sexual function questions were recorded at specific intervals. Acute grade 2 or less GU and GI toxicities were 48.5% and 39%, respectively; only 1 patient had acute grade 3 GU toxicity, which required catheterization but resolved with ibuprofen and tamsulosin. Late grade 2 or less GU and GI toxicities were 45% and 37%, respectively, with no late grade 3 toxicities reported. The incidence of erectile dysfunction after therapy was 23%. The actuarial 48-month biochemical freedom from relapse was 70% using the American Society for Therapeutic Radiology and Oncology (ASTRO) definition of failure.[67] This study is promising in that it demonstrates the feasibility of delivering hypofractionated radiotherapy to the prostate, acceptable GU and GI toxicity rates, and appropriate biochemical response. The small cohort size and limited follow-up, however, do warrant further clinical validation of hypofractionation before this is widely adopted as an option for the treatment of localized prostate cancer.

Cryoablation of the Prostate

Cryoablation destroys prostate tissue using extreme cold temperatures. The technique of cryotherapy was first described in the early 1960s by Cooper and Lee,[68] using a small-caliber vacuum-insulated liquid nitrogen cryoprobe, which enabled precise organ targeting. Although there are several theories to explain the mechanism of tissue injury using cryoablation, the most well-accepted hypothesis is that freezing tissue directly causes cellular death.[7,69] This is accomplished through two main mechanisms: direct cellular toxicity from disruption of the cellular

membrane by ice ball crystals and vascular compromise from thrombosis and ischemia.[69]

Gonder and Soanes[70] were the first to describe the use of cryoablation in the treatment of prostatic disease. A single cryoprobe was inserted transurethrally into the prostate, and the freezing process was monitored by DRE and by a temperature gauge placed in Denonvilliers' fascia. This method, unfortunately, was fraught with several complications, including urethral sloughing, urinary incontinence, and urethrorectal fistula. These complications were attributed to a lack of accurate monitoring of the freezing process. Starting in the 1980s with the advent of TRUS, improvements were made in prostate cryosurgery in terms of enabling real-time imaging of the prostate and using sonography to guide more precise placement of multiple cryoprobes. The introduction of a urethral warming catheter also helped to prevent urethral sloughing and resultant strictures.[71] Although these adjustments improved cryoablative surgery immensely, the continued incidence of rectourethral fistulae combined with a substandard oncologic outcome pushed cryotherapy again to the wayside. It was not until the late 1990s that cryoablation was again revisited as a formidable technique for prostate cancer treatment. The new gas-driven probes were smaller, and a brachytherapy template was used to facilitate more accurate placement of probes transperineally. Multiple temperature sensors are used for better control of the freeze zone, and a urethral warming catheter is always placed to protect the urethra.[72] Patient selection has also improved, with the optimal prostate size being less than 50 g.

After cryotherapy, PSA levels reach a nadir within 3 months of treatment. Although there are several studies that follow biochemical progression-free survival after cryotherapy, recurrence-free outcomes are difficult to interpret, because no clear definition of recurrence after cryotherapy has been established.[73,74] In addition, some patients in these studies received neoadjuvant hormone ablation, which further clouds the definition of freedom from biochemical progression.

In a pooled analysis by Long and colleagues,[75] with a median follow-up of 24 months, the actuarial 5-year biochemical disease-free survival (bDFS) rates were 60%, 45%, and 36% for low-, intermediate-, and high-risk patients, respectively, using a PSA threshold of 0.5 ng/mL to define failure (as is done in many surgical series), and 76%, 71%, and 45% using a threshold of 1.0 ng/mL to define failure. In an often cited multi-institutional study by Bahn and colleagues,[76] 590 patients were followed for a mean of 5.4 years. These investigators reported 7-year bDFS rates stratified by the same risk definitions as used by Long and colleagues,[75] employing several different definitions for treatment failure. Using an absolute PSA threshold of 0.5 ng/mL to define failure, the bDFS rates were 61%, 68%, and 61% for low-, intermediate-, and high-risk patients, respectively.[76] In another review by Katz and Rewcastle,[73] 5-year biochemical progression-free survival rates were compared among different forms of primary therapy for prostate cancer. Patients were stratified into low-, intermediate-, and high-risk groups, and biochemical progression was defined using the ASTRO criteria. According to this review, radical prostatectomy was superior in the low-risk group; however, in the intermediate- and high-risk groups, there was a decline in efficacy for all treatment modalities with the exception of cryotherapy, which had the highest PSA progression-free survival within the 5 years of follow-up currently available in the literature. Although encouraging, these results must be tempered, given the lack of long-term data regarding metastasis-free or disease-specific survival, which, again, ultimately precludes truly meaningful comparisons of these outcomes that have been reported in the radical prostatectomy and radiation therapy literature.

Radiation therapy is a common and effective treatment option for patients who have newly discovered localized prostate cancer. Despite the contemporary modifications of 3D-CRT and IMRT, recent data have demonstrated a biochemical failure rate of 63% after radiation therapy, with positive prostate biopsies in one third of these patients.[77,78] If detected early, prostate cancer cure may still be possible; however, treatment options are limited and have long been plagued with higher rates of morbidity. The recent advances in cryotherapy technology, however, afford decreased rates of treatment-associated morbidity and have rekindled interest in this treatment option for localized recurrence after radiation therapy failure.

Although there has been no established set of parameters to define salvage cryotherapy failure, most groups use PSA values of 0.5 ng/mL or greater or persistent disease diagnosed by prostate biopsy to define outcomes.[79] Bahn and colleagues[80] reported a bDFS rate of 59% at 7 years of follow-up using a cutoff value of PSA less than 0.5 ng/mL in 59 patients. Chin and colleagues[81] performed cryosurgery on 118 patients who had recurrent disease after radiation therapy. Seven patients were treated with a repeat procedure for persistent disease. One third of these patients maintained PSA values less than 0.5 ng/mL at 18.6 months of median follow-up. Of note, 10 patients ultimately went on to develop

metastatic disease. In the longest reported follow-up to date, Hamoui and colleagues[82] reported 10-year treatment outcomes of salvage cryotherapy for locally recurrent prostate cancer in 110 patients. After salvage cryotherapy, 78 patients (71.6%) developed biochemical failure (PSA $\geq$ 0.5 ng/mL), and among those patients, the 10-year disease-specific survival was 82.5%.

With the advent of third-generation cryotherapy technology, there has been a dramatic decrease in morbidity compared with that reported with first-generation cryosurgery. In fact, rectal and bladder complications are now rare (<0.5%) in patients undergoing primary treatment.[76,83,84] Third-generation cryosurgery is associated with an incontinence rate of up to 5.5% and urethral sloughing rates up to 6.7%, and up to 5.5% of patients have required transurethral resection of the prostate (TURP) for bladder outlet obstruction after cryotherapy.[76,84] In terms of complications, impotence remains a significant problem after cryosurgery,[74,85] although with the advent of targeted intervention strategies, these numbers are improving. In a study by Robinson and colleagues,[86] 13% of patients regained potency and an additional 34% remained sexually active with the assistance of erectile aids 3 years after cryoablation. Ellis and colleagues[87] reported potency rates of 41.4% at 1 year and 51.3% at 4 years when patients were placed on a penile rehabilitation program after total gland cryoablation.

The clear trend in contemporary reduction of complication rates applies equally to salvage cryoablation as well. Given the nature of retreatment, one would expect higher complication rates with salvage cryotherapy. For example, urinary incontinence, which was once an expected occurrence after prostate cryoablation, is now infrequent, with reported rates of less than 10%.[79] In one of the largest multicenter studies from the Cryo On-Line Data (COLD) registry, data from 279 patients were obtained after salvage prostate cryoablation. In terms of complications, these groups reported a combined incontinence rate (requiring pad use) of 4.4%, with another 5.8% reporting occasional leakage not requiring the use of absorbent pads. The rectal fistula rate was low at 1.2%.[88] Unfortunately, there were insufficient data to assess postcryoablation potency, but most current studies still report rates of greater than 80%.[79]

High-Intensity Focused Ultrasound

HIFU is a minimally invasive approach that uses US beams to treat prostatic disease. With this technique, a probe is inserted transrectally and a high-energy US beam is focused into the prostate. Acoustic energy absorbed by the prostate tissue is converted into thermal energy with intraprostatic temperatures reaching upward of 100°C.[89] This interaction produces coagulating heat, high pressure, cavitation bubbles, and chemically active free radicals; the result is a focal area of tissue destruction by way of coagulative necrosis.[90] HIFU of the prostate can be performed under spinal or general anesthesia with the patient lying on his side or in the dorsal lithotomy position. With the imaging and treatment probes placed transrectally, the prostate is imaged and a therapeutic plan is created. A series of adjacent target zones is mapped to each cross-sectional level of the prostate gland, and once activated, the machine automatically cycles through the outlined treatment plan. A monitoring device automatically deactivates the machine if the patient moves, and cooling fluid is circulated around the treatment probe to protect the rectal wall. Up to 3 months is required for necrosis to occur, and because the energy used is non-ionizing, treatment can be repeated.

HIFU is widely available in Europe (where most of the studies regarding its use in prostate cancer have been done), but outside of clinical trials, it is not as accessible in the United States. In a large, open-label, multicenter study in Europe, slightly more than 400 patients underwent HIFU for prostate cancer between 1995 and 1999. Of the 288 patients who underwent repeat biopsy after treatment, 87% were negative for carcinoma. Complications included urinary incontinence in 13.1% and rectourethral fistulas in 1.3%. Follow-up was relatively short at just longer than 13 months, and the treatment protocol evolved during the trial, making the interpretation of these results somewhat difficult.[91] In another early study by Beerlage and colleagues,[92] the first 49 of 111 patients were treated by selectively focusing the US beams to the prostate region believed to harbor the tumor. Of this selectively treated cohort, 72% had residual cancer on repeat biopsy (most likely reflecting the multifocal nature of prostate cancer), demonstrating the limitation of prostate-sparing HIFU. The remaining 62 patients received therapy to the entire prostate, yet the repeat biopsy rate was still relatively high at 32%. Significant side effects included urinary incontinence in 8.1%, rectourethral fistulas in 2.7%, and urethral stenosis in 1 patient. Initial results by Blana and colleagues[93] reported a 70% progression-free survival rate with a mean follow-up of 23 months, but the durability of responses has not been documented. In a more recent study, Uchida and colleagues[94] treated 503 patients between 1999 and 2006 with HIFU for T1-3N0M0 prostate cancer. The bDFR at 5 years for all patients was 63.5%, with the actual bDFR in the low-, intermediate-, and high-risk groups being 86.3%, 64.8%, and 31.3%, respectively. Negative prostate biopsy findings were found in 80.2%. Complications included urethral stricture, impotence, epididymitis, and urinary incontinence in 16%, 14%, 4%, and 0.8%, respectively.

In an effort to decrease complications, groups have continued to modify their techniques to spare tissue at the apex and near the neurovascular bundles. Gelet and colleagues[95] treated 102 patients, sparing tissue at the apex in an effort to improve continence rates (they also recommended sparing tissue near the neurovascular bundles to preserve potency in selected patients). At 19 months of follow-up, 22.5% of patients continued to have some form of urinary incontinence, although demonstrating 66% progression-free survival. Vallancien and colleagues[96] went as far as performing TURP before HIFU in an effort to minimize postoperative retention. Of the 30 patients treated, 73% had negative biopsies at 1 year, the urinary retention rate was lower than that of other studies (which, on average, occurs in 20% of patients) at 6.6%, and 1 patient developed urinary incontinence. The effect that these modifications may have on cure rates is unclear, and long-term biochemical, disease-specific, and overall survival data are not yet available.

SUMMARY

Over the past 2 decades, we have seen a more favorable stage and grade migration for renal and prostate cancer thanks to the ubiquitous use of abdominal imaging and PSA screening, respectively. Driven by patient preference and a more favorable oncologic prognosis at diagnosis, there has been a paradigm shift in the treatment of urologic cancers. Although the standard of care for most urologic malignancies continues to be surgical extirpation, ablation, in the form of needle-based or extracorporeal approaches, is quickly establishing itself as a viable primary treatment option. If there is anything to be learned from the pioneering studies that have been reviewed here, it is that there must be strict adherence to inclusion criteria for patient enrollment and that there are real limitations with each approach. It is only with this awareness that we can achieve maximal benefit while limiting the number of unnecessary complications and poor oncologic outcomes.

REFERENCES

1. American Cancer Society. Facts and figures, 2007.

2. Jayson M, Sanders H. Increased incidence of serendipitously discovered renal cell carcinoma. Urology 1998;51:203–5.

3. Chawla SN, Crispen PL, Hanlon AL, et al. The natural history of observed enhancing renal masses: meta-analysis and review of the world literature. J Urol 2006;175:425–31.

4. Van Poppel H. Conservative versus radical surgery for renal cell carcinoma. BJU Int 2004;94:766–8.

5. Uchida M, Imaide Y, Sugimoto K, et al. Percutaneous cryosurgery for renal tumors. Br J Urol 1995;75:132–6 [discussion: 136–7].

6. Chosy SG, Nakada SY, Lee FT, et al. Monitoring renal cryosurgery: predictors of tissue necrosis in swine. J Urol 1998;159:1370–4.

7. Hoffman NE, Bischof JC. The cryobiology of cryosurgical injury. Urology 2002;60 (Suppl 2A):40–49.

8. Gill IS, Novick AC. Renal cryosurgery. Urology 1999;54:215–9.

9. Baust JG, Gage AA. The molecular basis of cryosurgery. BJU Int 2005;95:1187–91.

10. Hedican SP, Wilkinson ER, Lee FT, et al. Cryoablation of advanced renal cancer has a survival advantage in a murine model compared to nephrectomy. J Urol 2004;171(4 Suppl) [abstract No. 778].

11. Larson TR, Robertson DW, Corica A, et al. In vivo interstitial temperature mapping of the human prostate during cryosurgery with correlation to histopathology outcome. Urology 2000;55:547–52.

12. Campbell SC, Krishnamurthi V, Chow G, et al. Renal cryosurgery: experimental evaluation of treatment parameters. Urology 1998;52:29–33.

13. Woolley ML, Schulsinger DA, Durand DB, et al. Effect of freezing parameters (freeze cycle and thaw process) on tissue destruction following renal cryoablation. J Endourol 2002;16:519–22.

14. Sung GT, Gill IS, Hsu TH, et al. Effect of intentional cryoinjury to the renal collecting system. J Urol 2003;170:619–22.

15. Janzen NK, Perry KT, Han KR, et al. The effects of intentional cryoablation and radio frequency ablation of renal tissue involving the collecting system in a porcine model. J Urol 2005;173:1368–74.

16. Gill IS, Novick AG, Meraney AM, et al. Laparoscopic renal cryoablation in 32 patients. Urology 2000;56:748–53.

17. Davol PE, Fulmer BR, Rukstalis DB. Long-term results of cryoablation for renal cancer and complex renal masses. Urology 2006;68:2–6.

18. Schwartz BF, Rewcastle JC, Powell T, et al. Cryoablation of small peripheral renal masses: a retrospective analysis. Urology 2006;68(Suppl 1A):14–8.

19. Lawatsch EJ, Langenstroer P, Byrd GF, et al. Intermediate results of laparoscopic cryoablation in 59

patients at the Medical College of Wisconsin. J Urol 2006;175:1225–9.

20. Cestari A, Sangalli M, Buffi N, et al. Laparoscopic renal cryoablation (LRC) of small renal masses: lessons learned from 104 cases in a 7-year experience. Eur Urol Suppl 2008;7(3):192.

21. Aron M, Kamoi K, Haber G-P, et al. Laparoscopic renal cryoablation: long-term oncologic outcomes with minimum 5-year follow-up. J Urol 2008;179(4 Suppl) [abstract No. 596].

22. Gill IS, Remer EM, Hasan WA, et al. Renal cryoablation: outcome at 3 years. J Urol 2005;173:1903–7.

23. Allaf ME, Bhayani SB, Rogers C, et al. Laparoscopic partial nephrectomy: evaluation of long-term oncologic outcome. J Urol 2004;172:871–3.

24. Desai MM, Aron M, Gill IS. Laparoscopic partial nephrectomy versus laparoscopic cryoablation for the small renal tumor. Urology 2005;66:23–8.

25. Hruby G, Reisiger K, Venkatesh R, et al. Comparison of laparoscopic partial nephrectomy and laparoscopic cryoablation for renal hilar tumors. Urology 2006;67:50–4.

26. Gupta A, Allaf ME, Kavoussi LR, et al. Computerized tomography guided percutaneous renal cryoablation with the patient under conscious sedation: initial clinical experience. J Urol 2006;175:447–53.

27. Atwell TD, Farrell MA, Leibovich BC, et al. Percutaneous renal cryoablation: experience treating 115 tumors. J Urol 2008;179:2136–41.

28. Bassignani MJ, Moore Y, Watson L, et al. Pilot experience with real-time ultrasound guided percutaneous renal mass cryoablation. J Urol 2004;171:1620–3.

29. Rehman J, Landman J, Lee D, et al. Needle-based ablation of renal parenchyma using microwave, cryoablation, impedance- and temperature-based monopolar and bipolar radiofrequency, and liquid and gel chemoablation: laboratory studies and review of the literature. J Endourol 2004;18:83–104.

30. Silverman SG, Tuncali K, Van Sonnenberg E, et al. Renal tumors: MR imaging-guided percutaneous cryotherapy—initial experience in 23 patients. Radiology 2005;236:716–24.

31. Sewell P, Shingleton W. Five-year treatment success and survival of patients treated with percutaneous IMRI guided and monitored renal cell carcinoma cryoablation. BJU Int 2004;94:106 [abstract MP-1609].

32. Lehman DS, Hruby GW, Phillips CK, et al. Laparoscopic renal cryoablation: efficacy and complications for larger renal masses. J Endourol 2008;22:1123–7.

33. Johnson DB, Solomon SB, Su LM, et al. Defining the complications of cryoablation and radiofrequency ablation of small renal tumors: a multi-institutional review. J Urol 2004;172:874–7.

34. Carvalhal EF, Gill IS, Meraney AM, et al. Laparoscopic renal cryoablation: impact on renal function and blood pressure. Urology 2001;58:357–61.

35. Finley DS, Beck S, Box G, et al. Percutaneous and laparoscopic cryoablation of small renal masses. J Urol 2008;180:492–8.

36. Cosman ER, Nashold BS, Ovelman-Levitt J. Theoretical aspects of radiofrequency lesions in the dorsal root entry zone. Neurosurgery 1984;15:945–50.

37. Corwin TS, Lindberg G, Traxer O, et al. Laparoscopic radiofrequency thermal ablation of renal tissue with and without hilar occlusion. J Urol 2001; 166:281–4.

38. Gill IS, Hsu TH, Fox RL, et al. Laparoscopic and percutaneous radiofrequency ablation of the kidney: acute and chronic porcine study. Urology 2000;56: 197–200.

39. Hoey MF, Mulier PM, Leveillee RJ, et al. Transurethral prostate ablation with saline electrode allows controlled production of larger lesions than conventional methods. J Endourol 1997;11:279–84.

40. Renshaw A. The natural history of incidentally detected small renal masses. Cancer 2004;101: 650–2.

41. Merkle EM, Shonk JR, Duerk JL, et al. MR-guided RF thermal ablation of the kidney in a porcine model. Am J Roentgenol 1999;173:645–51.

42. Jacomides L, Ogan K, Watumall L, et al. Laparoscopic application of radiofrequency energy enables in situ renal tumor ablation and partial nephrectomy. J Urol 2003;169:49–53.

43. Matsumoto ED, Johnson DB, Ogan K, et al. Short-term efficacy of temperature-based radiofrequency ablation of small renal tumors. Urology 2005;65:877–81.

44. Gervais DA, McGovern FJ, Arellano RS, et al. Radiofrequency ablation of renal cell carcinoma: part 1. Indications, results, and role in patient management over a 6-year period and ablation of 100 tumors. AJR Am J Roentgenol 2005;185:64–71.

45. Gervais DA, Arellano RS, McGovern FJ, et al. Radiofrequency ablation of renal cell carcinoma: part 2. Lessons learned with ablation of 100 tumors. AJR Am J Roentgenol 2005;185:72–80.

46. Stern JM, Svatek R, Park S, et al. Intermediate comparison of partial nephrectomy and radiofrequency ablation for clinical T1a renal tumors. BJU Int 2007;100:287–90.

47. Levinson AW, Agarwal D, Sroka M, et al. Long-term oncologic and overall outcomes of radiofrequency ablation in high-risk patients with solitary renal masses. J Urol 2008;179(Suppl 4):330.

48. Lucas SM, Stern JM, Adibi M, et al. Renal function outcomes in patients treated for renal masses smaller than 4 cm by ablative and extirpative techniques. J Urol 2008;179:75–80.

49. Traver MA, Werle DM, Clark PE, et al. Oncological efficacy and factors influencing the success of computerized tomography (CT)-guided percutaneous radiofrequency ablation (RFA) on renal neoplasms. J Urol 2006;175(Suppl):360.

50. Weiser AZ, Raj G, O'Connel M, et al. Complications after percutaneous radiofrequency ablation of renal tumors. Urology 2005;66:1176–80.

51. Weight CJ, Kaouk JH, Hegarty NJ, et al. Correlation of radiographic imaging and histopathology following cryoablation and radiofrequency ablation for renal tumors. J Urol 2008;179:1277–81.

52. Marcovich R, Aldana JP, Morgenstern N, et al. Optimal lesion assessment following acute radio frequency ablation of porcine kidney: cellular viability or histopathology? J Urol 2003;170:1370–4.

53. Neumann RA, Knobler RM, Pieczkowski F, et al. Enzyme histochemical analysis of cell viability after argon laser-induced coagulation necrosis of the skin. J Am Acad Dermatol 1991;25:991–8.

54. Michaels MJ, Rhee HK, Mourtzinos AP, et al. Incomplete renal tumor destruction using radio frequency interstitial ablation. J Urol 2002;168:2406–10.

55. Matlaga BR, Zagoria RJ, Woodruff RD, et al. Phase II trial of radio frequency ablation of renal cancer: evaluation of the kill zone. J Urol 2002;168:2401–5.

56. Stern J, Raman JD, Cadeddu JA. Absence of viable carcinoma in biopsies performed greater than 1-year following radiofrequency ablation of renal cortical tumors. J Urol 2008;179(4 Suppl):413.

57. Ankem MK, Nakada SY. Needle ablative nephron sparing surgery. BJU Int 2005;95(Suppl 2):46–51.

58. Liang P, Wang Y, Zhang D, et al. Ultrasound guided percutaneous microwave ablation for small renal cancer: initial experience. J Urol 2008;180:844–8.

59. Marberger M, Schatzl G, Kranston D, et al. Extracorporeal ablation of renal tumors with high intensity focused ultrasound. BJU Int 2005;95(Suppl 2):52–5.

60. Hacker A, Michel MS, Marlinghaus E, et al. Extracorporeally induced ablation of renal tissue by high-intensity focused ultrasound. BJU Int 2006;97: 779–85.

61. Ponsky LE, Crownover RL, Rosen MJ, et al. Initial evaluation of CyberKnife technology for extracorporeal renal tissue ablation. Urology 2003;61(3):498–501.

62. Ponsky LE, Mahadevan A, Gill IS, et al. Renal radiosurgery: initial clinical experience with histological evaluation. Surg Innov 2007;14(4):265–9.

63. Hong YM, Shanmugham L, La Rosa S, et al. CyberKnife radiosurgical ablation of primary renal tumors. Personal correspondence. Presented at World Congress of Endourology, November 30-December 3, 2008; Shanghai, China.

64. Bentzen SM, Ritter MA. The α/β ratio for prostate cancer: what is it, really? Radiother Oncol 2005;76:1–3.

65. King CR, Fowler JF. A simple analytic derivation suggests that prostate cancer α/β ratio is low. Int J Radiat Oncol Biol Phys 2001;51:213–4.

66. King CR, Lehmann J, Adler JR, et al. CyberKnife radiotherapy for localized prostate cancer: rationale and technical feasibility. Technol Cancer Res Treat 2003;2:25–9.

67. Madsen BL, His RA, Pham HT, et al. Stereotactic hypofractionated accurate radiotherapy of the prostate (SHARP), 33.5 Gy in five fractions for localized disease: first clinical trial results. Int J Radiat Oncol Biol Phys 2007;67:1099–105.
68. Cooper IS, Lee AS. Cryostatic congelation: a system for producing a limited, controlled region of cooling or freezing of biological tissue. J Nerv Ment Dis 1961;133:259–63.
69. Gage AA, Baust J. Mechanisms of tissue injury in cryosurgery. Cryobiology 1998;37:171–86.
70. Gonder MJ, Soanes WA, Shulman S. Cryosurgical treatment of the prostate. Invest Urol 1966;3:372–8.
71. Onik GM, Cohen JK, Reyes GD, et al. Transrectal ultrasound-guided percutaneous radical cryosurgical ablation of the prostate. Cancer 1993;72:1291–9.
72. Saliken JC, Donnelly BJ, Rewcastle JC. The evolution and state of modern technology for prostate cryosurgery. Urology 2002;60:26–33.
73. Katz AE, Rewcastle JC. The current and potential role of cryoablation as a primary therapy for localized prostate cancer. Curr Oncol Rep 2003;5:231–8.
74. Shinohara K. Prostate cancer cryotherapy. Urol Clin North Am 2003;30:725–36.
75. Long JP, Bahn D, Lee F, et al. Five-year retrospective, multi-institutional pooled analysis of cancer-related outcomes after cryosurgical ablation of the prostate. Urology 2001;57(3):518–23.
76. Bahn DK, Lee F, Badalament R, et al. Targeted cryoablation of the prostate: 7-year outcomes in the primary treatment of prostate cancer. Urology 2002;60:3–11.
77. Agarwal PK, Sadetsky N, Konety BR, et al. Treatment failure after primary and salvage therapy for prostate cancer: likelihood, patterns of care and outcomes. Cancer 2008;112:307–14.
78. Crook JM, Perry GA, Robertson S, et al. Routine biopsies following radiotherapy for prostate cancer: results for 226 patients. Urology 1995;45:624–32.
79. Babaian RJ, Donnelly B, Bahn D, et al. Best practice statement on cryosurgery for the treatment of localized prostate cancer. J Urol 2008;180:1993–2004.
80. Bahn DK, Lee F, Silverman P, et al. Salvage cryosurgery for recurrent prostate cancer after radiation therapy: a seven-year follow-up. Clin Prostate Cancer 2003;2:111–4.
81. Chin JL, Pautler SE, Mouraviev V, et al. Results of salvage cryoablation of the prostate after radiation: identifying predictors of treatment failure and complications. J Urol 2001;165:1937–41.
82. Hamoui O, Wiegand L, Pisters LL, et al. Ten-year treatment outcomes of salvage cryotherapy for locally recurrent prostate cancer. J Urol 2008;179(Suppl 4):253.
83. Donnelly BJ, Saliken JC, Ernst DS, et al. Prospective trial of cryosurgical ablation of the prostate: five year results. Urology 2002;60:645–9.
84. Ellis DS. Cryosurgery as a primary treatment for localized prostate cancer: a community hospital experience. Urology 2002;60:34–9.
85. Han K-R, Cohen JK, Miller RJ, et al. Treatment of organ-confined prostate cancer with third generation cryosurgery: preliminary multi-center experience. J Urol 2003;170:1126–30.
86. Robinson JW, Donnelly BJ, Saliken JC, et al. Quality of life and sexuality of men with prostate cancer 3 years after cryosurgery. Urology 2002;60(2 Suppl 1):12–8.
87. Ellis DS, Manny TB Jr, Rewcastle JC. Cryoablation as a primary treatment for localized prostate cancer followed by penile rehabilitation. Urology 2007;69:306–10.
88. Pisters LL, Rewcastle JC, Donnelly BJ, et al. Salvage prostate cryoablation: initial results from the cryo on-line data registry. J Urol 2008;180:559–65.
89. Madersbacher S, Padevilla M, Vingers L, et al. Effect of high-intensity focused ultrasound on human prostate cancer in vivo. Cancer Res 1995;55:3346–51.
90. Chapelon JY, Ribault M, Vernier F, et al. Treatment of localized prostate cancer with transrectal high intensity focused ultrasound. Eur J Ultrasound 1999;9:31–8.
91. Thuroff S, Chaussy C, Vallancien G, et al. High-intensity focused ultrasound and localized prostate cancer: efficacy results from the European Multicentric Study. J Endourol 2003;17:673–7.
92. Beerlage HP, Thuroff S, Debruyne FM, et al. Transrectal high-intensity focused ultrasound using the Ablatherm device in the treatment of localized prostate carcinoma. Urology 1999;54:273–7.
93. Blana A, Walter B, Rogenhofer S, et al. High-intensity focused ultrasound for the treatment of localized prostate cancer: 5-year experience. Urology 2004;63:297–300.
94. Uchida T, Nitta M, Hongo S, et al. High-intensity focused ultrasound for the treatment in 503 patients with localized prostate cancer. Urology 2007;70(3 Suppl 1):2.
95. Gelet A, Chapelon JY, Bouvier R, et al. Transrectal high intensity focused ultrasound for the treatment of localized prostate cancer: factors influencing the outcome. Eur Urol 2001;40:124–9.
96. Vallancien G, Prapotnich D, Cathelineau X, et al. Transrectal focused ultrasound combined with transurethral resection of the prostate for the treatment of localized prostate cancer: feasibility study. Urology 2004;171:2265–7.

Nanotechnology in Urology

Shihua Jin, MD[a], Vinod Labhasetwar, PhD[a,b],*

KEYWORDS

- Nanoparticles • Drug delivery • Cancer • Imaging
- Anticancer drugs

Nanomedicine is a new distinct scientific discipline that explores applications of nanoscale materials (1–1000 nm) for various biomedical applications. At nanoscale, the physical properties of materials are altered, as are their interactions with cells and tissue. This occurs primarily because of the significant difference in the surface area/volume ratio as materials are reduced to nanosized level.[1] Nanomedicine explores nanotechnology for monitoring, repair, and control of human biologic systems at cellular and molecular levels using engineered nanodevices and nanostructures.[2] Nanomedicine can improve diagnosis and treatment, and it can also be used in tissue engineering to replace some functions of human organs. The potential scope of nanotechnology in urology is wide-ranging, from prevention to early detection, treatment, prognosis, and symptom management.[3] The most common nanoscale drug delivery and imaging vehicles (nanocarriers) include polymeric nanoparticle, dendrimers, nanoshells, liposomes, nucleic acid–based nanoparticles, magnetic nanoparticles, and virus nanoparticles.[4] This article summarizes some of the emerging applications of nanomedicine in urology.

APPLICATION OF NANOTECHNOLOGY FOR DIAGNOSIS
Application of Nanotechnology for Imaging

Applications of nanotechnology in the diagnosis of genitourinary diseases have been extensively studied in recent years. Advances in nanotechnology have shown the promise of nanoparticles for noninvasive tumor imaging. Noninvasive imaging approaches, such as X-ray–based CT, positron emission tomography, single-photon emission CT, and MRI, are used as important tools for detection of human cancers. The development of tumor-targeted contrast agents based on nanoparticle formulations has been shown to increase the sensitivity and specificity of tumor imaging using currently available imaging modalities.[5] Superparamagnetic iron oxide or iron oxide nanoparticles are becoming increasingly attractive as the precursor for the development of target-specific MRI agents. Magnetic nanoparticles can shorten both T1 and T2 and enhance MRI contrast. T1 shortening processes require a close interaction between protons and T1 agents, however, which can be hindered by the thickness of the coating on the magnetic nanoparticles. The T2 shortening is caused by the large susceptibility difference between the particles and surrounding medium.[5]

Magnetic nanoparticles can extravasate into the interstitial space and subsequently transport to lymph nodes where they are taken up by macrophages. This can be used to detect lymph node metastasis.[6] Within the lymph nodes, lymphotropic superparamagnetic nanoparticles are internalized by macrophages and change magnetic properties detectable by MRI.[7] Renal carcinoma is the third most common genitourinary tumor.[8] The lymphatic metastasis is associated with the patient's survival; it is important to improve the detection of nodal metastases. MRI is widely used to diagnose renal cancer. Although it provides images with excellent anatomic details and soft tissue contrast, it is relatively insensitive to detect lymph node metastases.[9] Lymphotrophic nanoparticle-enhanced MRI (LNMRI) has

[a] Department of Biomedical Engineering, Lerner Research Institute, Cleveland Clinic, 9500 Euclid Avenue, Cleveland, OH 44195, USA
[b] Taussig Cancer Center, Cleveland Clinic, Cleveland, OH 44195, USA
* Corresponding author. Department of Biomedical Engineering/ND-20, Cleveland Clinic, 9500 Euclid Avenue, Cleveland, OH 44195.
E-mail address: labhasv@ccf.org (V. Labhasetwar).

Urol Clin N Am 36 (2009) 179–188
doi:10.1016/j.ucl.2009.02.005
0094-0143/09/$ – see front matter © 2009 Elsevier Inc. All rights reserved.

been used to identify malignant nodal involvement in patients with renal neoplasm. In one study, monocrystalline iron oxide magnetic nanoparticles were administrated by intravenous method, and imaging was performed before, immediately after, and 24 hours after administration. LNMRI showed high sensitivity (100%) and specificity of detection of lymph note metastasis (95.7%).[10]

Prostate cancer is one of the most common cancers in North America.[11] After the diagnosis of prostate cancer, accurate detection of lymph node metastases is essential to determine the extent of the disease to select appropriate therapy. Patients with local prostate cancer can receive radical prostatectomy, watchful waiting, or radiotherapy; however, patients with advanced or metastatic prostate cancer require an adjuvant androgen-deprivation therapy. Nanoparticles are used to detect the nodal metastases in patients with prostate cancer. In one study, all patients with nodal metastases were identified by MRI with lymphotropic superparamagnetic nanoparticles, and node-by-node analysis showed MRI with nanoparticles had a significantly higher sensitivity than conventional method (90.5% versus 35.4%; $P<.001$).[6] LNMRI is also used to detect the metastases within retroperitoneal nodes in patients with testicular cancer; the sensitivity, specificity, and accuracy of LNMRI for malignant lymph node involvement were 88.2%, 92%, and 90.4%, respectively. The sensitivity, specificity, and accuracy of size criteria for detecting malignant nodes were 70.5%, 68%, 69%, respectively.[11] These clinical trials suggest a promising future of applications of LNMRI in urology.

Recently, Jain and colleagues[12–14] have developed biocompatible magnetic nanoparticles with dual functional properties. The iron-oxide core is first coated with oleic acid and then oleic acid–coated particles are stabilized with plutonic F127 to make them dispersible in aqueous vehicle. Plutonic prevents protein binding and particles aggregation, which reduces their rapid clearance by the reticuloendothelial system, keeping nanoparticles in systemic circulation to allow their extravasation into tumor tissue. Doxorubicin (base form) and paclitaxel were shown to load these nanoparticles with high efficiency (75%–95%), and the loaded drugs are released over 2 weeks, sustaining the drug effect. Further, a combination of drugs can be loaded in these nanoparticles for synergistic activity. These multifunctional nanoparticles have greater advantage as compared with conventional magnetic nanoparticles because they can be used for both drug delivery and imaging applications (**Fig. 1**).

Semiconductor quantum dots are nanometer-scale, light-emitting particles, which have some unique optical and electronic properties, such as size-tunable light emission, improved signal brightness, enhanced stability of the fluorescent signal, and the ability to simultaneously excite multiple fluorescent colors.[15] These characteristics allow quantum dots to have broad absorption, narrow and symmetric emission spectra, long-term photostability, and continuous absorption spectra, and they are easy to use as probes for multicolor imaging compared with conventional dyes.[16,17] Gao and colleagues[18] developed a bioconjugated quantum dot probe suitable for in vivo targeting and imaging in mice. The conjugated quantum dots are modified with an amphiphilic tribolck copolymer for in vivo protection, antibody to target prostate-specific membrane antigen (PSMA), and multiple polyethylene glycol (PEG) molecules to improve biocompatibility and circulation. Imaging study in vivo demonstrated that quantum dots probes can be targeted to prostate tumor sites in mice through both passive and active mechanism, but passive targeting is much slower and less efficient than active targeting.

Application of Nanotechnology for Detection of Single Nucleotide Polymorphism

Progress in nanotechnology allowed detection of single-nucleotide polymorphisms in genes related to cancer, genetic disease, and nitrification.[19–22] Autosomal-dominant polycystic kidney disease is a genetic disease of humans. Autosomal-dominant polycystic kidney disease is characterized by enlarged polycystic kidneys and results in end-stage renal disease. Autosomal-dominant polycystic kidney disease is caused by mutations of two genes: PKD1 and PKD2.[23,24] Son and colleagues[25] have developed a rapid, accurate, and inexpensive nanoparticle-DNA–based assay to detect PKD single-nucleotide polymorphism mutations in hybridizations-in-solution platform. The Fe3O4/Eu:Gd2O3 and Fe3O4/Tb:Gd2O3 core-shell nanoparticles were used to capsulate DNA. The PKD single-nucleotide polymorphisms from kidney tissue and blood samples can be detected without a polymerase chain reaction step, which is convenient. The sensitivity of this method is very high and for blood genomic DNA, only 0.02 to 0.05 mL of whole blood sample is needed for detection.

Application of Nanosensor for Bacterial Detection

Basu and colleagues[26] developed a quick and sensitive procedure for bacterial detection in

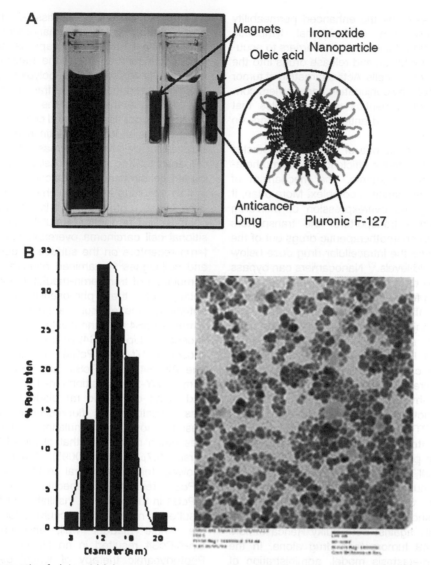

Fig. 1. (*A*) Schematic of oleic acid (pluronic)–coated iron oxide magnetic nanoparticles. (*B*) Particle size analysis of magnetic nanoparticles. Mean diameter of the core is approximately 12 nm, whereas hydrodynamic diameter is around 190 nm. (*From* Jain TK, Reddy MK, Morales MA, et al. Biodistribution, clearance, and biocompatibility of iron oxide magnetic nanoparticles in rats. Mol Pharmaceutics 2008;5:316–27; with permission.)

case of kidney infection. The procedure is based on both optical and electrochemical studies. Detection method used gold nanowire devices in conjunction with a linker arm attached to specific *Escherichia coli* antibodies. The study showed that the biosensor can detect each of 50 *E coli* cells with the sensor area of 0.178 cm.

APPLICATION OF NANOTECHNOLOGY FOR TREATMENT
Nanocarrier Delivery of Drugs for Treatment of Urologic Cancers

Nanoscale vehicles have been extensively investigated to delivery anticancer drugs. The most common examples of the nanoscale delivery vehicles include polymeric nanoparticles, dendrimers, nanoshells, liposomes, nucleic acid–based nanoparticles, magnetic nanoparticles, and virus nanoparticles.[27] Current chemotherapeutic drugs not only kill cancer cells, but also healthy cells and cause significant toxicity to patients. The nanocarrier-based delivery of anticancer drugs to tumor tissue can be achieved by either passive or active targeting; hence, these methods of drug delivery can increase the effect of drug while reducing side effects. Tumors tissue has leaky blood vessels and poor lymphatic drainage. Although free drugs may diffuse nonspecifically, a nanocarrier can extravasate into the tumor tissue by way of the leaky vessels by the enhanced permeability and retention. The dysfunctional lymphatic drainage in tumor facilitates nanocarriers to accumulate in tumor tissue and release drugs into the vicinity of the tumor cells. Active targeting of tumor cells is achieved by conjugating nanocarriers containing chemotherapeutics with molecules that bind to overexpressed antigens or receptors on the target cell.[28]

Drug resistance is one of the major obstacles limiting the therapeutic efficiency of chemotherapeutic or biologic agents. The mechanism of cancer drug resistance is complex. More often, it is caused by the overexpression of multidrug drug resistance transporters; the transporters actively pump chemotherapeutic drugs out of the cell and reduce the intracellular drug dose below lethal threshold levels.[27] Nanocarriers can bypass the multidrug drug resistance by preventing anticancer drugs from encountering the transporters. Sahoo and Labhasetwar[29] studied cytotoxicity of transferrin-conjugated and unconjugated paclitaxel-loaded nanoparticles in vitro in drug-resistant cell lines. They found the conjugated nanoparticle can overcome drug resistance by sustaining intracellular drug retention.

7-Ethyl-10-hydroxy-camptothecin (SN-38) is a biologically active metabolite of irinotecan hydrochloride (CPT-11) and has potent antitumor activity. Sumitomo and colleagues[30] used SN38-incorporated polymeric micelles, NK012, to treat the renal cell carcinoma model established by inoculating murine Renca cells and human renal cancer cells SKP-9. Compared with CPT-11, NK012 was shown to have significantly higher antitumor activity against both bulky Renca tumors and SKRC-49 tumors than drug alone. In the pulmonary metastasis model, administration of NK012 enhanced and prolonged distribution of free SN-38 in metastatic lung tissues; the concentration of SN-38 in nonmetastatic lung tissues was much lower. NK012 treatment decreased the metastatic nodule number significantly. These results demonstrate the significant advantages of polymeric micelle-based drug carriers and the authors suggested that NK012 would be effective in treating disseminated renal cancer with irregular vascular architectures.

Current treatment of superficial bladder cancer consists of transurethral tumor resection and chemotherapy. Chemotherapy usually follows surgery to reduce tumor recurrence or progression. Intravesical chemotherapy can selectively deliver drugs to bladder while minimizing systemic exposure. However, the response of intravesical chemotherapy is incomplete, and variable among patients; this is partly caused by the inability of drug to penetrate bladder tissue. Chemotherapeutic drugs loaded with nanocarriers provide more efficient and specific approaches to treat bladder cancer than drug alone. Paclitaxel for clinical use is dissolved in polyoxyl compound; however, it reduces the free fraction of paclitaxel and consequently lowers the drug penetration into the bladder tissue. Lu and colleagues[31] developed paclitaxel-loaded gelatin nanoparticles for intravesical delivery to increase the penetration of paclitaxel into bladder tissue. The paclitaxel-loaded gelatin nanoparticles can release the drug rapidly, resulting in much higher drug concentrations in the urothelium and lamina propria than paclitaxel in Cremophor formulation. Bladder transitional cell carcinoma overexpresses the transferrin receptors on the surface of cells. Derycke and colleagues[32] examined penetration and accumulation of transferrin-mediated liposomal targeting of the photosensitizer, aluminum phthalocyanine tetrasulfonate (AlPcS4), in bladder tumor. AlPcS4 was encapsulated in unconjugated liposomes (Lip-AlPcS4) or transferrin-conjugated liposomes (Tf-Lip–AlPcS4). The accumulation of free AlPcS4, Lip-AlPcS4, and Tf-Lip–AlPcS4 in human AY-27 transitional-cell carcinoma cells and in an orthotopic rat bladder tumor model was visualized by fluorescence microscopy. Results showed accumulation of Tf-Lip–AlPcS4 was much more than that of Lip-AlPcS4 (384.1 versus $3.7 \mu M$; $P = .0095$). The in vivo study showed that intravesical instillation of Tf-Lip–AlPcS4 resulted in specific accumulation of AlPcS4 in tumor tissue, instillation of free AlPcS4 resulted in nonselective accumulation throughout the whole bladder wall, and instillation of Lip-AlPcS4 resulted in no tissue accumulation. Photodynamic therapy of AY-27 cells showed Tf-Lip–AlPcS4 had high cytotoxicity. The results suggested that transferrin-mediated liposomal targeting of photosensitizing drugs is a promising potential tool for photodynamic therapy of superficial bladder tumors. Submucosal injection of doxorubicin-loaded liposome in bladder was shown to result in better distribution of drug and prolonged retention through the bladder wall and regional lymphoid nodes compared with free drug. The result suggests the therapeutic use of nanocarrier not only in superficial bladder cancer but also in invasive bladder cancer and regional lymphoid node metastasis.[33]

Because of its high mobility, prostate cancer always causes great interest to researchers. There are several examples of applications of chemotherapeutic-drug loaded nanocarriers for treating prostate cancer. Doxorubicin-loaded micelle and curcumin-loaded liposomes have been shown to improve the efficacy over free drugs.[34,35] It has been shown that A10 2′-fluoropyrimidine RNA aptamer (Apt) can bind to the PSMA. A combination of Apt and antibody against PSMA (J591) conjugated to nanoparticles was shown significantly to improve the uptake of nanoparticles by PSMA (+) prostate cancer cells (**Fig. 2**).[36–38] In another approach, the fact that transferrin receptors are overexpressed on the surface of prostate cancer cells was used to improve drug delivery. Sahoo and colleagues[28] used transferring-conjugated sustained-release paclitaxel-loaded biodegradable nanoparticles to treat prostate cancer. The in vivo experiment in subcutaneous animal model by direct intratumoral injection of transferrin-conjugated nanoparticles showed complete tumor regression compared with paclitaxel–polyoxyl compound and paclitaxel-loaded nanoparticle without transferrin (**Fig. 3**). The efficacy of

transferrin-conjugated nanoparticles is suggested to be caused by enhanced cellular drug uptake and sustained drug retention in tumor tissue. Direct intratumoral injection of drug-loaded nanoparticles can be effective in the treatment of localized tumor, such as prostate or kidney tumors, and could be a preferred option over surgical intervention to remove tumor.

The possibility of thermal therapy of prostate cancer with nanocarriers is another interesting approach, particularly to treat cancer refractory to chemotherapy. Kawai and colleagues[39] examined the hyperthermic effect of magnetic particles in rat prostate cancer. Magnetic liposomes generate heat in an alternating magnetic field. The tumor temperature can increase to 45°C, whereas the body temperature remains at around 38°C. Significant tumor regression was observed in the hyperthermic group. Immunohistochemical staining

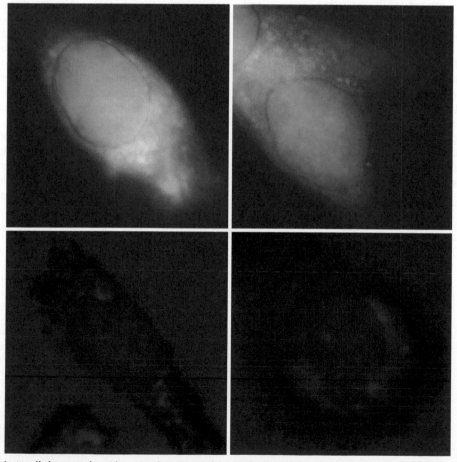

Fig. 2. NP-Apt cellular uptake. The nitrobenzoxazole (NBD) dyes (green) were encapsulated into PLGA-PEG-aptamer triblock nanoparticles. Left two pictures are LNCaP (PSMA-positive) cells, right two pictures are PC3 (PSMA-negative) cells. Cells were incubated with 50 μg of NBD encapsulated PLGA-PEG-aptamer nanoparticles for 30 minutes. (*From* Gu F, Zhang L, Teply BA, et al. Precise engineering of targeted nanoparticles by using self-assembled biointegrated block copolymers. Proc Natl Acad Sci U S A 2008;105:2586–91; with permission. Copyright © 2008 National Academy of Sciences, USA.)

showed the presence of CD3, CD4, and CD8 immunocytes in the tumor tissues of the rats exposed to hyperthermia. Heat shock protein 70 also appeared in the viable area at its boundary with the necrotic area. Further study showed magnetic liposomes plus alternating magnetic field heat therapy suppressed tumor growth in bone microenvironment; however, almost half of the animals that received magnetic liposomes plus alternating magnetic field treatment died. This method has some side effects and needs further study.[40] Gold nanoshells are designed to absorb near-infrared light that strongly generates heat and provides optically guided hyperthermic ablation. Laser-activated gold nanoshells have been shown to kill human prostate cancer cell PC-3 and C4-2 in vitro,[41] and in vivo study with ectopic murine prostate cancer model with laser-activated gold nanoshells caused 93% necrosis and regression in the high dose of gold nanoshell–treated mice.[42]

Several clinical trials of nanocarrier-based delivery of chemotherapeutic drugs are underway. One multi-institutional phase II trial of pegylated-liposome doxorubicin in the treatment of locally advanced unresectable or metastatic transitional cell carcinoma of the urothelial tract showed clinical response rate and favorable toxicity profile.[43] Liposomal doxorubicin was used to treat hormone-refractory prostate cancer, which is a challenge to urologists. The phase I study in which liposome-encapsulated doxorubicin was used to treat patients with advanced, androgen-independent prostate cancer did not show clinical response, but that may be because of the low

dosage.[44] In another prospective randomized phase II trial, however, patients with symptomatic hormone-refractory prostate cancers were treated with pegylated liposomal doxorubicin at 25 mg/m^2 every 2 weeks for 12 cycles (group A) or 50 mg/m^2 every 4 weeks for 6 cycles (group B). Decrease of prostate-surface antigen level was observed in 25.8% patients in group B, the mean time to disease progression was 6.5 months, patients in group B had a significantly higher rate of pain relief, and the mean 1-year survival rate was also significantly higher. Toxicity types differed significantly between groups A and B, but no dose-limiting cardiotoxicities or hematotoxicities were found.[45]

Nanocarrier Delivery of Drug for Noncancer Diseases

Nanocarrier delivery of drug not only can be used to treat cancer but also benign diseases. The effect of liposomes prepared from various natural and synthetic lipids on attenuating hyperactivity in bladder irritation was studied. Liposome of uncharged zwitterionic phospholipids significantly attenuated the irritation and decreased bladder contrast frequency caused by protamine sulfate but empty liposomes were not able to achieve the same effect.[46]

Effect of intraurethral application of prostaglandin E_1–loaded liposome was compared with that of intracavernosal injection of prostaglandin E_1 for treating psychogenic and organic erectile dysfunction. The intraurethral application of

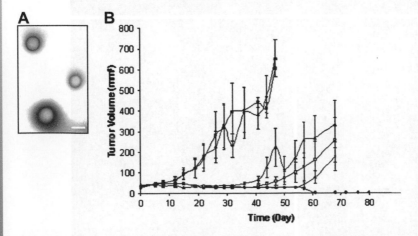

Fig. 3. (A) Paclitaxel-loaded PLGA nanoparticles. Bar indicates 100 nm. (B) Antitumor activity of Tx-NPs-Tf (paclitaxel-loaded transferrin conjugated nanoparticles) in a murine prostate tumor model. PC3 cells (2 × 10^6 cells) were implanted subcutaneously in athymic nude mice. Tumor nodules were allowed to grow to diameter of about 50 mm^3 before receiving different formulations as a single-dose treatment. Tx-NPs-Tf (•, 24 mg/kg; □, 12 mg/kg); Tx-NPs (X, 24 mg/kg); Tx–polyoxyl compound formulation (▲, 24 mg/kg); (◆) control NPs and (■) polyoxyl compound formulation. Data are means ± SEM, N = 6. *P<.005 Tx-NPs-Tf versus Tx-NPs and Tx–polyoxyl compound groups. (Fig. A From Sahoo SK, Labhasetwar V. Enhanced antiproliferative activity of transferrin-conjugated paclitaxel-loaded nanoparticles is mediated via sustained intracellular drug retention. Mol Pharmaceutics 2005;2:373–83; with permission; Fig. B From Sahoo SK, Ma W, Labhasetwar V. Efficacy of transferrin-conjugated paclitaxel-loaded nanoparticles in a murine model of prostate cancer. Int J Cancer 2004;112:335–40; with permission.)

liposomal prostaglandin E_1 was not effective in patients with organic erectile dysfunction. In 60% of patients with psychogenic erectile dysfunction, however, it was effective enough. It might be a convenient and painless therapeutic alternative for selective groups of patients.[47] Foldvari and colleagues[48] tested the effect of transdermal delivery of liposome-encapsulated prostaglandin E_1 in patients with erectile dysfunction. The study was performed in five patients in a double-blind, placebo-controlled fashion. Application of two transdermal prostaglandin E_1 formulations caused peak systolic flow velocities in the deep cavernosal arteries of patients to increase significantly. The highest mean peak systolic flow velocity was achieved at 45 minutes after application. Formulation of liposome with encapsulated prostaglandin E_1 showed sevenfold increase mean peak flow velocity compared with baseline values following transdermal application of the formulation, and could be a promising approach for the treatment of erectile dysfunction.

Significantly improved survival of rats with renal transplantation was shown following intravenous administration of bilayer liposome-encapsulated methylprednisolone once a week. Daily administration of the same dose of free drug could result in similar survival, but urine analysis showed a consistently higher protein excretion and retention of creatinine and urea in the free-drug group. Compared with free methylprednisolone, liposome-encapsulated methylprednisolone may selectively inhibit T-cell activation and cytokine production. The expression of CD45RC, CD25, interleukins-2, -7, and -12, tumor necrosis factor-α, and interferon-γ was strongly inhibited in the drug-encapsulated group.[49]

Nanocarrier for Delivery of Genes

Gene therapy refers to the transfer and expression of genes of therapeutic applications in the target cells and is regarded as a potential revolution in medicine.[50] The application of gene therapy promises progress in understanding physiologic roles of genes and in treating diseases at the genetic level. The ectopic expression of foreign genes is the most critical aspect for the success of in vivo gene expression and therapy. The vectors, which protect the ectopic genetic material and ferry it to the cells, are classified into two categories: viral and nonviral.[51] Viral vectors have efficient cell-entry mechanism; however, these viral vectors have several major restrictions, such as limited DNA-carrying capacity, lack of target-cell specificity, immunogenicity, and the risk of insertional mutagenesis.[52] Nonviral vectors are relatively simple to synthesize and have fewer risks than their viral counterparts. In addition, the nonviral vectors have no limitation on the size and number of the genetic inserts.[51] Nanocarriers are promising used as nonviral vectors.

Prabha and Labhasetwar[53] studied the parameters that influence the efficacy of nanoparticle-mediated gene transfection. The results showed the DNA loading in nanoparticle and its release, and surface properties of nanoparticles are the critical determinant in nanoparticle-mediated gene transfection. Larchian and colleagues[54] developed a liposome-mediated immune gene therapy using interleukin-2 and B7.1 in a MBT-2 mouse bladder cancer model. The study showed that the liposome-mediated transfection is safe, simple, and highly effective compared with retroviral system. Herpes simplex virus thymidine kinase (HSV-tk) gene delivered by folate-linked, lipid-based nanoparticles can achieve high transfection efficiency and selectivity, inhibiting tumor growth following intratumoral injection into prostate cancer.[55]

APPLICATION OF NANOTECHNOLOGY IN TISSUE ENGINEERING OF UROLOGY

The epidemic of end-stage renal disease continues worldwide; nearly 900,000 patients are currently on dialysis or surviving with a functioning kidney transplantation.[56] The most common treatment of end-stage renal disease is intermittent hemodialysis. Hemodialysis has high mortality and morbidity, however, for long-term use. Nissenson and colleagues[56] applied nanotechnology to develop a renal replacement device, the human nephron filter, which might significantly improve the current outcomes and quality of life of end-stage renal disease patients. The human nephron filter consists of two membranes operating in series within one cartridge. The first membrane, the G membrane, mimics the function of the glomerulus. Plasma ultrafiltrate generated by using convective transport contains all solutes approaching the molecular weight of albumin. The second membrane is the molecularly engineered T membrane, which mimics the function of the renal tubules. The human nephron filter could provide the equivalent of 30 mL/min of glomerular filtration rate if operated for 12 hours per day (**Fig. 4**). The instrument is wearable and can permit full mobility and improve patient quality of life significantly.

Pattison and colleagues[57,58] developed three-dimensional, porous, degradable poly lactic acid-co-glycolide and poly ether urethane scaffolds

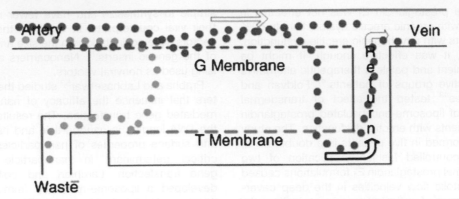

Fig. 4. Blood flows across the G membrane, which creates an ultrafiltrate, which then passes over the T membrane. The needed solutes and water passed through molecularly engineered pores is returned to the blood, whereas the remainder of the ultrafiltrate is collected in the drainage bag. (*From* Nissenson AR, Ronco C, Pergamit G, et al. Continuously functioning artificial nephron system: the promise of nanotechnology. Hemodial Int 2005;9:210–7; with permission.)

having nano-rough surface topographies. Human bladder smooth muscle cells seeded on these scaffolds showed increased cell adhesion, growth, and protein production compared with those seeded on the conventional, microdimensional scaffolds. The results suggested the nano-dimensional polymeric scaffolds are promising replacement materials for human bladder wall.

SUMMARY

Translational nanomedicine is undergoing rapid transition from development and evaluation in laboratory animals to clinical practices. In the future, it is anticipated that nanotechnology can provide urologists a new point of view to understand the mechanism of disease, tools for early diagnosis of the disease, and effective modality for treatment.

REFERENCES

1. Asiyanbola B, Soboyejo W. For the surgeon: an introduction to nanotechnology. J Surg Educ 2008;65(2): 155–61.
2. Shergill IS, Rao A, Arya M, et al. Nanotechnology: potential applications in urology. BJU Int 2006; 97(2):219–20.
3. Alexis F, Rhee JW, Richie JP, et al. New frontiers in nanotechnology for cancer treatment. Urol Oncol 2008;26(1):74–85.
4. Wang X, Yang L, Chen ZG, et al. Application of nanotechnology in cancer therapy and imaging. CA Cancer J Clin 2008;58(2):97–110.
5. Sun C, Lee JS, Zhang M. Magnetic nanoparticles in MR imaging and drug delivery. Adv Drug Deliv Rev 2008;60(11):1252–65.
6. Harisinghani MG, Barentsz J, Hahn PF, et al. Noninvasive detection of clinically occult lymph-node metastases in prostate cancer. N Engl J Med 2003; 348(25):2491–9.
7. Wunderbaldinger P, Josephson L, Bremer C, et al. Detection of lymph node metastases by contrast-enhanced MRI in an experimental model. Magn Reson Med 2002;47(2):292–7.
8. Jemal A, Siegel R, Ward E, et al. Cancer statistics, 2008. CA Cancer J Clin 2008;58(2):71–96.
9. Guimaraes AR, Tabatabei S, Dahl D, et al. Pilot study evaluating use of lymphotrophic nanoparticle-enhanced magnetic resonance imaging for assessing lymph nodes in renal cell cancer. Urology 2008;71(4):708–12.
10. Manyak MJ, Javitt M, Kang PS, et al. The evolution of imaging in advanced prostate cancer. Urol Clin North Am 2006;33(2):133–46, v.
11. Harisinghani MG, Saksena M, Ross RW, et al. A pilot study of lymphotrophic nanoparticle-enhanced magnetic resonance imaging technique in early stage testicular cancer: a new method for noninvasive lymph node evaluation. Urology 2005;66(5):1066–71.
12. Jain TK, Morales MA, Sahoo SK, et al. Iron oxide nanoparticles for sustained delivery of anticancer agents. Mol Pharmaceutics 2005;2(3):194–205.
13. Jain TK, Reddy MK, Morales MA, et al. Biodistribution, clearance, and biocompatibility of iron oxide magnetic nanoparticles in rats. Mol Pharmaceutics 2008;5(2):316–27.
14. Jain TK, Richey J, Strand M, et al. Magnetic nanoparticles with dual functional properties: drug delivery and magnetic resonance imaging. Biomaterials 2008;29(29):4012–21.
15. Chan WC, Nie S. Quantum dot bioconjugates for ultrasensitive nonisotopic detection. Science 1998; 281(5385):2016–8.

16. Shi C, Zhu Y, Cerwinka WH, et al. Quantum dots: emerging applications in urologic oncology. Urol Oncol 2008;26(1):86–92.

17. Smith AM, Ruan G, Rhyner MN, et al. Engineering luminescent quantum dots for in vivo molecular and cellular imaging. Ann Biomed Eng 2006;34(1):3–14.

18. Gao X, Cui Y, Levenson RM, et al. In vivo cancer targeting and imaging with semiconductor quantum dots. Nat Biotechnol 2004;22(8):969–76.

19. Bao YP, Huber M, Wei TF, et al. SNP identification in unamplified human genomic DNA with gold nanoparticle probes. Nucleic Acids Res 2005;33(2):e15.

20. Qin WJ, Yung LY. Nanoparticle-based detection and quantification of DNA with single nucleotide polymorphism (SNP) discrimination selectivity. Nucleic Acids Res 2007;35(17):e111.

21. Storhoff JJ, Marla SS, Bao P, et al. Gold nanoparticle-based detection of genomic DNA targets on microarrays using a novel optical detection system. Biosens Bioelectron 2004;19(8):875–83.

22. Zhou X, Zhou J. Improving the signal sensitivity and photostability of DNA hybridizations on microarrays by using dye-doped core-shell silica nanoparticles. (Wash) Anal Chem 2004;76(18):5302–12.

23. Hateboer N, Veldhuisen B, Peters D, et al. Location of mutations within the PKD2 gene influences clinical outcome. Kidney Int 2000;57(4):1444–51.

24. Kozlowski P, Bissler J, Pei Y, et al. Analysis of PKD1 for genomic deletion by multiplex ligation-dependent probe assay: absence of hot spots. Genomics 2008;91(2):203–8.

25. Son A, Dhirapong A, Dosev DK, et al. Rapid and quantitative DNA analysis of genetic mutations for polycystic kidney disease (PKD) using magnetic/luminescent nanoparticles. Anal Bioanal Chem 2008;390(7):1829–35.

26. Basu M, Seggerson S, Henshaw J, et al. Nano-biosensor development for bacterial detection during human kidney infection: use of glycoconjugate-specific antibody-bound gold NanoWire arrays (GNWA). Glycoconj J 2004;21(8-9):487–96.

27. Peer D, Karp JM, Hong S, et al. Nanocarriers as an emerging platform for cancer therapy. Nat Nanotechnol 2007;2(12):751–60.

28. Sahoo SK, Ma W, Labhasetwar V. Efficacy of transferrin-conjugated paclitaxel-loaded nanoparticles in a murine model of prostate cancer. Int J Cancer 2004;112(2):335–40.

29. Sahoo SK, Labhasetwar V. Enhanced antiproliferative activity of transferrin-conjugated paclitaxel-loaded nanoparticles is mediated via sustained intracellular drug retention. Mol Pharmaceutics 2005;2(5):373–83.

30. Sumitomo M, Koizumi F, Asano T, et al. Novel SN-38-incorporated polymeric micelle, NK012, strongly suppresses renal cancer progression. Cancer Res 2008;68(6):1631–5.

31. Lu Z, Yeh TK, Tsai M, et al. Paclitaxel-loaded gelatin nanoparticles for intravesical bladder cancer therapy. Clin Cancer Res 2004;10(22):7677–84.

32. Derycke AS, Kamuhabwa A, Gijsens A, et al. Transferrin-conjugated liposome targeting of photosensitizer AlPcS4 to rat bladder carcinoma cells. J Natl Cancer Inst 2004;96(21):1620–30.

33. Kiyokawa H, Igawa Y, Muraishi O, et al. Distribution of doxorubicin in the bladder wall and regional lymph nodes after bladder submucosal injection of liposomal doxorubicin in the dog. J Urol 1999;161(2):665–7.

34. McNealy TL, Trojan L, Knoll T, et al. Micelle delivery of doxorubicin increases cytotoxicity to prostate carcinoma cells. Urol Res 2004;32(4):255–60.

35. Thangapazham RL, Puri A, Tele S, et al. Evaluation of a nanotechnology-based carrier for delivery of curcumin in prostate cancer cells. Int J Oncol 2008;32(5):1119–23.

36. Cheng J, Teply BA, Sherifi I, et al. Formulation of functionalized PLGA-PEG nanoparticles for in vivo targeted drug delivery. Biomaterials 2007;28(5):869–76.

37. Gu F, Zhang L, Teply BA, et al. Precise engineering of targeted nanoparticles by using self-assembled biointegrated block copolymers. Proc Natl Acad Sci U S A 2008;105(7):2586–91.

38. Patri AK, Myc A, Beals J Jr, et al. Synthesis and in vitro testing of J591 antibody-dendrimer conjugates for targeted prostate cancer therapy. Bioconjug Chem 2004;15(6):1174–81.

39. Kawai N, Ito A, Nakahara Y, et al. Anticancer effect of hyperthermia on prostate cancer mediated by magnetite cationic liposomes and immune-response induction in transplanted syngeneic rats. Prostate 2005;64(4):373–81.

40. Kawai N, Futakuchi M, Yoshida T, et al. Effect of heat therapy using magnetic nanoparticles conjugated with cationic liposomes on prostate tumor in bone. Prostate 2008;68(7):784–92.

41. Stern JM, Stanfield J, Lotany Y, et al. Efficacy of laser-activated gold nanoshells in ablating prostate cancer cells in vitro. J Endourol 2007;21:939–43.

42. Stern JM, Stanfield J, Kabbani W, et al. Selective prostate cancer thermal ablation with laser activated gold nanoshells. J Urol 2008;179(2):748–53.

43. Winquist E, Ernst DS, Jonker D, et al. Phase II trial of pegylated-liposomal doxorubicin in the treatment of locally advanced unresectable or metastatic transitional cell carcinoma of the urothelial tract. Eur J Cancer 2003;39(13):1866–71.

44. Flaherty KT, Malkowicz SB, Vaughn DJ. Phase I study of weekly liposome-encapsulated doxorubicin in patients with advanced, androgen-independent prostate cancer. Am J Clin Oncol 2004;27(2):136–9.

45. Heidenreich A, Sommer F, Ohlmann CH, et al. Prospective randomized phase II trial of pegylated

doxorubicin in the management of symptomatic hormone-refractory prostate carcinoma. Cancer 2004;101(5):948–56.

46. Tyagi P, Chancellor M, Yoshimura N, et al. Activity of different phospholipids in attenuating hyperactivity in bladder irritation. BJU Int 2008;101(5):627–32.

47. Engelhardt PF, Plas E, Hubner WA, et al. Comparison of intraurethral liposomal and intracavernosal prostaglandin-E1 in the management of erectile dysfunction. Br J Urol 1998;81(3):441–4.

48. Foldvari M, Oguejiofor C, Afridi S, et al. Liposome encapsulated prostaglandin E1 in erectile dysfunction: correlation between in vitro delivery through foreskin and efficacy in patients. Urology 1998; 52(5):838–43.

49. Binder J, Braeutigam R, Oertl A, et al. Methylprednisolone in bilayer liposomes prolongs cardiac and renal allograft survival, inhibits macrophage activation, and selectively modifies antigen presentation and T-helper cell function in rat recipients. Transplant Proc 1998;30(4):1051.

50. Verma IM, Somia N. Gene therapy: promises, problems and prospects. Nature 1997;389(6648): 239–42.

51. Roy I, Stachowiak MK, Bergey EJ. Nonviral gene transfection nanoparticles: function and applications in the brain. Nanomedicine 2008;4(2):89–97.

52. Mastrobattista E, van der Aa MA, Hennink WE, et al. Artificial viruses: a nanotechnological approach to gene delivery. Nat Rev Drug Discov 2006;5(2): 115–21.

53. Prabha S, Labhasetwar V. Critical determinants in PLGA/PLA nanoparticle-mediated gene expression. Pharm Res 2004;21(2):354–64.

54. Larchian WA, Horiguchi Y, Nair SK, et al. Effectiveness of combined interleukin 2 and B7.1 vaccination strategy is dependent on the sequence and order: a liposome-mediated gene therapy treatment for bladder cancer. Clin Cancer Res 2000;6(7):2913–20.

55. Hattori Y, Maitani Y. Folate-linked lipid-based nanoparticle for targeted gene delivery. Curr Drug Deliv 2005;2(3):243–52.

56. Nissenson AR, Ronco C, Pergamit G, et al. Continuously functioning artificial nephron system: the promise of nanotechnology. Hemodial Int 2005; 9(3):210–7.

57. Pattison M, Webster TJ, Leslie J, et al. Evaluating the in vitro and in vivo efficacy of nano-structured polymers for bladder tissue replacement applications. Macromol Biosci 2007;7(5):690–700.

58. Pattison MA, Wurster S, Webster TJ, et al. Three-dimensional, nano-structured PLGA scaffolds for bladder tissue replacement applications. Biomaterials 2005;26(15):2491–500.

Advances in Laser Technology in Urology

Jason Lee, MBBS, MClinEpid[a],
Troy R.J. Gianduzzo, MBBS, FRACS (Urol)[a,b],*

KEYWORDS

• Urology • Lasers • Laparoscopy
• Urolithiasis • Nephrectomy • Prostatectomy

Since the Ruby laser was first developed in 1960 as the first successful optical laser, laser energy has continued to be developed and used in industry and medicine alike. Laser use in urology, however, has been limited largely until the last decade. The unique properties of laser energy have now led to its widespread use within urology, particularly in the treatment of benign prostatic hyperplasia (BPH), urolithiasis, stricture disease, and novel laparoscopic applications. This article details laser developments in each of these areas.

UROLITHIASIS

The first major general use of laser energy in urology has been in the treatment of stone disease. A number of lasers have been trialed for laser lithotripsy, of which the holmium:yttrium-aluminum-garnet (Ho:YAG) laser is the most commonly used. The Ho:YAG laser produces fragmentation of stones by a predominantly photo-thermal mechanism and requires direct contact of the laser tip with the stone. Ho:YAG lasers operate at a wavelength of 2100 nm, which is predominantly absorbed by water, hence making it important to keep the laser fiber close to the calculus when firing. The distance between the fiber and the stone is bridged by a laser-induced vapor channel (the "Moses effect"), which allows direct irradiance of the stone and an increase in temperature. This results in chemical breakdown of the stone, which reduces the mechanical strength of the calculus, allowing the vapor bubble and interstitial water expansion to achieve fragmentation.[1] Because of this unique mechanism, the Ho:YAG laser is associated with least propulsive effect and minimizes stone migration during treatment. The Ho:YAG laser is normally used at frequencies ranging from 5 to 10 Hz; however, recent in vitro studies have been performed examining the effectiveness of high-frequency Ho:YAG stone fragmentation in the order of 20 to 40 Hz, which Chawla and colleagues[2] describe as the "popcorn effect." This has potential advantages in that direct contact of the laser fiber on the stone is not required, such as in the situation of multiple small fragments in a lower pole calyx. The laser fiber can be positioned near the fragments, away from urothelium, and continuously fired, relying on the retropulsion of the stones and continuous irrigation within the confined space to move the stones in front of the laser fiber and achieve final fragmentation at the end of a procedure.

A recent review on the use of the Ho:YAG for ureteric stones indicates that stone clearance rates with the Ho:YAG were related to the location of the stone and whether the stone was impacted in the ureteral mucosa. Multivariate analysis of 543 patients indicated that the stone-free rate for impacted stones in the proximal ureter was only 67.2%.[3] A prospective analysis of 697 patients undergoing Ho:YAG lithotripsy demonstrated lower stone clearance rates for proximal ureteric stones (70.3%) compared with distal (100%) and mid ureteric calculi (97.9%).[4] Breda and colleagues[5] report their single institution

[a] Department of Urology, Royal Brisbane and Women's Hospital, Butterfield Street, Herston Q 4029, Brisbane, Australia
[b] Department of Urology, Wesley Medical Centre, Suite 16, Level 2, 40 Chasely Street, Auchenflower Q 4066, Brisbane, Australia
* Corresponding author. Department of Urology, Wesley Medical Centre, Suite 16, Level 2, 40 Chasely Street, Auchenflower Q 4066, Brisbane, Australia.
E-mail address: troy@gianduzzo.net (T.R.J. Gianduzzo).

Urol Clin N Am 36 (2009) 189–198
doi:10.1016/j.ucl.2009.02.004

experience of 51 patients undergoing flexible ureteroscopy and Ho:YAG laser lithotripsy with ureteric access sheath for multiple intrarenal stones. The overall stone-free rate was 92.2%, with a mean of 1.3 primary treatments per patient. Stone clearance was higher in stones under 2 cm. Studies comparing the complication rates of Ho:YAG and electrohydraulic lithotripsy have indicated the overall safety of the Ho:YAG laser, with overall complication rates of 1% to 2% and stricture rates of 0.35% to 0.72%. The Ho:YAG laser has also been shown to be safe and efficacious in patients in whom extracorporeal shock wave lithotripsy may be unsuitable, such as pregnant patients or those with a coagulopathy.[3,6]

The frequency-doubled double-pulse neodymium:YAG (FREDDY) laser has also been described and is a solid-state laser with wavelengths of 1064 and 532 nm, which fragments stones by generation of a plasma bubble.[7] The fragmentation ability of the FREDDY laser has been assessed using calculi of varying types from the human urinary tract, in an in vitro setting. It was found that the FREDDY laser was able to fragment a variety of calcium, uric acid, and struvite stones with a mean time to fragmentation of 2.5 ± 4.6 minutes.[8] A comparative in vitro study assessing the retropulsion and fragmentation of the FREDDY laser with the Ho:YAG laser and a pneumatic lithotripter found that the highest retropulsion occurred with the pneumatic lithotripter. The FREDDY laser caused significantly more retropulsion than the Ho:YAG laser. Stone fragmentation, measured as stone weight loss, was significantly greater with the FREDDY laser compared with the Ho:YAG laser.[9] Initial clinical experience of the FREDDY laser in 26 patients and 29 stones found that 18 patients were stone-free in 3 months. Fragmentation was ineffective for cysteine stones and was poor for a calcium oxalate monohydrate stone. One ureteral perforation occurred in the case of an impacted ureteral stone.[10] The FREDDY laser is not able to fragment cysteine stones and is also not able to coagulate, incise, or vaporize tissue; however, the FREDDY laser seems be a low-cost alternative for laser lithotripsy for noncysteine stones.

BENIGN PROSTATIC HYPERPLASIA

A variety of lasers are available for laser prostatectomy, with success initially involving the Ho:YAG laser and more recently the potassium titanyl phosphate (KTP) laser, the lithium triborate laser (LBO), and the semiconductor diode (SCDs) lasers.

Holmium:Yttrium-Aluminum-Garnet Laser

The Ho:YAG laser can be used for a variety of methods of treating BPH including holmium enucleation (HoLEP), holmium ablation, and holmium resection of the prostate. The absorption depth in prostatic tissue is 0.4 mm and results in the prostatic tissue being heated to temperatures above 100°C, causing vaporization without deep coagulation.[11] Kuntz and Ahyai[12,13] have published two separate randomized controlled trials, one comparing HoLEP with transurethral resection of the prostate (TURP) and the other with open prostatectomy. Initially, 100 patients were randomized to either HoLEP or TURP. At 36 months postprocedure peak flow rate (Qmax) and American Urological Association symptom scores were not statistically different between the two groups, whereas postvoid residual was significantly better in the HoLEP group (20.2 versus 8.4 mL). There were no blood transfusions in the HoLEP group versus two transfusions in the TURP group. The HoLEP group also had significantly shorter catheter times (1 day versus 2 days for TURP). Late complications at 36 months were similar.[12] In a further randomized analysis these same authors compared open prostatectomy with HoLEP for prostates greater than 100 g. There was a follow-up period of 5 years; however, 46 patients (38.3%) were lost to follow-up or were excluded. Mean American Urological Association symptom scores, postvoid residual, and Qmax were not significantly different between the two groups at 5-year follow-up. There were no blood transfusions in the HoLEP group versus 13.3% in the open prostatectomy group. Retrospective matched-pair analysis of open prostatectomy and those who had HoLEP with morcellation showed operative times were not significantly different. The number of patients requiring reoperation in the 5-year follow-up period were similar.[13]

Gilling and colleagues[14] reported on their mean of 6-year follow-up with HoLEP, which was derived from patients who were contactable from three previous randomized controlled trials. Seventy-one patients were eligible, and of these 38 patients were available for analysis, 19 could not be located, and 14 had died since their surgery. Outcome measures including International Prostate Symptom Score, quality of life score, and Qmax all showed durable improvement at 6 years postprocedure. One patient required a repeat HoLEP procedure at 5 years and one patient needed an urethrotomy at 6 months. Although limited, these results seem to indicate that HoLEP offers sustained improvement in voiding symptoms up to 6 years. The use of HoLEP in anticoagulated patients was examined by a retrospective review of 83 patients.[15] A total of 14 patients underwent surgery without cessation of anticoagulant and 34 had low-molecular-weight heparin substitution. Mean prostate size was 82.4 g. The blood transfusion rate was 14.2% in the fully anticoagulated patients, 14.7% in the low-molecular-weight heparin substitution group, and 3% in those who temporarily ceased anticoagulation. The retrospective nature of the study and variety of anticoagulants and timing of their cessation make the results difficult to interpret. The blood transfusion rate with HoLEP in this series is less than the 30% transfusion rate reported by Parr and coworkers,[16] however, who examined 12 patients who had TURP without withdrawal of warfarin therapy.

Potassium Titanyl Phosphate and Lithium Triborate Lasers ·

The KTP and LBO laser are used for photoselective vaporization of the prostate (PVP), with the newer 120-W LBO representing the latest advancement over the older 80-W KTP system. These lasers operate at a wavelength of 532 nm, at which there is maximal absorption by hemoglobin and minimal absorption by water, and remove prostatic tissue by vaporization. There is limited long-term data regarding the 120-W LBO system, with the largest experience being prospective and multicenter from the International Greenlight Laser User group.[17] Their data reported in 2008 are limited by short follow-up (mean, 4.2 months). They found significant improvement in International Prostate Symptom Score, Qmax, and postvoid residual in the subgroups of patients with preoperative urinary retention; on anticoagulants (35 aspirin, 22 warfarin, 13 clopidogrel, 2 on both aspirin and clopidogrel); and those with large prostates (>80 mL). The short follow-up makes it difficult to assess complications, such as urethral stricture or bladder neck stricture.

Intraoperative bleeding complications were evident in seven patients (2.9%) in the no anticoagulation group who required electrocautery to control bleeding, versus one patient (1.5%) in the anticoagulation group. In the early postoperative phase (mean, 12 weeks), there were two patients requiring blood transfusion, whereas two patients needed reoperation for insufficient voiding and 14 patients required recatheterization for urinary retention.[17] The effect of anticoagulants on patients having PVP has also been examined in 116 men on oral anticoagulants (71 on aspirin, 9 on clopidogrel, and 36 on coumarin derivatives) compared with 92 men without anticoagulants.

No anticoagulants were ceased at any stage. No patients in either group required a blood transfusion perioperatively.[18]

Spaliviero and colleagues[19] reported on 70 consecutive patients who underwent LBO laser PVP, and further analyzed them on the basis of whether they passed a voiding trial 2 hours post-procedure (catheter negative) or passed a trial of void the following morning (catheter positive). Overall, 49 patients were catheter negative and 21 were catheter positive. No patients failed the postoperative morning trial of void. Overall voiding outcomes in the two groups were improved from baseline out to 24 weeks follow-up. Qmax in the catheter-positive group improved from 8 mL per second at baseline to 21 mL per second at 24 weeks, and in the catheter-negative group improved from 10 mL per second at baseline to 24 mL per second at 24 weeks. Two patients in the catheter-positive group required temporary catheterization within 30 days for acute urinary retention.

The long-term outcomes of the 80-W KTP laser and the initial 60-W prototype have been well reported in the literature, with a number of trials with up to 5-year follow-up demonstrating sustained clinical improvement in symptom scores and urinary flow rates.[20,21] A nonrandomized comparative trial of the 80-W KTP laser and TURP with up to 24-months follow-up was recently reported by Ruszat and colleagues.[22] Sustained improvements in voiding parameters, which were comparable between the two groups, were noted. There were significantly fewer intraoperative bleeding complications and blood transfusions in the PVP group; however, the PVP group had a higher reoperation rate of 6.7% versus 3.9% for TURP, which did not reach statistical significance on chi-square testing.[22] A second comparative trial of the 80-W KTP laser and TURP was performed by Bouchier-Hayes and colleagues.[23] Of the 44 patients who had 12-month follow-up, there was no significant difference between the two groups regarding International Prostate Symptom Score, Qmax, or postvoid residual volume, although the authors note that the results are preliminary because the study was underpowered.

PVP and holmium ablation of the prostate were compared in a prospective, randomized trial of 109 patients who had lower urinary tract symptoms with a prostate size less than 60 g. After 12-months follow-up, both groups demonstrated significant improvements in International Prostate Symptom Score and Qmax compared with baseline. Hospital stay was 0.8 days in the holmium ablation of the prostate group and 0.9 days in the PVP group. Operative time was significantly longer in the holmium ablation of the prostate group (69.8 versus 55.5 minutes) and there were no major intraoperative complications in either group.[24] A randomized prospective study compared the 80-W KTP laser with transvesical open enucleation for prostatic adenomas greater than 80 mL in size. Of 125 randomized patients there were no differences in International Prostate Symptom Score or Qmax. There were five patients in the PVP group in whom a resectoscope was required to control hemostasis during the procedure. A total of eight patients in the open prostatectomy group required a perioperative blood transfusion, compared with zero patients in the PVP group.[25]

One of the criticisms of PVP and other laser ablative techniques is the lack of tissue for histologic examination. Biers and colleagues[26] reviewed data from the Royal Hampshire County Hospital from 1996 to 2006 and noted that the TURP-detected cancer rate fell from 22% in 1996 to 1997 to 1.5%-5.6% per year from 2001 to 2006. TURP-diagnosed cancers are mainly from the transitional zone and were found to have a mean Gleason score of 5.7. Most TURP-diagnosed cancers were allocated to active surveillance (82%) with 18% started on hormonal therapy. There were no prostate cancer progressions requiring radical prostatectomy or prostate cancer–related deaths in this group over a mean follow-up period of 49.2 months.

Thulium Laser

The thulium laser has a tunable wavelength between 1.75 and 2.22 μm, and for use in the prostate is tuned to a wavelength near the maximal absorption of laser energy into water. This results in high absorption of the laser energy into the prostate and tissue vaporization and a shallow penetration depth.[27] Wendt-Nordahl and colleagues[28] used a 2-μm continuous-wave thulium laser in an ex vivo model using an isolated, blood-perfused porcine kidney. They compared it with TURP and PVP using the 80-W KTP laser. The thulium laser had a faster tissue ablation rate than the KTP laser at 6.56 ± 0.69 g per minute versus 3.99 ± 0.48 g per minute, respectively. The hemostatic properties of the two lasers were similar. In comparison with TURP, the thulium laser had slower tissue ablation but superior hemostatic properties, with bleeding for both the thulium and KTP laser noted to be 100 times less compared with TURP. Clinical studies are limited at this stage; however, a prospective randomized controlled trial of thulium continuous-wave versus Ho:YAG

enucleation of the prostate found no differences in efficacy or complication rates at 12 months.[29] Xia and colleagues[30] described the tangerine technique in which the prostatic lobes are dissected off the capsule, yielding tissue for histologic analysis and compared it with TURP. Urodynamic findings and symptom scores at 1 year in both groups showed significant improvement from baseline and were not statistically different. Catheterization time, hospital stay, and hemoglobin drop were all significantly less in the thulium group. Operative time was similar in the two groups. One patient had stress incontinence and one patient had a urethral stricture in the thulium group compared with three urethral strictures in the TURP group.

Semiconductor Diode Lasers

The 980-nm SCD laser uses a wavelength that has the highest simultaneous absorption in hemoglobin and water, which is theorized to provide both hemostatic and ablative properties. Using an ex vivo porcine kidney model, Wendt-Nordahl and colleagues[31] compared a 980-nm SCD laser with TURP and an 80-W KTP laser. The authors found that the SCD laser had a faster tissue ablation rate of 7.24 ± 1.48 g per 10 minutes compared with 3.99 ± 0.48 g per 10 minutes for the KTP laser. TURP had the fastest tissue ablation rate at 8.28 ± 0.38 g per 10 minutes. The bleeding rate for both the SCD laser and the KTP laser was approximately 100 times less than for TURP. A prototype 50-W diode laser prototype operating at wavelength of 1470 nm was trialed in 10 patients with bladder outlet obstruction secondary to BPH. The 1470-nm wavelength is well absorbed by both hemoglobin and water. Based on urodynamic findings and symptom scores, the study concluded that the 1470-nm SCD laser seemed to be feasible and effective for relieving bladder outflow obstruction in BPH, up to the follow-up time of 1 year; however, two patients required TURP within 2 months because they were not satisfied with their outcome.

STRICTURES AND URETEROPELVIC JUNCTION OBSTRUCTION

The Ho:YAG laser is suited for endoureterotomy because it can make accurate incisions with a peripheral zone of thermal injury of less than 1 mm.[32] Ho:YAG use in ureteropelvic junction obstruction has been described in a single-institution, prospective series of 64 patients comparing Ho:YAG endopyelotomy (N = 37) with a fluoroscopically guided hot-wire balloon (N = 27) for use in both primary and secondary ureteropelvic junction obstruction of less than 2 cm in length.[33] The authors found that hospital stay, indwelling stent duration and long-term success rates (defined as resolution of symptoms and intravenous urography, diuretic renography, or both) were equivalent. The overall long-term success rate for hot-wire balloon was 77.8% versus 74.3% for the Ho:YAG laser. Two patients (7.4%) in the hot-wire balloon group required transfusion and embolization. There were no major complications in the Ho:YAG group.

The Ho:YAG laser has also been used as an endourologic alternative to traditional laparotomy and reimplantation in the management of ureterointestinal strictures. Watterson and colleagues[34] reported on a series of 23 patients with 24 strictures in patients with ileal conduit urinary diversion with no prior radiotherapy. By a percutaneous approach to the kidney they performed Ho:YAG endoureterotomy into the retroperitoneal fat with subsequent balloon dilatation. They had an overall success rate of 71% with a mean follow-up of 22 months, which compares with cold knife, balloon dilatation, and a hot-wire balloon whose success rates range from 33% to 65%. There have been limited reports regarding the use of the Ho:YAG laser for ureterovesical strictures in kidney transplant patients. In a small series of nine patients with ureterovesical strictures, six were treated with balloon dilatation and Ho:YAG laser endoureterotomy and the success rate was 67% with a mean follow-up of 58 months. The authors commented that all the failures in the laser endoureterotomy group were in patients whose strictures were greater than 10 mm.[35]

LASERS IN LAPAROSCOPY

Laser applications in laparoscopic urology remain experimental at this time. Laser tissue welding in laparoscopic pyeloplasty and laser laparoscopic partial nephrectomy (LPN) have been extensively investigated, although most recently laser applications in laparoscopic and robotic-assisted radical prostatectomy (RARP) have also been explored.

Laser Laparoscopic Pyeloplasty

Laser laparoscopic pyeloplasty has focused on laser welding to simplify pyeloureteral reconstruction. Laser welding uses the photothermal properties of laser light whereby laser energy is applied to a solder, typically 50% human albumin, in conjunction with laser wavelength–specific chromophores to facilitate laser light absorption. The resultant temperature increase denatures the solder and results in a coagulum that increases the strength at the repair site. Eden and

Coptcoat[36] examined laser welding, fibrin glue, and suture in the porcine model for pyeloureteral reconstruction. Both laser welding and fibrin glue produced supraphysiologic leak pressures but the fibrin glue was significantly faster to perform and easier to apply in comparison with laser welding. In a similar study, Wolf and coworkers[37] laparoscopically repaired 22 proximal ureterotomies in 14 pigs using fibrin glue, laser welding, suturing, or free suturing. The authors concluded that given the expense of laser systems, laser welding needs to be significantly superior to free suturing to justify its routine clinical use. Recently, Shumalinsky and colleagues[38] demonstrated successful laser welding of the pyeloureteral anastomosis in 10 farm pigs using a fiberoptic CO_2 laser soldering system. A unique, flexible, fiberoptic CO_2 laser delivery system, which included a real-time infrared thermal sensor that regulated the laser output within a 2°C to 3°C temperature range, was used. Successful tissue welding of the pyeloureteral anastomosis was demonstrated. Ultimately, however, laser welding of the pyeloureteral anastomosis has not demonstrated an advantage over standard suturing techniques and accordingly laser welding of the pyeloureteral anastomosis is not performed in routine clinical practice.

Laser Laparoscopic Partial Nephrectomy

Recently, LPN has been developed and offers equivalent oncologic and renal function outcomes but with improved convalescence compared with open partial nephrectomy.[39] LPN is a technically demanding procedure, however, that is difficult to master and requires hilar clamping with its associated warm ischemia. Laser LPN has been examined to allow excision of the tumor mass without hilar clamping while minimizing complex intracorporeal reconstruction. The Ho:YAG laser has been investigated in this regard. Lotan and colleagues[40] described the clinical use of the Ho:YAG laser in three cases of a complex cyst, a nonfunctioning lower-pole moiety in a duplex system in an 8-year-old boy, and a case of renal cell carcinoma. The hilum was not clamped in two of three cases. Fibrin glue or oxidized cellulose was required in each case. Blood loss was less than 50 mL in case 1 and less than 100 mL in case 2. In the third case, a 2.5-cm exophytic renal cell carcinoma was resected without hilar clamping and the estimated blood loss was 500 mL. In these cases, splattering was particularly troublesome when larger vessels were transected. In 2004 this same group performed five acute and five survival lower pole laser transperitoneal

LPNs in five pigs using the Ho:YAG laser.[40] Fibrin glue was applied to the cut surface to seal the collecting system. Blood loss was less than 50 mL for each procedure. Again, blood splattering and smoke generation were problematic.

Diode lasers have also been trialed. Ogan and colleagues[41] performed 10 laparoscopic transperitoneal partial nephrectomies in five 45- to 50-kg female farm pigs without hilar clamping using a 980-nm diode laser. The laser was insufficient for hemostasis in 3 of the 10 partial nephrectomies and adjunctive hemostatic clips were necessary to stop bleeding from larger vessels toward the center of the parenchyma. In 2003, this group examined the 810-nm pulsed diode laser combined with 50% liquid-albumin-indocyanine green solder to weld the parenchyma to achieve hemostasis and seal the collecting system.[42] Five survival and five acute heminephrectomies were assessed in five farm pigs. The renal pedicle was clamped and the heminephrectomy performed with scissors. The solder and the laser were then applied to the cut renal surface. The mean blood loss was 43.5 mL and the warm ischemia time 11.7 minutes. Two of the acute kidneys demonstrated minimal urine extravasation on ex vivo retrograde pyelography, although none of the survival kidneys demonstrated any clinically relevant urine leak.

Recently, high-power 532-nm wavelength laser systems have been investigated. Moinzadeh and colleagues[43] examined KTP laser LPN in the unclamped calf model using an 80-W system. Ablative vaporization of renal tissue was assessed in five subjects and wedge resection in seven. Eleven of the 12 procedures were performed without hilar clamping. The mean total operating time was 2.9 hours and the mean blood loss was 119 mL. The mean lasing time was 56 minutes. At 1-month follow-up there was no evidence of urine-leak on pyelography or arteriovenous fistula on arteriography. Smoke generation was noted and necessitated the use of a smoke evacuator system and two insufflators to counteract the loss of the pneumoperitoneum.

Hindley and colleagues[44] performed transperitoneal KTP laser LPN in four pigs. In this study an 80-W system was used without renal cooling or hilar clamping. The mean blood loss was less than 30 mL. In one procedure a 7-mm vein was transected that required a single laparoscopic clip to secure hemostasis. The authors report that the hemostatic properties of the KTP laser were excellent, but also noted that smoke production was a particular problem.

To overcome the issue of smoke production, Liu and colleagues[45] examined saline irrigation during KTP laser LPN in the porcine model. Fourteen LPNs were performed without hilar occlusion in four pigs with continuous saline irrigation to suppress smoke. Thirteen of the 14 partial nephrectomies were performed without hilar clamping and with successful suppression of smoke. The mean partial nephrectomy time was 13.14 minutes and the mean blood loss was 28.57 mL. Anderson and colleagues[46] examined the KTP laser LPN in six pigs. The hilum was clamped in all cases. The 80-W KTP laser was used at a setting of 80 W for tissue cutting and 30 W for coagulation delivered by a 365-μm fiber. Hemostasis was successful in all cases and no perioperative complications occurred. Mean blood loss was 80 mL, mean laser time was 35 minutes, and the mean warm ischemia time was 34 minutes. Urinary extravasation was noted in seven out of eight kidneys on retrograde pyelography. Saline irrigation eliminated smoke formation but slowed the time of resection. Hilar clamping decreased smoke formation and charring and greatly facilitated dissection. Smoke production, although less, was still a factor and a smoke evacuator was required at a suction rate of 5 L per minute.

The clinical applicability of laser robotic-assisted LPN was examined at the Cleveland Clinic in a pilot series of five patients (unpublished data). In this series a 120-W system was used in conjunction with a robotic unit to facilitate laser delivery. Specific purpose-built, prototype robotic instrumentation was engineered for this study. The laser beam was delivered by a purpose-built, end-firing 600-μm fiber using a laser system to a maximum setting of 80 W to excise the tumor mass. A CT-1 needle with 3-zero polyglactin suture was used to perform meticulous running repair of any collecting system defects. Hemostasis was problematic throughout the series and the laser did not coagulate the larger more centrally placed interlobar arteries. All cases required additional hemostatic maneuvers, such as clips, suture, Floseal, or surgical bolster. The mean blood loss for the series was 400 mL. One case required hilar clamping with 14 minutes of warm ischemia time and was also complicated by postoperative hemorrhage requiring embolization and a subsequent 4-unit blood transfusion. The intraoperative blood loss in the final patient was 1300 mL and a 2-unit intraoperative blood transfusion was required. Dissection proceeded slowly and mass excision times were in the order of 36 to 96 minutes. There was one focally positive margin. Laser transection resulted in significant charring of the renal parenchyma, which obscured the intrarenal dissection planes and it is likely that this was a major contributing factor to the focally positive margin. Smoke generation was problematic and high-flow insufflation at 40 L per minute in conjunction with active smoke evacuation by smoke suction units was required.

The 2013-nm thulium laser has been evaluated in both animal and clinical series. Bui and colleagues[47] 2007 assessed the 30-W thulium laser delivered by a 365-μm fiber passed through a flexible cystoscope in conjunction with continuous saline irrigation in a survival porcine model without hilar clamping. Laser LPN was completed successfully in all cases with an estimated blood loss of less than 50 mL with minimal smoke and minimal tissue charring. Fibrin glue was also applied to the exposed parenchyma. A limitation of this study is that only the renal cortex was treated and in the authors' initial nonsurvival pilot assessment they state that the laser was unable to control the more centrally placed larger medullary vessels near the hilum. In an open series Gruschwitz and colleagues[48] reported success with the thulium laser in five patients by an open loin approach. Operative time was reported in one patient and was stated to be less than 20 minutes. The authors state that the thulium laser can coagulate vessels up to 1.5 mm and because of the short operative time, minimal blood loss, and absence of clamping, the thulium laser may be useful in high-risk patients. At this time, however, the collective data are insufficient to support the routine use of laser energy during LPN.

Laser Laparoscopic and Robotic Radical Prostatectomy

Laser laparoscopic radical prostatectomy (LRP) has recently been investigated. Laser energy potentially allows for precise dissection with good hemostasis and minimal adjacent tissue injury. Monopolar and bipolar diathermy and ultrasonic shears (US) are known to affect cavernous nerve function.[49] In contrast, laser energy is a direct photonic beam that potentially allows precise dissection with good hemostasis and a minimum of adjacent tissue injury. These theoretical benefits in concert with the advantages of RARP by way of the highly magnified three-dimensional view, wristed instrumentation, complete absence of tremor, and fine movement scaling could theoretically allow for extremely fine and accurate dissection with a minimum of collateral damage and improved operative outcomes.

An initial series of neodymium (Nd):YAG laser nerve-sparing LRP in five patients observed an acute mean depth of injury of 615 μm to the neurovascular bundles.[50] A series of studies has since investigated the potential application of laser energy facilitating LRP.[51–53] Initially, the canine model was assessed for its suitability as a nerve-sparing radical prostatectomy model.[51] Next, the effects of the KTP laser on neurovascular bundle function was assessed and compared with cold scissor dissection.[52] In this assessment laparoscopic KTP laser dissection of the neurovascular bundles was found to be equivalent to cold scissor dissection and superior to US in preservation of cavernous nerve function.[52] Laparoscopic unilateral neurovascular bundle mobilization was performed in 36 dogs using KTP laser (N = 12), US (N = 12), or athermal technique (AT) using cold scissors and titanium clips (N = 12). KTP laser mobilization was performed using a 15-W laser unit. Peak penile intracavernosal pressure normalized against simultaneously recorded mean arterial pressure measurements (ICP%MAP) following cavernous nerve stimulation was recorded both before and following unilateral neurovascular bundles mobilization. The ICP%MAP following KTP laser dissection was comparable with that of cold scissor dissection both immediately postoperatively and at 1 month, whereas US dissection resulted in a significant decrease in the mean ICP%MAP response compared with both the KTP and AT groups (acute ICP%MAP: KTP 92%, AT 96%, US 49%; KTP versus AT $P = .54$, US versus KTP $P<.001$, US versus AT $P<.001$; chronic ICP%MAP: KTP 95%, AT 98%, US 58%; KTP versus AT $P = .71$, US versus. KTP $P = .02$, US versus AT $P = .02$). Histologic assessment of the prostate specimens from the laser group demonstrated a zone of laser-induced necrosis of 600 μm compared with a median of 1200 μm in the US group and 450 μm of crush injury in the AT group.

On the basis of these findings, laser RARP was then assessed.[53] Laser RARP was performed in 10 male dogs. Predissection and postdissection ICP%MAP were again recorded in response to cavernous nerve stimulation. Laser RARP was performed completely using the KTP and Nd:YAG lasers. Most of the dissection was performed using the KTP laser, whereas the Nd:YAG laser was used selectively for hemostasis of larger vessels as required. All 10 procedures were entirely completed with the use of laser energy. No additional hemostatic maneuvers, such as clips, US, or electrocautery, were required in any case. The median operative blood loss was 50 mL. The median postdissection ICP%MAP was slightly reduced; however, this was not statistically significant (preoperative ICP%MAP 99.3%; postoperative 77%; $P = .12$). Histologic assessment of the excised acute specimens demonstrated a zone of necrosis typically extending 0.5 to 1 mm from the cut edge of the prostatic fascia, extending focally to a maximum of 1.5 mm in some sections with areas of injured but nonnecrotic tissue of up to 2 mm beyond the cut edge. There were no laser-related complications.

Finally, KTP laser robotic-assisted LRP was performed in 10 patients as a phase 1 clinical assessment.[54] In this initial series complete laser RARP was performed successfully using a low-power 15-W laser unit. Additional hemostatic maneuvers using clips, sutures, or diathermy were required on an average of eight occasions per case. The mean perioperative values were operative time 217 minutes, blood loss 290 mL, hospital stay 39.9 hours, mean laser time 65.9 minutes, and laser energy 20,862 J. Eight patients had pT2 disease and two had pT3. All surgical margins were negative. There were no laser-related complications. There was one urine leak and one drain site infection.[54] From this series of studies it seems that laser RARP is feasible; however, it is unclear as to whether this offers any benefit over standard laparoscopic and robotic techniques. Certainly, thermal energy should be avoided wherever possible in the region of the neurovascular bundles in accordance with standard athermal dissection techniques. Whether laser energy offers any benefit during laparoscopic or RARP over current athermal practices remains to be seen and the application of this technology to LRP and RARP is unproved at this time.

SUMMARY

Lasers have become well established in urology, particularly in the treatment of urolithiasis and BPH such that laser use in these areas is becoming standard, accepted practice. Laparoscopic applications continue to be examined but remain unproved at this time. Laser LPN aims to provide a bloodless knife for excision of renal masses; however, hemostasis and smoke generation remain problematic. Although laser RARP seems feasible, further long-term assessments are required. It is likely that laser energy will continue to be increasingly developed and used in urology.

REFERENCES

1. Chan KF, Vassar GJ, Pfefer TJ, et al. Holmium:YAG laser lithotripsy: a dominant photothermal ablative mechanism with chemical decomposition of urinary calculi. Lasers Surg Med 1999;25(1):22–37.
2. Chawla SN, Chang MF, Chang A, et al. Effectiveness of high-frequency holmium:YAG laser stone fragmentation: the popcorn effect. J Endourol 2008; 22(4):645–50.
3. Seitz C, Tanovic E, Kikic Z, et al. Impact of stone size, location, composition, impaction, and hydronephrosis on the efficacy of holmium:YAG-laser ureterolithotripsy. Eur Urol 2007;52(6):1751–7.
4. Jiang H, Wu Z, Ding Q, et al. Ureteroscopic treatment of ureteral calculi with holmium: YAG laser lithotripsy. J Endourol 2007;21(2):151–4.
5. Breda A, Ogunyemi O, Leppert JT, et al. Flexible ureteroscopy and laser lithotripsy for multiple unilateral intrarenal stones. Eur Urol 2008 Jun 13; [Epub ahead of print].
6. Sofer M, Watterson JD, Wollin TA, et al. Holmium:YAG laser lithotripsy for upper urinary tract calculi in 598 patients. J Urol 2002;167(1):31–4.
7. Delvecchio FC, Auge BK, Brizuela RM, et al. In vitro analysis of stone fragmentation ability of the FREDDY laser. J Endourol 2003;17(3):177–9.
8. Zorcher T, Hochberger J, Schrott KM, et al. In vitro study concerning the efficiency of the frequency-doubled double-pulse Neodymium:YAG laser (FREDDY) for lithotripsy of calculi in the urinary tract. Lasers Surg Med 1999;25(1):38–42.
9. Marguet CG, Sung JC, Springhart WP, et al. In vitro comparison of stone retropulsion and fragmentation of the frequency doubled, double pulse Nd:YAG laser and the holmium:YAG laser. J Urol 2005; 173(5):1797–800.
10. Dubosq F, Pasqui F, Girard F, et al. Endoscopic lithotripsy and the FREDDY laser: initial experience. J Endourol 2006;20(5):296–9.
11. Kuntz RM. Current role of lasers in the treatment of benign prostatic hyperplasia (BPH). Eur Urol 2006; 49(6):961–9.
12. Ahyai SA, Lehrich K, Kuntz RM. Holmium laser enucleation versus transurethral resection of the prostate: 3-year follow-up results of a randomized clinical trial. Eur Urol 2007;52(5):1456–63.
13. Kuntz RM, Lehrich K, Ahyai SA. Holmium laser enucleation of the prostate versus open prostatectomy for prostates greater than 100 grams: 5-year follow-up results of a randomised clinical trial. Eur Urol 2008;53(1):160–6.
14. Gilling PJ, Aho TF, Frampton CM, et al. Holmium laser enucleation of the prostate: results at 6 years. Eur Urol 2008;53(4):744–9.
15. Elzayat EA, Elhilali MM. Holmium laser enucleation of the prostate (HoLEP): the endourologic alternative to open prostatectomy. Eur Urol 2006;49(1): 87–91.
16. Parr NJ, Loh CS, Desmond AD. Transurethral resection of the prostate and bladder tumour without withdrawal of warfarin therapy. Br J Urol 1989;64(6):623–5.
17. Woo H, Reich O, Bachmann A, et al. Outcome of Greenlight HPS 120-W laser therapy in specific patient populations: those in retention, on anticoagulants and with large prostates (≥80ml). European Urology Supplements 2008;7:378–83.

18. Ruszat R, Wyler S, Forster T, et al. Safety and effectiveness of photoselective vaporization of the prostate (PVP) in patients on ongoing oral anticoagulation. Eur Urol 2007;51(4):1031–8 [discussion: 1038–41].

19. Spaliviero M, Araki M, Page JB, et al. Catheter-free 120W lithium triborate (LBO) laser photoselective vaporization prostatectomy (PVP) for benign prostatic hyperplasia (BPH). Lasers Surg Med 2008; 40(8):529–34.

20. Malek RS, Kuntzman RS, Barrett DM. Photoselective potassium-titanyl-phosphate laser vaporization of the benign obstructive prostate: observations on long-term outcomes. J Urol 2005;174(4 Pt 1): 1344–8.

21. Ruszat R, Seitz M, Wyler SF, et al. GreenLight laser vaporization of the prostate: single-center experience and long-term results after 500 procedures. Eur Urol 2008;54(4):893–901.

22. Ruszat R, Wyler SF, Seitz M, et al. Comparison of potassium-titanyl-phosphate laser vaporization of the prostate and transurethral resection of the prostate: update of a prospective non-randomized two-centre study. BJU Int 2008;102:1432–9.

23. Bouchier-Hayes DM, Anderson P, Van Appledorn S, et al. KTP laser versus transurethral resection: early results of a randomized trial. J Endourol 2006;20(8): 580–5.

24. Elzayat E, Elhilali M. Holmium laser ablation (HoLAP) versus photoselective vaporization (PVP) of the prostate: a prospective randomized trial. J Urol 2008;179(4 Suppl 1):675–6.

25. Alivizatos G, Skolarikos A, Chalikopoulos D, et al. Transurethral photoselective vaporization versus transvesical open enucleation for prostatic adenomas >80ml: 12-mo results of a randomized prospective study. Eur Urol 2008;54(2):427–37.

26. Biers SM, Oliver HC, King AJ, et al. Does laser ablation prostatectomy lead to oncological compromise? BJU Int 2008;103(4):454–7.

27. Fried NM, Murray KE. High-power thulium fiber laser ablation of urinary tissues at 1.94 microm. J Endourol 2005;19(1):25–31.

28. Wendt-Nordahl G, Huckele S, Honeck P, et al. Systematic evaluation of a recently introduced 2-microm continuous-wave thulium laser for vaporesection of the prostate. J Endourol 2008;22(5): 1041–5.

29. Gordon S, Watson G. Thulium laser enucleation of the prostate. European Urology Supplements 2006; 5(6):310.

30. Xia SJ, Zhuo J, Sun XW, et al. Thulium laser versus standard transurethral resection of the prostate: a randomized prospective trial. Eur Urol 2008; 53(2):382–9.

31. Wendt-Nordahl G, Huckele S, Honeck P, et al. 980-nm Diode laser: a novel laser technology for vaporization of the prostate. Eur Urol 2007;52(6):1723–8.

32. Patel RC, Newman RC. Ureteroscopic management of ureteral and ureteroenteral strictures. Urol Clin North Am 2004;31(1):107–13.

33. Ponsky LE, Streem SB. Retrograde endopyelotomy: a comparative study of hot-wire balloon and ureteroscopic laser. J Endourol 2006;20(10): 823–6.

34. Watterson JD, Sofer M, Wollin TA, et al. Holmium:YAG laser endoureterotomy for ureterointestinal strictures. J Urol 2002;167(4):1692–5.

35. Gdor Y, Gabr AH, Faerber GJ, et al. Holmium: yttrium-aluminum-garnet laser endoureterotomy for the treatment of transplant kidney ureteral strictures. Transplantation 2008;85(9):1318–21.

36. Eden CG, Coptcoat MJ. Assessment of alternative tissue approximation techniques for laparoscopy. Br J Urol 1996;78(2):234–42.

37. Wolf JS Jr, Soble JJ, Nakada SY, et al. Comparison of fibrin glue, laser weld, and mechanical suturing device for the laparoscopic closure of ureterotomy in a porcine model. J Urol 1997;157(4):1487–92.

38. Shumalinsky D, Lobik L, Cytron S, et al. Laparoscopic laser soldering for repair of ureteropelvic junction obstruction in the porcine model. J Endourol 2004;18(2):177–81.

39. Novick AC. Laparoscopic and partial nephrectomy. Clin Cancer Res 2004;10(18 Pt 2):6322S–7S.

40. Lotan Y, Gettman MT, Ogan K, et al. Clinical use of the holmium:YAG laser in laparoscopic partial nephrectomy. J Endourol 2002;16(5):289–92.

41. Ogan K, Wilhelm D, Lindberg G, et al. Laparoscopic partial nephrectomy with a diode laser: porcine results. J Endourol 2002;16(10):749–53.

42. Ogan K, Jacomides L, Saboorian H, et al. Sutureless laparoscopic heminephrectomy using laser tissue soldering. J Endourol 2003;17(5):295–300.

43. Moinzadeh A, Gill IS, Rubenstein M, et al. Potassium-titanyl-phosphate laser laparoscopic partial nephrectomy without hilar clamping in the survival calf model. J Urol 2005;174(3):1110–4.

44. Hindley RG, Barber NJ, Walsh K, et al. Laparoscopic partial nephrectomy using the potassium titanyl phosphate laser in a porcine model. Urology 2006; 67(5):1079–83.

45. Liu M, Rajbabu K, Zhu G, et al. Laparoscopic partial nephrectomy with saline-irrigated KTP laser in a porcine model. J Endourol 2006;20(12): 1096–100.

46. Anderson JK, Baker MR, Lindberg G, et al. Large-volume laparoscopic partial nephrectomy using the potassium-titanyl-phosphate (KTP) laser in a survival porcine model. Eur Urol 2007;51(3):749–54.

47. Bui MH, Breda A, Gui D, et al. Less smoke and minimal tissue carbonization using a thulium laser for laparoscopic partial nephrectomy without hilar clamping in a porcine model. J Endourol 2007; 21(9):1107–11.

48. Gruschwitz T, Stein R, Schubert J, et al. Laser-supported partial nephrectomy for renal cell carcinoma. Urology 2008;71(2):334–6.

49. Ong AM, Su LM, Varkarakis I, et al. Nerve sparing radical prostatectomy: effects of hemostatic energy sources on the recovery of cavernous nerve function in a canine model. J Urol 2004; 172(4 Pt 1):1318–22.

50. Gianduzzo TR, Chang CM, El-Shazly M, et al. Laser nerve-sparing laparoscopic radical prostatectomy: a feasibility study. BJU Int 2007;99(4): 875–9.

51. Gianduzzo TR, Colombo JR, El-Gabry E, et al. Anatomical and electrophysiological assessment of the canine periprostatic neurovascular anatomy: perspectives as a nerve sparing radical prostatectomy model. J Urol 2008; 179(5):2025–9.

52. Gianduzzo T, Colombo JR Jr, Haber GP, et al. Laser nerve-sparing laparoscopic radical prostatectomy: effects of potassium-titanyl-phosphate laser on cavernous nerve function in a survival canine model. J Urol 2007;177(4):804.

53. Gianduzzo T, Colombo JR Jr, Haber GP, et al. Laser robotically assisted nerve-sparing radical prostatectomy: a pilot study of technical feasibility in the canine model. BJU Int 2008;102(5):598–602.

54. Gianduzzo T, Kaouk J, Colombo JR, et al. KTP Laser robotic nerve-sparing radical prostatectomy: development and initial clinical experience. Engineering and Urology Society 22nd Annual Meeting May 2007: abstract 212.

Regenerative Medicine and Tissue Engineering in Urology

Anthony Atala, MD

KEYWORDS

- Tissue engineering • Regenerative medicine
- Biomaterials • Bladder • Kidney
- Stem cells • Reconstruction • Therapeutic cloning

Congenital disorders, cancer, trauma, infection, inflammation, iatrogenic injuries, or other conditions of the genitourinary system can lead to organ damage or complete loss of function. Both situations usually necessitate eventual reconstruction or replacement of the damaged organs. Currently, reconstruction may be performed with native non-urologic tissues (skin, gastrointestinal segments, or mucosa from multiple body sites), homologous tissues from a donor (cadaver fascia or cadaver or living donor kidney), heterologous tissues or substances (bovine collagen), or artificial materials (silicone, polyurethane, or polytetrafluoroethylene). All these materials often lead to various complications after reconstruction, however, because the implanted tissue is rejected or because inherently different functional parameters cause a mismatch in the system. For example, replacement of bladder tissue with gastrointestinal segments can be problematic because of the opposite ways in which these two tissues handle solutes—urologic tissue normally excretes material, and gastrointestinal tissue generally absorbs the same materials. This mismatched state can lead to metabolic complications in addition to infection and other issues.[1] Therefore, the replacement of lost or deficient urologic tissues with functionally equivalent ones would certainly improve the outcome of reconstructive surgery in the genitourinary system. This goal may soon be attainable with the use of tissue engineering techniques.

TISSUE ENGINEERING STRATEGIES FOR UROGENITAL REPAIR

Tissue engineering uses the principles of cell transplantation, materials science, and biomedical engineering to develop biologic substitutes that can restore and maintain normal function of damaged or lost tissues and organs. Tissue engineering may involve injection of functional cells into a nonfunctional site to stimulate regeneration. It can also involve the use of natural or synthetic matrices, often termed *scaffolds*, which encourage the body's natural ability to repair itself and assist in determination of the orientation and direction of new tissue growth. Often, tissue engineering uses a combination of these techniques. For example, matrices seeded with cells can be implanted into the body to encourage the growth or regeneration of functional tissue.

Use of Cells in Urogenital Tissue Engineering Applications

Often, when cells are used for tissue engineering, donor tissue is dissociated into individual cells, which are then implanted directly into the host or expanded in culture, attached to a support matrix, and reimplanted after expansion. The implanted tissue can be heterologous, allogeneic, or autologous. Ideally, this approach allows lost tissue function to be restored or replaced in toto and with limited complications.[2–7]

Department of Urology, Wake Forest Institute for Regenerative Medicine, Wake Forest University School of Medicine, Fifth Floor, Watlington Hall, Medical Center Boulevard, Winston-Salem, NC 27157, USA
E-mail address: aatala@wfubmc.edu

Urol Clin N Am 36 (2009) 199–209
doi:10.1016/j.ucl.2009.02.009
0094-0143/09/$ – see front matter © 2009 Published by Elsevier Inc.

An area of concern has been the source of cells for regeneration, however. The concept of creating engineered tissue constructs involves obtaining cells from the organ to be replaced and expanding these cells in vitro so that sufficient quantities are available for the implantation technique chosen. A major concern has been that, in certain cases, there may not be enough normal cells present in the diseased organ to begin this expansion process. This may not be the case; for example, one study has shown that cultured neuropathic bladder smooth muscle cells possess and maintain different characteristics than normal smooth muscle cells in vitro, as demonstrated by growth assays, contractility, and adherence tests in vitro.[8] Despite these differences, when neuropathic smooth muscle cells were cultured in vitro and then seeded onto matrices and implanted in vivo, the tissue-engineered constructs showed the same properties as the constructs engineered with normal cells.[9] It is known that genetically normal progenitor cells, which are the reservoirs for new cell formation and are present even in diseased tissue, are programmed to give rise to normal tissue, regardless of whether they reside in normal or diseased tissues. Therefore, the stem cell niche, and its role in normal tissue regeneration, remains a fertile area of ongoing investigation.

Stem Cells

Most current strategies for tissue engineering depend on a sample of autologous cells from the diseased organ of the host. For many patients with extensive end-stage organ failure, however, a tissue biopsy may not yield enough normal cells for expansion and transplantation. In other instances, primary autologous human cells cannot be expanded from a particular organ, such as the pancreas. In these situations, pluripotent human embryonic stem cells are envisioned as an ideal source of cells because they can differentiate into nearly any replacement tissue in the body.

Embryonic stem cells exhibit two remarkable properties: the ability to proliferate in an undifferentiated but still pluripotent state (self-renewal) and the ability to differentiate into a large number of specialized cell types.[10] They can be isolated from the inner cell mass of the embryo during the blastocyst stage, which occurs 5 days after fertilization. These cells have been maintained in the undifferentiated state for at least 80 passages when grown using current published protocols.[11] In addition, many protocols for differentiation into specific cell types in culture have been published. Many uses of these cells are currently banned in

the United States, however, because of the ethical dilemmas that are associated with the manipulation of embryos in culture.

Adult stem cells have the advantage of avoiding some of the ethical issues associated with embryonic cells, and, unlike embryonic cells, they do not transdifferentiate into a malignant phenotype; thus, there is a diminished risk for teratoma formation should the cells be implanted in vivo. Adult stem cells are limited for clinical use, however, because expansion to the large quantities needed for tissue engineering is difficult.

Fetal stem cells derived from amniotic fluid and placenta have recently been described and represent a novel source of stem cells.[12,13] The cells express markers consistent with human embryonic stem cells, such as OCT4 and SSEA-4, but they do not form teratomas. The cells are multipotent and are able to differentiate into cells from all three germ layers. In addition, the cells have high replicative potential and could be stored for future self-use, without the risks for rejection and without ethical concerns.

Therapeutic Cloning

Nuclear cloning, which has also been called nuclear transplantation and nuclear transfer, involves the introduction of a nucleus from a donor cell into an enucleated oocyte to create an embryo with a genetic makeup identical to that of the donor. Two types of nuclear cloning, reproductive cloning and therapeutic cloning, have been described. Banned in most countries for human applications, reproductive cloning is used to generate an embryo that has the identical genetic material as its cell source to produce offspring that are genetically identical to the donor. Conversely, therapeutic cloning is used to generate early-stage embryos that are used in vitro. They are explanted in culture to produce embryonic stem cell lines that are genetically identical to the source. These autologous stem cells have the potential to become almost any type of cell in the adult body, and thus would be useful in tissue and organ replacement applications (Fig. 1).[14] A particularly useful application for these cells would be in the treatment of end-stage kidney disease, for which there is limited availability of immunocompatible tissue transplants.

Biomaterials for Genitourinary Tissue Construction

Biomaterials in genitourinary tissue engineering function as an artificial extracellular matrix (ECM) and are used to replace biologic and mechanical functions of native ECM found in tissues in the

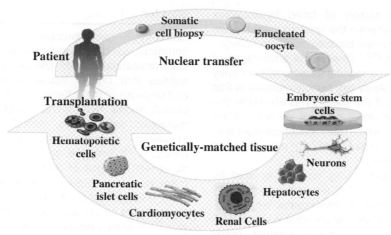

Fig. 1. Strategy for therapeutic cloning and tissue engineering.

body. Biomaterials facilitate the localization and delivery of cells or bioactive factors (eg, cell adhesion peptides, growth factors) to desired sites in the body and define a three-dimensional space for the formation of new tissues with appropriate structure. They also serve as a guide for the development of new tissues with appropriate function.[15,16] Direct injection of cell suspensions without such matrices has been used in some cases; however, without this scaffold function, it is difficult to control the localization of transplanted cells.[17,18]

The ideal biomaterial should be biocompatible, promote cellular interaction and tissue development, and possess the proper mechanical and physical properties found in the tissue to be generated. Generally, three classes of biomaterials have been used for the engineering of genitourinary tissues: naturally derived materials, such as collagen and alginate; acellular tissue matrices, such as bladder submucosa and small-intestinal submucosa (SIS); and synthetic polymers, such as polyglycolic acid (PGA), polylactic acid, and poly(lactic-co-glycolic acid). Although synthetic polymers can be produced reproducibly on a large scale with controlled properties of strength, degradation rate, and microstructure, naturally derived materials and acellular tissue matrices have the potential advantage of biologic recognition, which can lessen host-versus-graft reactions.

Vascularization of Engineered Tissue

Limitations of nutrient and gas exchange currently restrict tissue-engineered implants to a volume of approximately 3 mm^3.[19] Therefore, to achieve the goals of engineering large complex tissues and organs, vascularization of the regenerating cells is essential.

Three approaches have been used to encourage the vascularization of bioengineered tissue. First, incorporation of angiogenic factors in the bioengineered tissue has been used to attract host capillaries and to enhance neovascularization of the implanted tissue. Second, some studies have investigated the effects of seeding endothelial cells with other cell types in the bioengineered tissue. Finally, prevascularization of the matrix before cell seeding has been attempted. There are many obstacles to overcome before large tissue-engineered solid organs are produced, but recent developments in angiogenesis research may provide important knowledge and essential materials to accomplish this goal.

TISSUE ENGINEERING OF SPECIFIC UROLOGIC AND GENITAL STRUCTURES
Urethra

Various strategies have been proposed over the years for the regeneration of urethral tissue. Woven meshes of PGA have been used to reconstruct urethras in dogs.[20] Also, PGA has been used as a cell transplantation vehicle to engineer tubular urothelium in vivo.[2] SIS without cells was used as an onlay patch graft for urethroplasty in rabbits.[21] Finally, a homologous graft of acellular urethral matrix was also used in a rabbit model.[22]

Bladder-derived acellular collagen matrix has proved to be a suitable graft for repair of urethral defects in rabbits. In the rabbit model, the neourethras created with these matrices demonstrated a normal urothelial luminal lining and organized muscle bundles shortly after repair.[21,22] These results were confirmed clinically in a series of patients with a history of failed hypospadias reconstruction, wherein the urethral defects were repaired with human bladder acellular collagen matrices (**Fig. 2**).[23,24] One of the advantages of this material over nongenital tissue grafts currently used for urethroplasty (eg, buccal mucosa) is that the material is "off the shelf." This eliminates the necessity of additional surgical procedures for graft harvesting, which may decrease operative time, and the potential morbidity attributable to the harvest procedure.

These techniques using nonseeded acellular matrices were successfully applied experimentally and clinically for onlay urethral repairs. When tubularized urethral repairs were attempted experimentally, however, adequate urethral tissue regeneration was not achieved and complications ensued, such as graft contracture and stricture formation.[25] Tubularized collagen matrices seeded with cells have performed better in animal studies. In a rabbit model, entire urethral segments were resected and urethroplasties were performed with tubularized collagen matrices seeded with autologous cells or without cells. The tubularized collagen matrices seeded with autologous cells formed new tissue that was histologically similar to native urethral tissue.[26] The tubularized collagen matrices without cells lead to poor tissue development, fibrosis, and stricture formation.

Bladder

Currently, gastrointestinal segments are commonly used for bladder replacement or repair. Gastrointestinal tissues are designed to absorb solutes that urinary tissue excretes, however, and because of this difference in function, multiple complications may ensue, such as infection, metabolic disturbances, urolithiasis, perforation, increased mucus production, and malignancy.[1,27,28] Because of the problems encountered with the use of gastrointestinal segments, numerous investigators have attempted alternative reconstructive procedures for bladder replacement or repair. The use of tissue expansion,[29,30] seromuscular grafts,[31–36] matrices for tissue regeneration,[37–45] and tissue engineering with cell transplantation has been investigated.

Bladder Replacement Using Tissue Engineering

Cell-seeded allogeneic acellular bladder matrices have been used for bladder augmentation in dogs. A group of experimental dogs underwent a trigone-sparing cystectomy and were randomly assigned to one of three groups. One group underwent closure of the trigone without a reconstructive procedure, another group underwent reconstruction with a nonseeded bladder-shaped

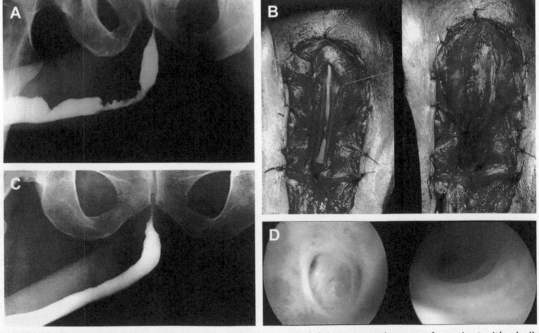

Fig. 2. Tissue engineering of the urethra using a collagen matrix. (*A*) Representative case of a patient with a bulbar stricture. (*B*) Urethral repair. Strictured tissue is excised, preserving the urethral plate on the left side, and matrix is anastomosed to the urethral plate in an onlay fashion on the right. (*C*) Urethrogram 6 months after repair. (*D*) Cystoscopic view of urethra before surgery on the left side and 4 months after repair on the right side.

biodegradable scaffold, and the last group underwent reconstruction using a bladder-shaped biodegradable scaffold that was seeded with autologous urothelial and smooth muscle cells.[46]

The cystectomy-only and nonseeded controls maintained average capacities of 22% and 46% of preoperative values, respectively. An average bladder capacity of 95% of the original precystectomy volume was achieved in the cell-seeded tissue-engineered bladder replacements, however (**Fig. 3**). The subtotal cystectomy reservoirs that were not reconstructed and the polymer-only reconstructed bladders showed a marked decrease in bladder compliance (10% and 42% of total compliance, respectively). The compliance of the cell-seeded tissue-engineered bladders was almost no different from preoperative values (106%). Histologically, the nonseeded scaffold bladders presented a pattern of normal urothelial cells with a thickened fibrotic submucosa and a thin layer of muscle fibers. The retrieved tissue-engineered bladders showed normal cellular organization, consisting of a trilayer of urothelium, submucosa, and muscle.[46]

A clinical experience involving engineered bladder tissue for cystoplasty reconstruction was conducted starting in 1999. A small pilot study of seven patients was reported, using a collagen scaffold seeded with cells with or without omentum coverage or a combined PGA-collagen scaffold seeded with cells and omental coverage (**Fig. 4**). The patients reconstructed with the engineered bladder tissue created with the PGA-collagen cell-seeded scaffolds showed increased compliance, decreased end-filling pressures, increased capacities, and longer dry periods (**Fig. 5**).[6] Although the experience is promising in terms of showing that engineered tissues can be implanted safely, it is just a start in terms of accomplishing the goal of engineering fully functional bladders. Further experimental and clinical work is being conducted.

Ureters

Ureteral nonseeded matrices have been used as a scaffold for the ingrowth of ureteral tissue in rats. These matrices promoted regeneration of the ureteral wall components.[47] Ureteral replacement

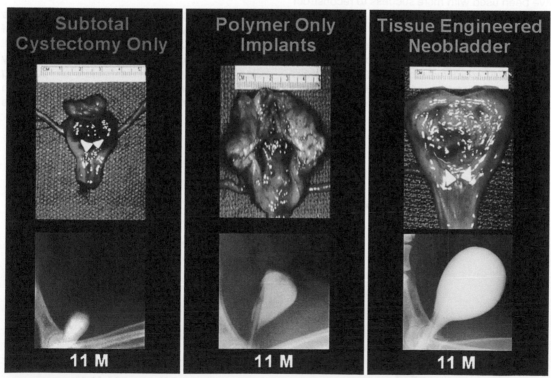

Fig. 3. Gross specimens and cystograms at 11 months of the cystectomy-only nonseeded controls and cell-seeded tissue-engineered bladder replacements in dogs. The cystectomy-only bladder had a capacity of 22% of the preoperative value and a decrease in bladder compliance to 10% of the preoperative value. The nonseeded controls showed significant scarring, with a capacity of 46% of the preoperative value and a decrease in bladder compliance to 42% of the preoperative value. An average bladder capacity of 95% of the original precystectomy volume was achieved in the cell-seeded tissue-engineered bladder replacements, and the compliance showed almost no difference from preoperative values that were measured when the native bladder was present (106%).

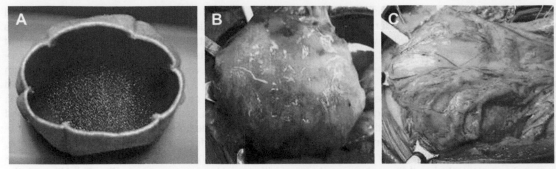

Fig. 4. Construction of an engineered human bladder. (*A*) Bladder-shaped scaffold seeded with cells before implantation in the patient. (*B*) Engineered bladder anastomosed to native bladder tissue with running 4-0 polyglycolic sutures. (*C*) Implanted bladder covered with fibrin glue and omentum.

with polytetrafluoroethylene grafts was also attempted in dogs but with poor functional results.[48] In a more recent study, nonseeded acellular collagen matrices were tubularized and used to replace 3-cm segments of canine ureters. The nonseeded acellular matrix tube was not able to replace the segment of the ureter successfully.[49]

Cell-seeded biodegradable polymer scaffolds have been used with more success to reconstruct ureteral tissues. In one study, urothelial and smooth muscle cells isolated from bladders and expanded in vitro were seeded onto tubular PGA scaffolds and implanted subcutaneously into athymic mice. After implantation, the urothelial cells proliferated to form a multilayered lining of the tubular structure, whereas the smooth muscle

cells organized into multilayered structures surrounding the urothelial cells. Abundant angiogenesis was evident. The degradation of the polymer scaffolds resulted in the eventual formation of natural urothelial tissues. This approach was expanded to replacement of ureters in dogs.

KIDNEY

The kidney is the most challenging organ in the genitourinary system to reconstruct because of its extremely complex structure and function. Concepts for a bioartificial kidney are currently being explored. Some investigators are pursuing the replacement of isolated kidney function parameters using extracorporeal units, whereas

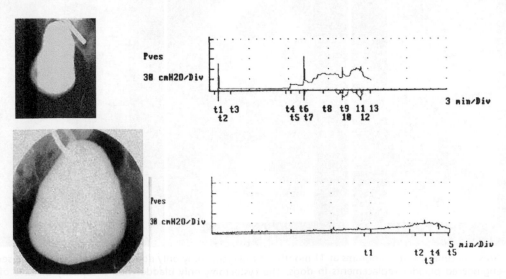

Fig. 5. Cystograms and urodynamic studies of a patient before and after implantation of the tissue-engineered bladder. Before surgery, a cystogram indicates an irregular and misshapen bladder. Additionally, abnormal bladder pressures during bladder filling were measured by means of a urodynamic study (*top*). After surgery, these findings were significantly improved. A larger bladder appears on the cystogram, and bladder filling pressures are within normal ranges (*bottom*). Pves, intravesicular pressure.

others are aiming to replace total renal function with tissue-engineered bioartificial renal structures.

Ex Vivo Functioning Renal Units

Dialysis is currently the most common form of renal replacement therapy. The relatively high morbidity and mortality resulting from this process have spurred investigators to seek alternative solutions, however. In an attempt to assess the viability and physiologic functionality of a cell-seeded device to replace the filtration, transport, metabolic, and endocrinologic functions of the kidney, a synthetic hemofiltration device and a device that contained tissue-engineered porcine renal tubules were incorporated into an extracorporeal perfusion circuit, and this was introduced into acutely uremic dogs. Levels of potassium and blood urea nitrogen were controlled during treatment with the device. The fractional reabsorption of sodium and water was possible. Active transport of potassium, bicarbonate, and glucose and a gradual ability to excrete ammonia were observed. These results demonstrated the feasibility of an extracorporeal assist device that is reinforced by the use of proximal tubular cells.[50]

Using similar techniques, a tissue-engineered bioartificial kidney consisting of a conventional hemofiltration cartridge in series with a renal tubule assist device containing human renal proximal tubule cells was used in patients with acute renal failure in the intensive care unit. The initial clinical experience with this bioartificial kidney suggests that renal tubule cell therapy may provide a dynamic and individualized treatment program as assessed by acute physiologic and biochemical indices.[51]

Creation of Functional Renal Structures in Vivo

Another approach to improve renal function involves the augmentation of renal tissue with kidney cells expanded in vitro and used for subsequent autologous transplantation. Most recently, an attempt was made to reconstitute renal epithelial cells for the generation of functional nephron units. Renal cells were harvested and expanded in culture. The cells were seeded onto a tubular device constructed from a polycarbonate membrane, which was connected at one end to a Silastic catheter that terminated in a reservoir. The device was implanted in athymic mice. Histologic examination of the implanted devices over time revealed extensive vascularization with formation of glomeruli and highly organized tubule-like structures. Immunocytochemical

staining confirmed the renal phenotype. Additionally, yellow fluid was collected from inside the implant, and its creatinine and uric acid concentrations were consistent with the makeup of dilute urine. Further studies have shown the formation of renal structures in cows using nuclear transfer techniques (**Fig. 6**).[52] The expansion of this system to larger three-dimensional structures is the next challenge awaiting researchers in the urogenital tissue engineering field.

GENITAL TISSUES
Reconstruction of Corporal Smooth Muscle

One of the major components of the phallus is corporal smooth muscle. The creation of autologous functional and structural corporal tissue de novo would be beneficial in cases of congenital abnormality of the genitals and in other situations in which reconstruction is functionally and aesthetically necessary. To look at the functional parameters of engineered corpora, acellular corporal collagen matrices were obtained from donor rabbit penile tissue, and autologous corpus cavernosal smooth muscle and endothelial cells were harvested, expanded, and seeded on the matrices. The entire rabbit corpora was removed and replaced with the engineered structures. The experimental corporal bodies demonstrated intact structural integrity by cavernosography and showed similar intracorporeal pressures by cavernosometry when compared with the normal controls. Rabbits that received scaffolds without cells failed to achieve normal erectile function throughout the study period. Mating activity in the animals with the cell-seeded corpora seemed normal by 1 month after implantation, however. The presence of sperm was confirmed during mating, and sperm was present in all rabbits with the engineered corpora. The female rabbits that mated with the animals implanted with engineered corpora conceived and delivered healthy pups. Animals implanted with the matrix alone were unable to demonstrate normal mating activity and failed to ejaculate into the vagina.[53,54]

Engineered Penile Prostheses

Although silicone is an accepted biomaterial for penile prostheses, biocompatibility is a concern.[55,56] Use of a natural prosthesis composed of autologous cells may be advantageous. In a recent study, the feasibility of applying engineered cartilage rods in situ was investigated.[57] Autologous chondrocytes were harvested from rabbit ear and expanded in culture. The cells were seeded onto biodegradable poly-L-lactic acid–coated PGA polymer rods and then

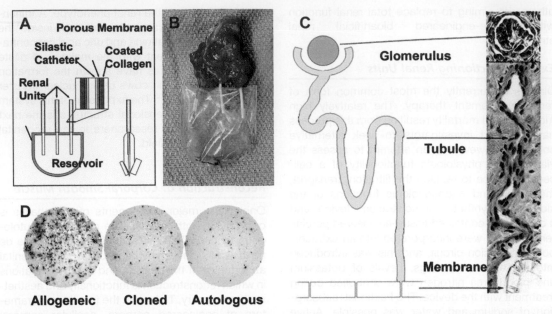

Fig. 6. Combining therapeutic cloning and tissue engineering to produce kidney tissue. (*A*) Illustration of the tissue-engineered renal unit. (*B*) Renal unit seeded with cloned cells 3 months after implantation shows the accumulation of urine-like fluid. (*C*) There was a clear unidirectional continuity between the mature glomeruli, their tubules, and the polycarbonate membrane. (*D*) Enzyme-linked immunospot analyses of the frequencies of T cells that secrete interferon-γ after primary and secondary stimulation with allogeneic renal cells, cloned renal cells, or nuclear donor fibroblasts.

implanted into the corporal spaces of rabbits. Examination at retrieval showed the presence of well-formed milky-white cartilage structures within the corpora at 1 month, and the polymer scaffolding had degraded by 2 months. There was no evidence of erosion or infection in any of the implantation sites. Subsequent studies were performed to assess the long-term functionality of the cartilage penile rods in vivo. To date, the animals have done well and can copulate and impregnate their female partners without problems.

Female Genital Tissues

Congenital malformations of the uterus may have profound implications clinically. Patients who have cloacal exstrophy and intersex disorders may not have sufficient uterine tissue present for future reproduction. We investigated the possibility of engineering functional uterine tissue using autologous cells. Autologous rabbit uterine smooth muscle and epithelial cells were harvested and expanded in culture. These cells were seeded onto preconfigured uterine-shaped biodegradable polymer scaffolds, and these were used for subtotal uterine tissue replacement in the corresponding autologous animals. On retrieval

6 months after implantation, histologic, immunocytochemical, and Western blot analyses confirmed the presence of normal uterine tissue components. Biomechanical analyses and organ bath studies showed that the functional characteristics of these tissues were similar to those of normal uterine tissue. Breeding studies using these engineered uteri are currently being performed.

Similarly, several pathologic conditions, including congenital malformations and malignancy, can adversely affect normal vaginal development or anatomy. To investigate tissue engineering methods of generating vaginal tissue for use in these situations, vaginal epithelial and smooth muscle cells of female rabbits were harvested, grown, and expanded in culture. These cells were seeded onto biodegradable polymer scaffolds, and the cell-seeded constructs were then implanted into nude mice for up to 6 weeks. Immunocytochemical, histologic, and Western blot analyses confirmed the presence of vaginal tissue phenotypes. Electrical field stimulation studies in the tissue-engineered constructs showed similar functional properties to those of normal vaginal tissue. When these constructs were used for autologous total vaginal replacement, patent vaginal structures were noted in the tissue-engineered specimens, whereas the non–cell-seeded structures were noted to be stenotic.[58]

Other Applications of Genitourinary Tissue Engineering

Fetal tissue engineering
The prenatal diagnosis of fetal abnormalities is now more common and more accurate. Improvements in prenatal diagnosis have led to demand for novel interventions designed to reverse potentially life-threatening processes before birth. Having a ready supply of urologic-associated tissue for immediate surgical reconstruction of congenital malformations at birth may be advantageous. Theoretically, once the diagnosis of the pathologic condition is confirmed prenatally, a small tissue biopsy could then be obtained under ultrasound guidance. These biopsy materials could then be processed expanded in vitro. Using tissue engineering techniques, in vitro-reconstituted structures could then be readily available at the time of birth for reconstruction.

Injectable therapies
Urinary incontinence and vesicoureteral reflux are common conditions affecting the genitourinary system. Currently, injectable bulking agents are one treatment used clinically for these conditions, but biocompatibility of current synthetic bulking agents is a concern. The ideal substance for endoscopic treatment of reflux and incontinence should be injectable, nonantigenic, nonmigratory, volume stable, and safe for human use. Animal studies have shown that chondrocytes (cartilage cells) can be easily harvested and combined with alginate in vitro, and the resulting suspension can be easily injected cystoscopically. The elastic cartilage tissue formed as a result of the injection is able to correct vesicoureteral reflux without any evidence of obstruction. This technology has been applied in humans for the correction of vesicoureteral reflux in children and for urinary incontinence in adults (see **Fig. 4**).[59,60]

Utilizing cell therapy techniques, the use of autologous smooth muscle cells has been explored for urinary incontinence and vesicoureteral reflux applications. The potential use of injectable cultured myoblasts for the treatment of stress urinary incontinence has also been investigated.[61,62] The use of injectable muscle precursor cells has also been investigated for use in the treatment of urinary incontinence attributable to irreversible urethral sphincter injury or maldevelopment.[63] A clinical trial involving the use of muscle-derived stem cells to treat stress urinary incontinence has also been performed with good

results. Biopsies of skeletal muscle were obtained, and autologous myoblasts and fibroblasts were cultured. Under ultrasound guidance, myoblasts were injected into the rhabdosphincter and fibroblasts mixed with collagen were injected into the submucosa. One year after injection, the thickness and function of the rhabdosphincter had significantly increased and all patients were continent.[64] These are the first demonstrations of the replacement of sphincter muscle tissue and its innervation by the injection of muscle precursor cells.

In addition, injectable muscle-based gene therapy and tissue engineering were combined to improve detrusor function in a bladder injury model and may potentially be a novel treatment option for urinary incontinence.[65]

Patients with testicular dysfunction require androgen replacement for somatic development. Conventional treatment for testicular dysfunction consists of periodic intramuscular injections of chemically modified testosterone or application of a transdermal testosterone patch. Long-term nonpulsatile testosterone therapy is not optimal, however, and can cause multiple problems, including erythropoiesis and bone density changes.

A system was designed in which Leydig cells were microencapsulated for controlled testosterone replacement. Purified Leydig cells were isolated and encapsulated in an alginate-poly-L-lysine solution. The encapsulated Leydig cells were injected into castrated animals, and serum testosterone was measured serially; the animals were able to maintain testosterone levels in the long term.[66] These studies suggest that microencapsulated Leydig cells may be able to replace or supplement testosterone in situations in which anorchia or testicular failure is present.

SUMMARY

Tissue engineering efforts are currently being undertaken for every type of tissue and organ within the urinary system. Most of the effort expended to engineer genitourinary tissues has occurred within the past decade. Tissue engineering techniques require a cell culture facility designed for human application. Personnel who have mastered the techniques of cell harvest, culture, and expansion in addition to polymer design are essential for the successful application of this technology. Before these engineering techniques can be applied to humans, further studies need to be performed in many of the tissues described. Recent progress suggests that engineered urologic tissues and cell therapy may have clinical applicability.

REFERENCES

1. McDougal WS. Metabolic complications of urinary intestinal diversion. J Urol 1992;147:1199–208.
2. Atala A, Vacanti JP, Peters CA, et al. Formation of urothelial structures in vivo from dissociated cells attached to biodegradable polymer scaffolds in vitro. J Urol 1992;148:658–62.
3. Atala A, Cima LG, Kim W, et al. Injectable alginate seeded with chondrocytes as a potential treatment for vesicoureteral reflux. J Urol 1993;150:745–7.
4. Atala A, Freeman MR, Vacanti JP, et al. Implantation in vivo and retrieval of artificial structures consisting of rabbit and human urothelium and human bladder muscle. J Urol 1993;150:608–12.
5. Atala A, Kim W, Paige KT, et al. Endoscopic treatment of vesicoureteral reflux with a chondrocyte-alginate suspension. J Urol 1994;152:641–3.
6. Atala A, Bauer SB, Soker S, et al. Tissue-engineered autologous bladders for patients needing cystoplasty. Lancet 2006;367:1241–6 [see comment].
7. Atala A. Tissue engineering, stem cells, and cloning for the regeneration of urologic organs. Clin Plast Surg 2003;30:649–67.
8. Lin HK, Cowan R, Moore P, et al. Characterization of neuropathic bladder smooth muscle cells in culture. J Urol 2004;171:1348–52.
9. Lai JY, Yoon CY, Yoo JJ, et al. Phenotypic and functional characterization of in vivo tissue engineered smooth muscle from normal and pathological bladders. J Urol 2002;168:1853–7.
10. Brivanlou AH, Gage FH, Jaenisch R, et al. Stem cells. Setting standards for human embryonic stem cells. Science 2003;300:913–6 [see comment].
11. Thomson JA, Itskovitz-Eldor J, Shapiro SS, et al. Embryonic stem cell lines derived from human blastocysts. Science 1998;282:1145–7 [see comment] [erratum appears in Science 1998 Dec 4;282(5395):1827].
12. De Coppi P, Bartsch G Jr, Siddiqui MM, et al. Isolation of amniotic stem cell lines with potential for therapy. Nat Biotechnol 2007;25:100–6 [see comment].
13. De Coppi P, Callegari A, Chiavegato A, et al. Amniotic fluid and bone marrow derived mesenchymal stem cells can be converted to smooth muscle cells in the cryo-injured rat bladder and prevent compensatory hypertrophy of surviving smooth muscle cells. J Urol 2007;177:369–76.
14. Hochedlinger K, Rideout WM, Kyba M, et al. Nuclear transplantation, embryonic stem cells and the potential for cell therapy. Hematol J 2004;5(Suppl 3):S114–7.
15. Kim BS, Baez CE, Atala A. Biomaterials for tissue engineering. World J Urol 2000;18:2–9.
16. Kim BS, Mooney DJ. Development of biocompatible synthetic extracellular matrices for tissue engineering. Trends Biotechnol 1998;16:224–30.
17. Ponder KP, Gupta S, Leland F, et al. Mouse hepatocytes migrate to liver parenchyma and function indefinitely after intrasplenic transplantation. Proc Natl Acad Sci U S A 1991;88:1217–21.
18. Brittberg M, Lindahl A, Nilsson A, et al. Treatment of deep cartilage defects in the knee with autologous chondrocyte transplantation. N Engl J Med 1994; 331:889–95 [see comment].
19. Folkman J, Hochberg M. Self-regulation of growth in three dimensions. J Exp Med 1973;138:745–53.
20. Olsen L, Bowald S, Busch C, et al. Urethral reconstruction with a new synthetic absorbable device. An experimental study. Scand J Urol Nephrol 1992;26:323–6.
21. Kropp BP, Ludlow JK, Spicer D, et al. Rabbit urethral regeneration using small intestinal submucosa onlay grafts. Urology 1998;52:138–42.
22. Sievert KD, Bakircioglu ME, Nunes L, et al. Homologous acellular matrix graft for urethral reconstruction in the rabbit: histological and functional evaluation. J Urol 2000;163:1958–65.
23. Atala A, Guzman L, Retik AB. A novel inert collagen matrix for hypospadias repair. J Urol 1999;162: 1148–51.
24. Chen F, Yoo JJ, Atala A. Acellular collagen matrix as a possible "off the shelf" biomaterial for urethral repair. Urology 1999;54:407–10.
25. le Roux PJ. Endoscopic urethroplasty with unseeded small intestinal submucosa collagen matrix grafts: a pilot study. J Urol 2005;173:140–3.
26. Roger EDF, James JY, Anthony A. Urethral replacement using cell seeded tubularized collagen matrices. J Urol 2002;168:1789–93.
27. Kaefer M, Hendren WH, Bauer SB, et al. Reservoir calculi: a comparison of reservoirs constructed from stomach and other enteric segments. J Urol 1998;160:2187–90 [see comment].
28. Kaefer M, Tobin MS, Hendren WH, et al. Continent urinary diversion: the Children's Hospital experience. J Urol 1997;157:1394–9.
29. Lailas NG, Cilento B, Atala A. Progressive ureteral dilation for subsequent ureterocystoplasty. J Urol 1996;156:1151–3.
30. Satar N, Yoo JJ, Atala A. Progressive dilation for bladder tissue expansion. J Urol 1999;162:829–31.
31. Blandy JP. Ileal pouch with transitional epithelium and anal sphincter as a continent urinary reservoir. J Urol 1961;86:749–67.
32. Blandy JP. The feasibility of preparing an ideal substitute for the urinary bladder. Ann R Coll Surg Engl 1964;35:287–311.
33. Harada N, Yano H, Ohkawa T, et al. New surgical treatment of bladder tumours: mucosal denudation of the bladder. Br J Urol 1965;37:545–7.
34. Oesch I. Neourothelium in bladder augmentation. An experimental study in rats. Eur Urol 1988;14:328–9.
35. Salle JL, Fraga JC, Lucib A, et al. Seromuscular enterocystoplasty in dogs. J Urol 1990;144:454–6.

36. Cheng E, Rento R, Grayhack JT, et al. Reversed seromuscular flaps in the urinary tract in dogs. J Urol 1994;152:2252–7.

37. Yoo JJ, Meng J, Oberpenning F, et al. Bladder augmentation using allogenic bladder submucosa seeded with cells. Urology 1998;51:221–5.

38. Probst M, Dahiya R, Carrier S, et al. Reproduction of functional smooth muscle tissue and partial bladder replacement. Br J Urol 1997;79:505–15.

39. Sutherland RS, Baskin LS, Hayward SW, et al. Regeneration of bladder urothelium, smooth muscle, blood vessels and nerves into an acellular tissue matrix. J Urol 1996;156:571–7.

40. Piechota HJ, Dahms SE, Nunes LS, et al. In vitro functional properties of the rat bladder regenerated by the bladder acellular matrix graft. J Urol 1998; 159:1717–24.

41. Badylak SF, Lantz GC, Coffey A, et al. Small intestinal submucosa as a large diameter vascular graft in the dog. J Surg Res 1989;47:74–80.

42. Kropp BP, Cheng EY, Lin HK, et al. Reliable and reproducible bladder regeneration using unseeded distal small intestinal submucosa. J Urol 2004;172:1710–3.

43. Kropp BP, Rippy MK, Badylak SF, et al. Regenerative urinary bladder augmentation using small intestinal submucosa: urodynamic and histopathologic assessment in long-term canine bladder augmentations. J Urol 1996;155:2098–104.

44. Portis AJ, Elbahnasy AM, Shalhav AL, et al. Laparoscopic augmentation cystoplasty with different biodegradable grafts in an animal model. J Urol 2000;164:1405–11.

45. Landman J, Olweny E, Sundaram CP, et al. Laparoscopic mid sagittal hemicystectomy and bladder reconstruction with small intestinal submucosa and reimplantation of ureter into small intestinal submucosa: 1-year followup. J Urol 2004;171:2450–5.

46. Oberpenning F, Meng J, Yoo JJ, et al. De novo reconstitution of a functional mammalian urinary bladder by tissue engineering. Nat Biotechnol 1999;17:149–55 [see comment].

47. Dahms SE, Piechota HJ, Nunes L, et al. Free ureteral replacement in rats: regeneration of ureteral wall components in the acellular matrix graft. Urology 1997;50:818–25.

48. Baltaci S, Ozer G, Ozer E, et al. Failure of ureteral replacement with Gore-Tex tube grafts. Urology 1998;51:400–3 [see comment].

49. Osman Y, Shokeir A, Gabr M, et al. Canine ureteral replacement with long acellular matrix tube: is it clinically applicable? J Urol 2004;172:1151–4.

50. Humes HD, Buffington DA, MacKay SM, et al. Replacement of renal function in uremic animals with a tissue-engineered kidney. Nat Biotechnol 1999;17:451–5 [see comment].

51. Humes HD, Weitzel WF, Bartlett RH, et al. Renal cell therapy is associated with dynamic and individualized responses in patients with acute renal failure. Blood Purif 2003;21:64–71.

52. Lanza RP, Chung HY, Yoo JJ, et al. Generation of histocompatible tissues using nuclear transplantation. Nat Biotechnol 2002;20:689–96 [see comment].

53. Yoo JJ, Park HJ, Atala A. Tissue-engineering applications for phallic reconstruction. World J Urol 2000;18:62–6.

54. Yoo JJ, Atala A. Tissue engineering of genitourinary organs. Ernst Schering Res Found Workshop 2002;105–27.

55. Nukui F, Okamoto S, Nagata M, et al. Complications and reimplantation of penile implants. Int J Urol 1997;4:52–4.

56. Thomalla JV, Thompson ST, Rowland RG, et al. Infectious complications of penile prosthetic implants. J Urol 1987;138:65–7.

57. Yoo JJ, Park HJ, Lee I, et al. Autologous engineered cartilage rods for penile reconstruction. J Urol 1999; 162:1119–21.

58. De Filippo RE, Yoo JJ, Atala A. Engineering of vaginal tissue in vivo. Tissue Engineering 2003;9: 301–6.

59. Diamond DA, Caldamone AA. Endoscopic correction of vesicoureteral reflux in children using autologous chondrocytes: preliminary results. J Urol 1999; 162:1185–8.

60. Bent AE, Tutrone RT, McLennan MT, et al. Treatment of intrinsic sphincter deficiency using autologous ear chondrocytes as a bulking agent. Neurourol Urodyn 2001;20:157–65.

61. Yokoyama T, Huard J, Chancellor MB. Myoblast therapy for stress urinary incontinence and bladder dysfunction. World J Urol 2000;18:56–61.

62. Chancellor MB, Yokoyama T, Tirney S, et al. Preliminary results of myoblast injection into the urethra and bladder wall: a possible method for the treatment of stress urinary incontinence and impaired detrusor contractility. Neurourol Urodyn 2000;19:279–87.

63. Yiou R, Yoo JJ, Atala A. Restoration of functional motor units in a rat model of sphincter injury by muscle precursor cell autografts. Transplantation 2003;76:1053–60.

64. Strasser H, Berjukow S, Marksteiner R, et al. Stem cell therapy for urinary stress incontinence. Exp Gerontol 2004;39:1259–65.

65. Huard J, Yokoyama T, Pruchnic R, et al. Muscle-derived cell-mediated ex vivo gene therapy for urological dysfunction. Gene Ther 2002;9:1617–26.

66. Machluf M, Orsola A, Boorjian S, et al. Microencapsulation of Leydig cells: a system for testosterone supplementation. Endocrinology 2003;144: 4975–9.

Articles of Interest

The following articles provide comparative research data but reference products by brand names. These articles are not included in the required articles for the CME post-test for this issue.

Any questions can be directed to John Owen, PhD, Office of Continuing Medical Education, University of Virginia School of Medicine, Charlottesville, Virginia. JAO2B@hscmail.mcc.virginia.edu

Intraoperative Tissue Characterization and Imaging

Sijo Parekattil, MD, Lawrence L. Yeung, MD, Li-Ming Su, MD*

KEYWORDS

- Imaging • Intraoperative • Tissue characterization
- Neurovascular bundle • Testis

As surgical operative technology improves, surgeons today have the ability to visualize fine structures and detailed anatomy. There are a number of advances that have been made to optimize patient outcomes with better tissue characterization in urologic procedures. This article focuses on advances in intraoperative imaging and tissue characterization for various urologic procedures. Each modality is presented with its corresponding applications in urology. The following techniques are covered: optical coherence tomography (OCT); confocal fluorescent microscopy (CFM); near-infrared fluorescence imaging; elastography; intraoperative ultrasonography (including Doppler, duplex flow, and high-resolution three-dimensional imaging); and the Cavermap neurovascular bundle (NVB) surgical mapping aid.

OPTICAL COHERENCE TOMOGRAPHY

OCT is an imaging technique that provides real-time, high-resolution, atraumatic, cross-sectional imaging of tissues. One OCT system has been used in urologic applications (bladder cancer detection and staging and NVB mapping).[1–6] The device is comprised of an 8F catheter fiberoptic probe with a computer console. The fiberoptic probe allows for it to be integrated into laparoscopic instruments or other flexible devices. OCT is similar to B-mode ultrasonography, but instead of measuring the backscattering of acoustic waves, it measures the backscattering of near-infrared light. Unlike ultrasound, however, OCT does not require direct probe contact with the tissue or a transducing medium, decreasing interference with the operative instruments in the surgical field. Image resolution as fine as 1 to 15 μm can be achieved with a maximal penetration depth of 1.6 mm, which allows for imaging of microscopic structures, such as the cavernous nerves, lymphatics, blood vessels, and fascial planes.

The superficial imaging characteristics of OCT make it ideally suited for possible assessment of depth of penetration of bladder cancer within the

Department of Urology, University of Florida, 1600 SW Archer Road, PO Box 100247, Gainesville, FL 32610–0247, USA
* Corresponding author.
E-mail address: sulm@urology.ufl.edu (L-M. Su).

Urol Clin N Am 36 (2009) 213–221
doi:10.1016/j.ucl.2009.02.008

bladder wall. A number of groups have evaluated the use of OCT as an adjunct to conventional cystoscopy to assess better the stage and grade of bladder cancers.[3,5,7] Specific attention has been paid to the use of OCT in assessing the depth of penetration of bladder tumors beyond the basement membrane (or lamina propria). **Fig. 1** illustrates some representative images by Hermes and colleagues[3] of OCT being used to assess bladder lesions (benign versus carcinoma in situ versus invasive carcinoma). At the present time, resection of these lesions is still performed, and so the added value of this imaging to current pathology evaluation may be questioned. The potential of using the OCT images in lieu of pathologic examination in terms of planning further treatment for these patients, however, is intriguing.

Rais-Bahrami and colleagues[6] and Fried and colleagues[2] demonstrated the use of OCT in imaging of the cavernous nerve and periprostatic tissue in the rat model. The rat model proved to be an ideal model for imaging because the cavernous nerve exists as a large, visible structure with minimal intervening vasculature or fat. To confirm the course of the cavernous nerve in the rat, the nerve was identified and stimulated with simultaneous intracorporeal pressure measurements and penile length and girth measurements taken. Hematoxylin-eosin–stained histologic specimens of the cavernous nerve and periprostatic tissues were then compared with the OCT images obtained from the same location on the prostate and were found to correlate well (**Fig. 2**).[6]

Rais-Bahrami and colleagues[6] and Aron and colleagues[1] both reported on the use of OCT to image human ex vivo prostatectomy specimens immediately after removal. Rais-Bahrami and colleagues[6] found the OCT images of human cavernous nerve and prostatic tissue to be similar to that of the rat in that there was good histologic correlation with the OCT images. Identification of the NVB proved to be more difficult, however, compared with the rat prostate because of the presence of more periprostatic blood vessels and fat resulting in a degradation of the OCT resolution. Aron and colleagues[1] also found that identification of the NVBs required an experienced operator to distinguish them from adipose tissue, small vessels, and lymphatics.

Although OCT has been used to aid in the intraoperative identification and preservation of the NVB,[1] success has yet to be validated by potency results. Future improvements in the technology resulting in greater depth of penetration and resolution may make OCT more feasible for intraoperative identification of the cavernous nerve during nerve-sparing prostatectomies or for localization of cavernous nerve endings to allow for a precise nerve graft anastomosis.

There is also preliminary work on the use of OCT for testicular seminiferous tubule imaging. In men who have nonobstructive azoospermia, testicular sperm extraction is used to retrieve sperm to achieve pregnancies with assisted reproductive techniques. Unfortunately, sperm retrieval is only successful in about 50% to 60% of these cases.[8] This has driven the development of "imaging-assisted" testicular sperm extraction to improve retrieval rates, using such techniques as microscopic assisted testicular sperm extraction[8] and power Doppler ultrasound assisted guidance.[9] OCT with its high-resolution images may improve sperm retrieval rates by better identifying isolated foci of spermatogenesis in these men with nonobstructive azoospermia.

CONFOCAL FLUORESCENT MICROSCOPY

CFM is a new technology that has been described for use in gastroenterology, dermatology, pulmonology, and urology and provides such incredibly detailed resolution that it allows for in vivo differentiation of cancerous and normal tissue.[10–14] CFM can also provide enough resolution to allow distinction between some differentiated and undifferentiated cancers.[15]

Koenig and colleagues[13] have demonstrated the use of CFM for endoscopic microscopy of the bladder and opened the possibility of using this technology for real-time in vivo assessment of bladder lesions. CFM allowed imaging of cellular details of the entire urothelium. The superficial umbrella cells, intermediary and basal cells, capillary vessel network, and layers of the lamina propria could all be clearly identified similar to histologic sections of the tissue. Currently, the CFM system provides imaging only on horizontal tissue planes. With three-dimensional software reconstruction, however, the production of real-time three-dimensional noninvasive histologic imaging with flexible fibers that could be passed through the working channel of the cystoscope is likely to become available in the near future.

CFM has also been used to provide real-time in vivo images of peripheral nerves and deep-brain structures in rats genetically engineered to express a fluorescent protein in all sensory and motor neurons.[16] CFM allows for enough spatial resolution to produce images down to the axonal level. A commercially available unit uses CFM technology, and is composed of a laser scanning unit, a small fiberoptic probe, and an image processing unit. Real-time images can be produced up to 12 frames per second, and the probe allows

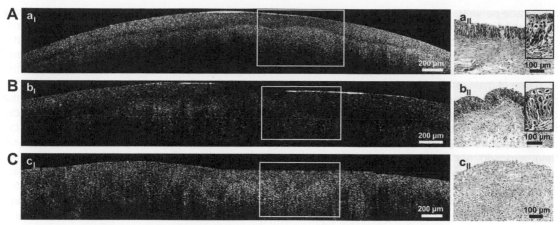

Fig. 1. (*A–C*) CT images of healthy tissue (a_I), carcinoma in situ (b_I), and incipient invasive transitional cell carcinoma (c_I, flat lesion) are correlated with histologic findings (a_{II}–c_{II}). (*From* Hermes B, Spoler F, Naami A, et al. Visualization of the basement membrane zone of the bladder by optical coherence tomography: feasibility of noninvasive evaluation of tumor invasion. Urology 2008;72:677; with permission.)

for a lateral resolution of 3.5 μm with a depth of penetration of 15 μm. Compared with such technologies as ultrasonography or OCT, CFM requires the use of a fluorescent dye applied and diffused within the tissue being studied to help resolve, differentiate, and augment tissue characteristics.

Boyette and colleagues[17] have used CFM technology along with injection of a fluorescent

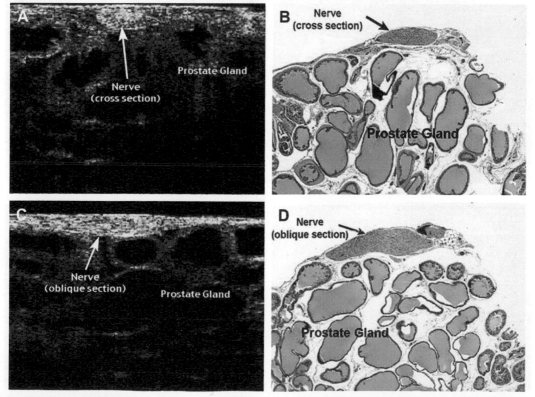

Fig. 2. CT imaging and histologic (hematoxylin-eosin) correlation of rat cavernous nerves in cross-section (*A, B*) and in oblique section (*C, D*) overlying prostate glandular tissue. (*From* Rais-Bahrami S, Levinson AW, Fried NM, et al. Optical coherence tomography of cavernous nerves: a step toward real-time intraoperative imaging during nerve-sparing radical prostatectomy. Urology 2008;72:198; with permission.)

retrograde nerve tracer to provide in vivo real-time images of the cavernous nerve in rats. A recombinant β subunit of cholera toxin conjugated to a fluorescent compound served as the fluorescent nerve tracer and was injected into the corpus cavernosum of male rats to allow for retrograde transport along the cavernous nerves. They found that optimal imaging of the cavernous nerve was obtained after allowing for 9 days of retrograde transport along the nerve. The cavernous nerves were then exposed and imaged using CFM, which produced exceptional images, even allowing for visualization of the branching of the cavernous nerve (**Fig. 3**). Confirmation that the nerves being imaged were actually the cavernous nerve was obtained by electrical stimulation of the fluorescent nerve with simultaneous intracavernosal pressure monitoring.

Although CFM technology produces striking images in the rat model, there are limitations to the technology that need to be overcome before successful application in humans. The depth of penetration of the probe is only 15 μm, which

works well for the rat model. As was encountered in translating OCT technology from the rat to human model, however, the greater amount of periprostatic fat, vessels, and lymphatics in the human model may hinder the view of structures, such as the cavernous nerve. Another major limitation to the technology is the need for injection of a fluorescent nerve tracer and waiting for retrograde transport to the cavernous nerve. Although transport in the rat model took 9 days, it has been estimated that it may take up to 45 days for optimal imaging to be obtained in the human because of the four to five times greater distance from the penis to the cavernous nerve the tracer has to travel.[17] Finally, although short-term safety of the injected tracer composed of the β subunit of cholera toxin was demonstrated in the rat model, long-term studies need to be performed in humans before the technology can become mainstream.

CFM has also been used to detect DNA abnormalities within spermatozoa in a noninvasive

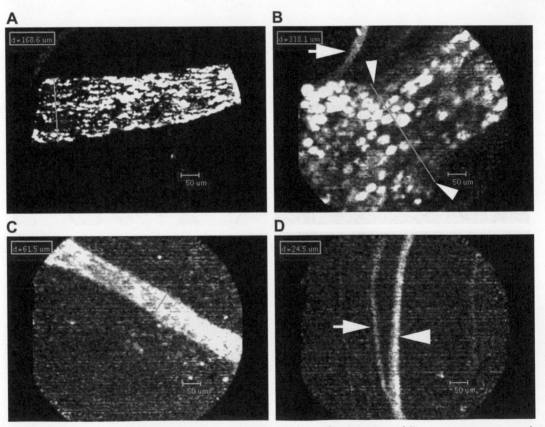

Fig. 3. (*A–D*) CFM images of rat cavernous nerves obtained 9 days after injection of fluorescent nerve tracer into corpus cavernosum. Fig. 3D demonstrates accessory nerve branching into larger and smaller bundles. (*From* Boyette LB, Reardon MA, Mirelman AJ, et al. Fiberoptic imaging of cavernous nerves in vivo. J Urol 2007;178:2694–700; with permission.)

manner.[18] This again brings about the possibility of using such imaging technology in men with nonobstructive azoospermia to identify areas within the testicle that may harbor pockets of spermatogenesis. The depth of penetration for imaging may be a limiting factor in truly performing a noninvasive scanning of the entire testicle, but as the technology improves, there are likely to be further applications for this modality.

NEAR-INFRARED FLUORESCENCE IMAGING

Golijanin and colleagues[19] have developed the concept of using an injectable fluorescent nerve tracer to localize the cavernous nerve. After injection of a fluorescent dye called indocyanine green into the rat penis and allowing time for retrograde transport to the cavernous nerves, they used a near-infrared fluorescence intraoperative imaging system composed of a laser used to illuminate fluorescent tissue and a camera sensitive to infrared fluorescence to capture images. Nerves were positively identified at 6, 8, 12, 18, 24, and 36 hours after indocyanine green injection. Maximal nerve fluorescence was noted at 18 and 24 hours postinjection.

The main advantage of near-infrared fluorescence using indocyanine green as a fluorescing agent over CFM with injection of a fluorescent compound is the significantly shorter time required for retrograde transport of the fluorescing agent. Nevertheless, further studies are required to determine the length of time needed for adequate transport of indocyanine green from the penis to the cavernous nerves in the human model. The downside to using indocyanine green as a fluorescing agent is that the agent contains iodine, however, which limits its use to patients without an allergy to iodine.

ELASTOGRAPHY

Elastography is an ultrasound-based imaging technique using remote palpation or quasistatic compression for imaging tissue elasticity. Pathologic changes in biologic tissue correlate with changes in the tissue mechanical properties. Elastography strives to assess these mechanical changes to detect areas within an organ, such as the prostate, which may harbor areas of cancer. Elastography is essentially a technique of measuring tissue strain in response to external compression. Areas in the prostate with malignancy tend to have irregular-shaped lesions compared with benign lesions that tend to be more symmetric and smooth.[20] As these areas of tissue are compressed, tissue strain varies in these regions. This strain in the tissue can be measured by specific ultrasound scanning modes. By using multiple arrays of these ultrasound transducers, a three-dimensional image of lesions within the prostate can be developed by mapping out areas of the prostate that have varying tissue strain.

Patil and colleagues[21] have performed some three-dimensional modeling work on prostatic tissue to detect irregularly shaped inclusion bodies (representing cancer nodules) that were placed into prostate models. The elastography device comprises a specialized ultrasound probe with arrays of imaging and tracking transducers capable of generating three-dimensional reconstructions of any regions within the prostate with different tissue characteristics. This modality potentially may be used real-time intraoperatively to identify regions within the prostate that harbor cancer. Identifying the location of prostate cancer nodules within the prostate during radical prostatectomy, especially during the NVB release, may be helpful in minimizing the risk of positive surgical margins.

Souchon and colleagues[22] have used elastography imaging during real-time in vivo high-intensity focused ultrasound therapy for prostate cancer. **Fig. 4** illustrates the imaging characterization of elastography. This particular use of elastography may be quite promising in that ultrasound technology is used in this setting both for imaging and therapy.

Emelianov and colleagues[23] have shown that elastography can also be used to identify renal pathology, which opens up the potential of its use real-time during renal procedures accurately to identify tumor margins. Pareek and colleagues[24] have performed real-time elastography of the kidney during radiofrequency ablation of renal lesions to delineate tumor margins better with very promising results. In this particular application, elastography provided a more accurate delineation of the ablated tumor margin than conventional imaging modalities, such as CT (because the ablated area does not differ real-time).

INTRAOPERATIVE ULTRASONOGRAPHY AND DOPPLER IMAGING
Real-Time Transrectal Ultrasonography

Ukimura and colleagues[25] described a technique to provide real-time intraoperative transrectal ultrasound (TRUS) imaging of the prostate and periprostatic tissues and vessels to assist with dissection to compensate for the muted tactile feedback present when performing laparoscopic radical prostatectomy. As opposed to screening TRUS, intraoperative TRUS combines prostate needle biopsy results with real-time imaging,

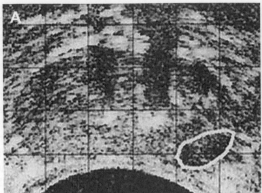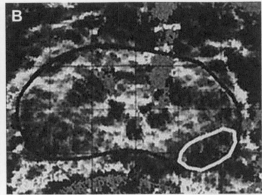

Fig. 4. Sonogram (*A*) and elastogram (*B*) of the prostate (*black outline*) and the tumor (*white outline*). (*From* Souchon R, Rouviere O, Gelet A, et al. Visualisation of HIFU lesions using elastography of the human prostate in vivo: preliminary results. Ultrasound Med Biol 2003;29:1007; with permission.)

allowing the ultrasonographer to direct the surgeon to a wider plane of dissection in areas suspicious for cancer, such as near hypoechoic lesions or regions where the biopsies were positive near the capsule. They reported the potential advantages of real-time TRUS imaging to be that it (1) identifies the anatomic course of the NVB; (2) measures the adequacy of NVB preservation; (3) identifies the apical margin of the prostate; (4) aids in the dissection of the posterior bladder neck, vas deferens, seminal vesicle, and release of the rectal wall; and (5) identifies any hypoechoic bulging nodule to help in avoiding positive surgical margins.[26] They found that their positive surgical margin rates decreased from 29% to 9% (*P* = .0002) with the use of intraoperative TRUS during laparoscopic radical prostatectomy and were able to map the course of the NVB using TRUS by tracing the arterial flow within the NVB.[25] Based on the previous findings by Lepor and colleagues[27] documenting the lateral location of the cavernous nerve within the NVB with relation to the vascular supply, it was theorized that if the vascular supply in the NVB is preserved after the nerve-sparing dissection as demonstrated by Doppler waveform analysis using TRUS, then the cavernous nerves should be spared. They were also able to report on the diameter of the NVB and the number of visible vessels within the NVB before and after the dissection to evaluate the quality of the nerve-sparing dissection and found a decrease in the number of visible vessels from 2.6 to 1.1 and a decrease in cross-sectional area of the NVB by 11%.[26] These findings have yet to be correlated, however, with any improvement in potency rates after nerve-sparing laparoscopic radical prostatectomy.

Another serious limitation to the use of TRUS during laparoscopic radical prostatectomy is that it is operator dependent and requires an experienced and dedicated ultrasonographer. This person is positioned between the patient's legs for most of the operation and is constantly involved with interpretation of the ultrasound and laparoscopic pictures simultaneously. The additional, highly trained, personnel required may also translate into a significant increase in the cost of the operation. In addition, the use of TRUS during robot-assisted laparoscopic prostatectomy poses an additional challenge because the robot is situated between the patient's legs where the TRUS operator normally sits. This may limit the use and widespread adoption of intraoperative TRUS because most prostatectomies in the United States are being performed with robot-assistance at the time of this writing.

Real-Time Doppler Imaging of the Testicle

Herwig and colleagues[28,29] have demonstrated the use of real-time intraoperative color Doppler ultrasound to improve sperm retrieval rates in men who have nonobstructive azoospermia who are undergoing testicular sperm extraction. Areas within the testicle with better blood perfusion seem to harbor areas of spermatogenesis more frequently than areas with less perfusion (**Fig. 5**). Intraoperative color Doppler ultrasound of the testicle is performed at the time of surgery and a small 22-gauge needle is placed into the location of highest flow. The tunica of the testicle is then opened, and a sampling of this tissue is performed. Additional verification of blood flow velocity in this area is performed using laser Doppler measurements (the phase shift in the Doppler reading is recorded as a measure of blood flow). Retrieval of sperm in high-flow regions of the

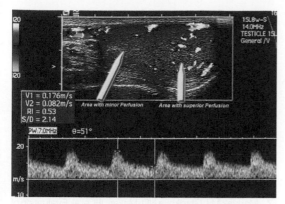

Fig. 5. Contrast-enhanced color Doppler ultrasound of left testicle of patient. Arrows indicate areas of major and minor perfusion. (*From* Herwig R, Tosun K, Schuster A, et al. Tissue perfusion-controlled guided biopsies are essential for the outcome of testicular sperm extraction. Fertil Steril 2007;87:1071; with permission.)

testicle was as high as 72% versus 13% in low-flow areas ($P = 0.008$).

The authors are investigating the development of alternative techniques for blood flow measurement using Doppler technology. Direct Doppler waveform analysis and phase shift recordings may have some promise in predicting locations within the testicle that are likely to harbor spermatogenesis.

Real-Time Doppler Mapping of the Renal Vessels

Hyams and colleagues[30] have used real-time laparoscopic Doppler ultrasonography of the renal hilum before dissection to assist in accurate localization of crossing vessels in pyeloplasty cases. Their group has also found this of benefit during nephrectomy and partial nephrectomy cases.

The authors' preliminary evaluation of the laparoscopic Doppler probe during robotic-assisted laparoscopic pyeloplasty is promising. Mean duration of cases without Doppler assistance was 223 minutes (range, 90–300 minutes). Mean duration with Doppler assistance was 168 minutes (range, 60–210 minutes). This difference was statistically significant ($P = 0.03$). Subjectively, the intraoperative Doppler allowed the surgeon to identify where the crossing vessel was located before the ureteropelvic junction dissection and was a useful teaching tool for resident training.

NEUROVASCULAR BUNDLE SURGICAL MAPPING AID

The CaverMap Surgical Aid (Blue Torch Corporation, Norwood, Massachusetts) was developed to assist in intraoperative localization of the cavernosal nerves by provoking an erectile response through electrical stimulation of the nerve. It has been shown that electrical stimulation of the cavernous nerve may cause very small changes in tumescence or detumescence of the penis, which may not be visible, but yet still physiologically detectable. The CaverMap device was designed to measure changes in penile girth as little as 0.5%. The system is composed of a control unit, a hand-held nerve stimulator, and a tumescence sensor placed around the penis to measure changes in circumference. Mapping of the cavernous nerve is performed by placing the nerve stimulation probe on tissues suspected to contain the cavernous nerve and using detected changes in penile tumescence during stimulation to, in theory, affirm correct identification of its location (see **Fig. 5**) The CaverMap can then be used after removal of the prostate to assess the continuity and integrity of the cavernous nerves by proximal stimulation of the nerves and again assessing penile tumescence. It can also be used to localize the distal end of a severed nerve to facilitate nerve graft anastamosis.

In concept, the CaverMap Surgical Aid seems to provide a sound solution to precise intraoperative cavernous nerve localization to achieve optimal cavernous nerve preservation during nerve-sparing radical prostatectomy. Practically, however, results using the CaverMap have been fraught with inconsistency. Klotz and Herschorn[31] reported a 94% potency rate (16 of 17 patients) after use of CaverMap for intraoperative nerve identification. They also report a 19% overall positive margin rate (five patients) in that study that included patients with clinical stage T1c and T2a–c disease. Only three (12%) of the patients had positive margins confined to the apex or lateral margin, however, and it is conceivable that the nerve-sparing approach may have altered the margin status. For the other two patients with positive margins, one had positive margins with seminal vesicle invasion, and the other had extensive positive margins with positive lymph nodes. It is possible that the nerve-sparing approach did not alter the final outcome in those two patients.

Klotz and Herschorn[31] then performed a prospective, randomized, multicenter study using the CaverMap-assisted nerve-sparing prostatectomy technique and compared it with conventional nerve-sparing techniques. They found that, at 1 year, the CaverMap group had a significant improvement in nocturnal tumescence compared with the conventional nerve-sparing group (greater than 60% tumescence for mean of 15.9 minutes versus 2.1 minutes, respectively) as measured by an instrument used to measure penile tumescence and rigidity.[32] The improved nocturnal tumescence, however, did not translate into a significant difference in the ability to have an erection sufficient for intercourse (71% versus 62%; $P = .17$). Kim and colleagues[33] reported that although they had a 77% positive CaverMap response rate, their overall potency rate was only 18% at 1 year. Furthermore, Walsh and colleagues[34] indicated that the CaverMap device should not be used to determine if a structure should be excised or not because they found the device to have a low specificity of 54%. This variability and lack of precision was also supported by Holzbeierlein and colleagues,[35] who showed that stimulation of an area on the anterior bladder wall far away from the NVB resulted in tumescence almost half the time. Although the CaverMap device had promising results early, efforts to duplicate this has been met with inconsistency and lack of specificity. This may in part be caused by the difficulty in correctly placing the CaverMap probe directly on the nerves and the diffuse and variable nature of the NVB.

SUMMARY

Collaborations with biomedical engineers and radiologists have provided a rich opportunity to explore and expand optical technology and imaging techniques for intraoperative use during urologic surgery. As various imaging and tissue characterization modalities continue to evolve and refine, the surgeons of tomorrow will have a number of tools at their disposal to improve intraoperative surgical decision-making. Only through the application of evidence-based assessment and evaluation, however, will there be a firm understanding of the true impact of these new technologies on the field of urology.

REFERENCES

1. Aron M, Kaouk JH, Hegarty NJ, et al. Second prize: preliminary experience with the Niris optical coherence tomography system during laparoscopic and robotic prostatectomy. J Endourol 2007;21:814.
2. Fried NM, Rais-Bahrami S, Lagoda GA, et al. Imaging the cavernous nerves in the rat prostate using optical coherence tomography. Lasers Surg Med 2007;39:36.
3. Hermes B, Spoler F, Naami A, et al. Visualization of the basement membrane zone of the bladder by optical coherence tomography: feasibility of noninvasive evaluation of tumor invasion. Urology 2008;72:677.
4. Jesser CA, Boppart SA, Pitris C, et al. High resolution imaging of transitional cell carcinoma with optical coherence tomography: feasibility for the evaluation of bladder pathology. Br J Radiol 1999;72:1170.
5. Lerner SP, Goh AC, Tresser NJ, et al. Optical coherence tomography as an adjunct to white light cystoscopy for intravesical real-time imaging and staging of bladder cancer. Urology 2008;72:133.
6. Rais-Bahrami S, Levinson AW, Fried NM, et al. Optical coherence tomography of cavernous nerves: a step toward real-time intraoperative imaging during nerve-sparing radical prostatectomy. Urology 2008;72:198.
7. Manyak MJ, Gladkova ND, Makari JH, et al. Evaluation of superficial bladder transitional-cell carcinoma by optical coherence tomography. J Endourol 2005;19:570.
8. Schlegel PN. Testicular sperm extraction: microdissection improves sperm yield with minimal tissue excision. Hum Reprod 1999;14:131.
9. Har-Toov J, Eytan O, Hauser R, et al. A new power Doppler ultrasound guiding technique for improved testicular sperm extraction. Fertil Steril 2004;81:430.
10. Gerger A, Hofmann-Wellenhof R, Langsenlehner U, et al. In vivo confocal laser scanning microscopy of melanocytic skin tumours: diagnostic applicability using unselected tumour images. Br J Dermatol 2008;158:329.
11. Hoffman A, Goetz M, Vieth M, et al. Confocal laser endomicroscopy: technical status and current indications. Endoscopy 2006;38:1275.
12. Hurlstone DP, Baraza W, Brown S, et al. In vivo real-time confocal laser scanning endomicroscopic colonoscopy for the detection and characterization of colorectal neoplasia. Br J Surg 2008;95:636.
13. Koenig F, Knittel J, Schnieder L, et al. Confocal laser scanning microscopy of urinary bladder after intravesical instillation of a fluorescent dye. Urology 2003;62:158.
14. Sutedja G. New techniques for early detection of lung cancer. Eur Respir J Suppl 2003;39:57s.
15. Kitabatake S, Niwa Y, Miyahara R, et al. Confocal endomicroscopy for the diagnosis of gastric cancer in vivo. Endoscopy 2006;38:1110.
16. Vincent P, Maskos U, Charvet I, et al. Live imaging of neural structure and function by fibred fluorescence microscopy. EMBO Rep 2006;7:1154.
17. Boyette LB, Reardon MA, Mirelman AJ, et al. Fiberoptic imaging of cavernous nerves in vivo. J Urol 2007;178:2694.
18. Tekola P, Baak JP, van Ginkel HA, et al. Three-dimensional confocal laser scanning DNA ploidy cytometry in thick histological sections. J Pathol 1996;180:214.
19. Golijanin D. Wood R. Madeb R, et al. Intraoperative visualization of cavernous nerves using near infrared fluorescence of indocyanine green in the rat. Available at: http://www.abstracts2view.com/aua_archive/view.php?nu=200696027. Abstract presented at American Urological Association Meeting, 2006.

20. Lee F, Littrup PJ, Torp-Pedersen ST, et al. Prostate cancer: comparison of transrectal US and digital rectal examination for screening. Radiology 1988; 168:389.

21. Patil AV, Garson CD, Hossack JA. 3D prostate elastography: algorithm, simulations and experiments. Phys Med Biol 2007;52:3643.

22. Souchon R, Rouviere O, Gelet A, et al. Visualisation of HIFU lesions using elastography of the human prostate in vivo: preliminary results. Ultrasound Med Biol 2003;29:1007.

23. Emelianov SY, Lubinski MA, Weitzel WF, et al. Elasticity imaging for early detection of renal pathology. Ultrasound Med Biol 1995;21:871.

24. Pareek G, Wilkinson ER, Bharat S, et al. Elastographic measurements of in-vivo radiofrequency ablation lesions of the kidney. J Endourol 2006;20:959.

25. Ukimura O, Magi-Galluzzi C, Gill IS. Real-time transrectal ultrasound guidance during laparoscopic radical prostatectomy: impact on surgical margins. J Urol 2006;175:1304.

26. Ukimura O, Gill IS, Desai MM, et al. Real-time transrectal ultrasonography during laparoscopic radical prostatectomy. J Urol 2004;172:112.

27. Lepor H, Gregerman M, Crosby R, et al. Precise localization of the autonomic nerves from the pelvic plexus to the corpora cavernosa: a detailed anatomical study of the adult male pelvis. J Urol 1985;133:207.

28. Herwig R, Tosun K, Pinggera GM, et al. Tissue perfusion essential for spermatogenesis and outcome of testicular sperm extraction (TESE) for assisted reproduction. J Assist Reprod Genet 2004;21:175.

29. Herwig R, Tosun K, Schuster A, et al. Tissue perfusion-controlled guided biopsies are essential for the outcome of testicular sperm extraction. Fertil Steril 2007;87:1071.

30. Hyams ES, Kanofsky JA, Stifelman MD. Laparoscopic Doppler technology: applications in laparoscopic pyeloplasty and radical and partial nephrectomy. Urology 2008;71:952.

31. Klotz L, Herschorn S. Early experience with intraoperative cavernous nerve stimulation with penile tumescence monitoring to improve nerve sparing during radical prostatectomy. Urology 1998;52:537.

32. Klotz L, Heaton J, Jewett M, et al. A randomized phase 3 study of intraoperative cavernous nerve stimulation with penile tumescence monitoring to improve nerve sparing during radical prostatectomy. J Urol 2000;164:1573.

33. Kim HL, Stoffel DS, Mhoon DA, et al. A positive caver map response poorly predicts recovery of potency after radical prostatectomy. Urology 2000;56:561.

34. Walsh PC, Marschke P, Catalona WJ, et al. Efficacy of first-generation Cavermap to verify location and function of cavernous nerves during radical prostatectomy: a multi-institutional evaluation by experienced surgeons. Urology 2001;57:491.

35. Holzbeierlein J, Peterson M, Smith JJ. Variability of results of cavernous nerve stimulation during radical prostatectomy. J Urol 2001;165:108.

Laparoendoscopic Single Site Surgery in Urology

Brian H. Irwin, MD[a,b], Pradeep P. Rao, MD[c], Robert J. Stein, MD[a,b], Mihir M. Desai, MD[a,b],*

KEYWORDS

- LESS • Laparoscopy • Robotics
- Single-port • Minimally invasive surgery

Over the past 30 years laparoscopy has expanded into a standard of care for the treatment of many benign and malignant conditions within the realm of surgical practice. Within urology, since Clayman's initial laparoscopic nephrectomy, laparoscopic and robotic-assisted surgery has impacted the entire spectrum of urologic surgery. Ongoing efforts to improve on the morbidity and cosmetic sequelae of laparoscopic surgery have stimulated the minimization of size and number of ports required during laparoscopic procedures. Laparoendoscopic single-site (LESS) surgery is a recently introduced term to describe various techniques that aim at performing laparoscopic surgery by consolidating all ports within a single skin incision, often concealed within the umbilicus. LESS surgery is not a new endeavor. Single-incision surgery has been performed anecdotally for decades in gynecology[1] and general surgery.[2] The recent exponential expansion of number and variety of clinical LESS cases has been facilitated by the introduction of new instrumentation and access devices and incorporation of novel approaches and new and existing robotic platforms into the repertoire. As such, within the past year nearly the entire gamut of extirpative and reconstructive urologic procedures has been performed using LESS surgery.

NOMENCLATURE

Various terminologies and acronyms have been used to describe surgical procedures that perform laparoscopic surgery through a single incision or surgical site (**Box 1**). To standardize terminology with regard to scientific communications and performance of clinical trials, LESS was proposed as a common nomenclature by a consortium comprised of experts from various surgical specialties. This term has also been endorsed by

a Department of Urology, Stevan B. Streem Center for Endourology, Glickman Urological and Kidney Institute, Cleveland Clinic, 9500 Euclid Avenue/Q10, Cleveland, OH 44195, USA
b Department of Urology, Center for Laparoscopic and Robotic Surgery, Glickman Urological and Kidney Institute, Cleveland Clinic, 9500 Euclid Avenue/Q10, Cleveland, OH 44195, USA
c Mamata Hospital, P43, Phase 2 MIDC, Dombivli East, Mumbai 421 203, India
* Corresponding author. Department of Urology, Stevan B. Streem Center for Endourology, Glickman Urological and Kidney Institute, Cleveland Clinic, 9500 Euclid Avenue/Q10, Cleveland, OH 44195, USA.
E-mail address: desaim1@ccf.org (M.M. Desai).

Urol Clin N Am 36 (2009) 223–235
doi:10.1016/j.ucl.2009.02.011
0094-0143/09/$ – see front matter © 2009 Elsevier Inc. All rights reserved.

Box 1
Acronyms used for laparoendoscopic single-site surgery procedures

E-NOTES: Embryonic natural orifice transumbilical endoscopic surgery

Minilaparoscopy

MISPORT: Minimally invasive single-port surgery

SILS: Single-incision laparoscopic surgery

SLiP: Single laparoscopic port procedure

SPA: Single-port access

SPELS: Single-port endoscopic and laparoscopic surgery

SPEARS: Single-port endoscopic and robotic surgery

SPE: Single-port endoscopic surgery

SPIs: Single-port intracorporeal surgery

SPLS: Single-port laparoscopic surgery

SPL: Single-port laparoscopy

SPS: Single-port surgery

TULAs: Translumenal laparoscopic-assisted surgery

TUPS: Transumbilical universal port surgery

---

the Urologic NOTES Working Group in a recent communication.[3] By combining these terms into a universal language, search engines can be applied more efficiently to the developing literature to promote the fast dissemination of ideas and results.

DEVELOPMENT AND EVOLUTION OF LAPAROENDOSCOPIC SINGLE-SITE SURGERY

The concept of LESS surgery has been around for many years and has been used across many surgical specialties. Gynecologists using a single-puncture laparoscope with an offset eyepiece[4] have performed tens of thousands of tubal ligations through the years.[5] More recently, single-incision techniques have been reported in the general surgery literature for insertion of peritoneal dialysis catheters in children using only an umbilical port for the laparoscope[6] and retroperitoneoscopic adrenalectomies using a large 4.5-cm trocar without insufflation.[7] A search of the historical literature produces many such published reports of what are now termed as LESS procedures.[8]

Natural orifice transluminal endoscopic surgery (NOTES) was first described in 2003 and has a similar philosophical basis as LESS surgery in terms of reduced morbidity and cosmetic appeal.[9]

There have been many reports of animal studies exploring various NOTES techniques, largely in the porcine model.[10] These are typically performed with flexible endoscopes with integral working channels for passage and manipulation of instruments introduced by way of the mouth, vagina, or rectum. Despite the relatively extensive laboratory experience, reported clinical cases remain few because of the unfamiliarity with instrumentation and optics. Most of the reported NOTES animal cases by urologists have been undertaken using a hybrid NOTES technique, using an additional 12-mm port in the umbilicus to aid in the surgery.[11] In contrast to the less familiar NOTES approaches, LESS procedures reduce the morbidity and improve on the cosmesis of laparoscopic surgery using more familiar laparoscopic instrumentation with equivalent results.

Since the initial reports of clinical successes, there have been a large number and variety of LESS surgeries reported in urology. The potential reasons for LESS gaining popularity in the future are multifactorial. Urologists are more familiar with surgery through the abdominal wall than they are approaching structures through a hollow viscus.[12] With the use of more familiar instruments, the learning curve with LESS may be shorter. The cosmetic benefits are maintained when a single umbilical incision is used because this can easily be hidden with careful closure.

LESS procedures are typically performed by a variation of one of two approaches. The first is single-site surgery, where more than one port, conventional or otherwise, can be used through common incision site. The second involves single-port surgery, where a single device, through which multiple instruments and optics can be passed, is used to access the peritoneal cavity. The access point for these surgeries may be in the umbilicus, an existing cicatrix on the abdomen, or extraumbilical; although this may be less cosmetic, at times it is necessary to complete the surgery.

INSTRUMENTS AND TECHNOLOGY

Improvements in access devices, optics, and instrumentation have driven the dissemination of this new format of laparoscopic surgery. A brief description of the various new devices that have been used follows (**Table 1**).

Access Devices

LESS surgery can be carried out through a variety of access devices. Conventional, albeit low-profile, laparoscopic trocars may be used in single-site surgery. Ports with a low external profile and of varying lengths are favored for these procedures to minimize the extracorporeal interaction of the devices causing limitation of movement internally. In addition, there have been reports of using shortened ports in the same way to reduce the intra-abdominal profile of the cannulae.[13]

Specific access devices used in single-port surgery allow multiple instruments to be passed through them at the same time. The best-known and most commonly used access system is the TriPort (Advanced Surgical Concepts, Wicklow, Ireland) (**Fig. 1**).[14] This Food and Drug Administration–approved device has two components: a retracting component, which consists of an inner and outer ring with a double-barreled plastic sleeve; and a multichannel valve, which has three valves made of a unique elastomeric material. These valves accommodate one 12-mm and two 5-mm instruments within the same working space. The size of the port is variable according to the size of the fascial incision and can range from 10 to 30 mm depending to the surgery to be carried out. There is a variation of this device called the Quad-Port, which has four working channels. It comes in two variations depending on the application for which it is intended (one 15-, one 12-, and two 5-mm ports; or four 12-mm ports). This device can be placed into incisions up to 50 mm in length and is useful for extirpative procedures in which a specimen needs to be removed. Both devices have a separate insufflation port through the valve housing; the valve housings can be removed to facilitate removal of a specimen through the retracting component. The TriPort can be placed by an open approach or after insufflation with an introducer, whereas the QuadPort must be placed with an open access technique.

The Uni-X Single Port Access Laparoscopic system (PNavel systems, Cleveland, Ohio), which has three working channels for 5-mm instruments, has also been used successfully for performing LESS procedures. It is placed by an open access technique and requires stitches to secure it in place to the fascia.

The use of a GelPort (Applied Medical, Rancho Santa Margarita, California) device by inserting three conventional laparoscopic ports through it to do a radical nephrectomy has been reported.[15] The advantage of this system is that it allows for the introduction of ports or instruments of varying shapes and sizes in different configurations directly through the gel. It can be placed into a larger incision allowing the surgeon to take advantage of the entire fascial incision required during extirpative procedures, such as radical and donor nephrectomy. The port can, however, balloon out during insufflation causing the

instruments to be pushed further from the operative field and the fulcrum to be less stable than is seen with the purpose-designed multichannel ports.

Other single-port devices are still in various stages of commercialization and there have been no published reports using these devices.

Instruments

The primary problems while doing LESS are loss of the triangulation, which is present with conventional laparoscopy, and the "chopsticks" effect with clashing of the closely situated instruments (**Fig. 2**). These can be overcome to some extent by using special instrumentation. Desai and colleagues[16] and Rane and colleagues[17] described the use of prototype fixed-shaft bent instruments to facilitate single-port surgery. Similar prototype instruments were also developed by PNavel systems for use with the Uni-X device.[18] Various newer actively articulating instruments are available. These companies have made a full spectrum of instruments available including endo-shears, needle drivers, graspers, and hook electrocauteries in these articulating series.[14] In contrast to instruments with a fixed curve, actively articulating instruments can be inserted through rigid trocars. Although these instruments are useful in overcoming issues of triangulation, they continue to lack sufficient strength to provide robust retraction and dissection.

Optics

A recurring problem encountered while performing LESS surgery is clashing of instruments and the camera as they are passed through a single fulcrum. Conventional laparoscopes have a large extracorporeal profile with a light cable perpendicular to the telescope, which exacerbates this problem. One elegant way of minimizing this problem is by using a lower profile camera system, such as one in which the video laparoscope is integrated with a coaxial light cable in line with the shaft of the telescope.[19] This is available in 5-mm size in 0-degree and 30-degree configurations. It is also available with a flexible actively deflectable tip. A videolaparoscope has also been developed that is currently available in a 10-mm diameter. Other special optics that may facilitate LESS surgery include a 45-degree telescope, which has a coaxial light guide attachment.

Intracorporeal and extracorporeal instrument clashing during LESS surgery often necessitates that the surgeon cross his or her hands, leading to the right-hand instrument going to the left side and vise versa. Because of this limitation of

Table 1
Currently available laparoendoscopic single-site surgery instrumentation

Instrument	Manufacturer	Comments
Access devices		
TriPort	Advanced Surgical Concepts, Wicklow, Ireland	12–25 mm incision Two 5-mm, one 12-mm port and one insufflation port Port introducer available
QuadPort	Advanced Surgical Concepts, Wicklow, Ireland	2.5–6 cm incision Two configurations available: four 12-mm ports or two 12-mm, one 5-mm and one 15-mm port
Uni-X	Pnavel Systems, Brooklyn, New York	Requires fascial suture to remain in place
Gel port	Applied Medical, Rancho Santa Margarita, California	Can accept instruments directly or ports Bulges away from patient with use Accommodates multiple instrument configurations Requires at least a 2.5-cm fascial incision
SILS Access	Covidien/Autosuture, Hamilton HM FX, Bermuda	Three foam insertion sites require low- profile ports Insufflation by tubing away from main port body
AirSeal	Surgiquest, Orange, Connecticut	Uses recirculated CO_2 to create seal, no gasket/valve No fulcrum for instruments Requires proprietary insufflator
Articulating instruments		
Roticulator series	Covidien/Autosuture, Hamilton HM FX, Bermuda	Fewer degrees of freedom Dissector, shears, grasper available Lower profile handle
RealHand series	Novare, Cupertino, California	One-handed locking mechanism More degrees of freedom Larger profile handle May be locked in straight position
Autonomy Laparo-Angle	Cambridge Endo, Framingham, Massachusetts	All instruments with locking mechanism More degrees of freedom Larger profile handle
Endoscope and camera systems		
EndoEYE	Olympus, Center Valley, Pennsylvania	Low-profile, in-line design Digital chip-on-the-tip technology, available in 0 degrees, 30 degrees, and flexible versions

(continued on next page)

Table 1 (continued)		
Instrument	**Manufacturer**	**Comments**
Magnetic Anchoring and Guidance System MAGS	In development	Inserted completely into abdominal cavity Secured and manipulated through abdominal wall by magnetic handle Current version with poor visibility and wireless not available
EYEMAX	Richard Wolf Medical Instruments, Vernon Hills, Illinois	Low-profile, in-line design Digital chip-on-the-tip technology only available in 10-mm diameter

movement, there is a distinct learning curve involved with attempting LESS procedures. To reduce this learning curve, research has focused on newer technologies to reduce the clashing of instruments and formal teaching and certifying protocols.

Park and colleagues[20] have developed a transabdominal magnetic anchoring and guidance system. This works as an intra-abdominal camera system in which the small camera device is introduced entirely into the abdominal cavity by a port and secured to the abdominal wall and manipulated through the use of an extracorporeal magnetic handle. Using this system, initial porcine nephrectomy was reported in the literature[21] and the first clinical cases have been performed.[22]

LESS is an exciting new technology and has provided a stimulus for improving instrumentation and optics that should also help conventional laparoscopy.

ROBOTICS

With the advent and unprecedented adoption of surgical robotics has come the natural hybridization of the technology with LESS surgery. Kaouk and colleagues[23] reported on the use of the DaVinci-S (Intuitive Surgical, Sunnyvale, California) robotic system in conjunction with a TriPort single-port access device to perform a radical prostatectomy, a pyeloplasty, and a radical nephrectomy for a 5.6-cm right-sided renal mass. A 12-mm three-dimensional camera and 5-mm grasping

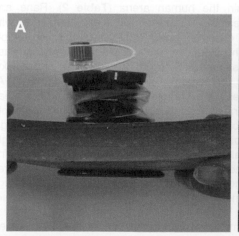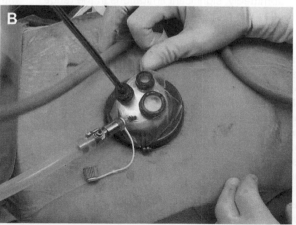

Fig. 1. The TriPort applied to a model abdominal wall (*A*) and as viewed from above (*B*). Note the presence of three working channels and an insufflation port.

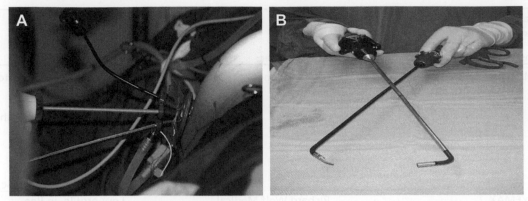

Fig. 2. LESS instrumentation. (*A*) Note instrument clashing, which is commonplace during LESS surgery, has been somewhat reduced with the use of a fixed bent instrument. (*B*) The surgeon's left hand holds an articulating dissector while the right holds a flexible camera device.

instrument were placed through the TriPort while an additional 8-mm port was placed alongside the port in the same incision for another robotic instrument. Using this platform they reported successful completion of all procedures without the need for the placement of additional ports. Operative times (radical prostatectomy = 5 hours, pyeloplasty = 4.5 hours, radical nephrectomy = 2.5 hours), estimated blood losses (radical prostatectomy = 250 mL, pyeloplasty = 80 mL, radical nephrectomy = 200 mL), and hospital length of stays (radical prostatectomy = 1.5 days, pyeloplasty = 2 days, radical nephrectomy = 2 days) were within the ranges of those reported with conventional laparoscopy. All patients had minimal pain at 1 week of follow-up with visual analog pain scale scores of 0. They stated that although there was significant "clashing" of the robotic arms, this platform provided a technique that might be more quickly learned than conventional single-port laparoscopy. Although there are, admittedly, significant limitations in the range of motion using the daVinci system for performing LESS surgery, development of purpose-specific robotic platforms, such as flexible robotics and miniature in vivo robotics, may allow for the performance of more complex procedures by a LESS approach in the future.

Flexible robotics may overcome many limitations with rigid systems particularly with LESS surgery. Through this technology a remotely controlled flexible endoscope along with flexible instrument passed through a working channel can be manipulated by a single incision or natural orifice to perform delicate tasks. Such a device has been used in both animal models and subsequent patient trials for performing ureterorenoscopic procedures for stone disease.[24] With this proof of concept and safety, such devices may provide future possibilities for intra-abdominal examination and manipulation by a single incision.

Microrobot development has started to allow for the performance of tasks by a small completely in vivo mini robot inserted either by a natural orifice or by a small single-site incision. Such robots have been developed for biopsy[25] and cholecystectomy[26] and have the potential for use in a large number of applications across many disciplines. Purpose-built single-port robotics have yet to be developed, but may allow for the introduction of articulating instruments in a manner that prevents inadvertent instrument collision and provides larger ranges of motion for more precise dissection, retraction, and reconstruction.

CLINICAL EXPERIENCE WITH UROLOGIC LAPAROENDOSCOPIC SINGLE-SITE PROCEDURES

The experience in clinical trials has expanded significantly since the application of the technique within the human arena (**Table 2**). Rane and colleagues[17] reported on their experience with five cases in which they performed two simple nephrectomies for end-stage kidney disease consequent to stone disease, one orchiopexy, one orchiectomy, and one ureterolithotomy. All cases were completed successfully with a mean operative time of 83 minutes and without complications. Raman and colleagues[12] reported single umbilical incision nephrectomy in four pigs (eight renal units) and three humans (two nonfunctioning kidneys and one renal mass). They used three standard 5-mm laparoscopic ports through a single umbilical incision for most of the dissection. One of the trocars was exchanged for a 12-mm port for transection of the hilar vessels with an endovascular stapler. The human procedures were performed in a mean time of 133 minutes with discharge on hospital day 2 in all cases. A 3-mm subxiphoid port was used in the only right-sided nephrectomy for liver retraction. The authors used an articulating grasper for the surgeon's left-hand instrument and a straight instrument in the right hand.

Two reports detailed the initial experience of LESS using single-port surgical platforms with multiple channels. Desai and colleagues[16] described its use during a simple nephrectomy and a pyeloplasty by a transumbilical approach (**Fig. 3**). A separate 2-mm port was used for the pyeloplasty procedure. Operative time was 220 minutes for the nephrectomy and 160 minutes for the pyeloplasty. Hospital stay was 1 and 2 days, respectively; no complications were noted.

In another trial, Kaouk and colleagues[18] reported on their experience with LESS procedures in 10 patients including nephrectomy (N = 1); sacrocolpopexy (N = 4); renal cryotherapy (N = 4); and renal biopsy (N = 1). The multichannel single port was used in all cases. A combination of bent and articulating instruments were used and no additional ports were placed. Mean operative time was 2.5 hours. Prolonged oxygen requirement and transfusion was noted in one patient who underwent cryotherapy.

After establishing that the techniques could be applied relatively safely within the human for benign diseases of the upper and lower urinary tracts, the indications for LESS have been carefully expanded to more complex procedures. Desai and colleagues[27] reported on their experience with reconstructive procedures performed transumbilically. They were able to carry out bilateral pyeloplasty in two patients and an ileal ureteral interposition (**Fig. 4**) and ureteral reimplantation with psoas hitch. A 2-mm needlescopic port and grasper were used in each case to aid in dissection and suturing. The single umbilical incision was slightly lengthened to perform the bowel reconstruction extracorporeally in the case of ileal ureter. No complications were reported.

Donor nephrectomy has traditionally been performed only by well-established techniques because of the need for conservative treatment of otherwise healthy altruistic donors. After substantial experience with LESS techniques, Gill and colleagues[28] reported on their initial experience with four LESS donor nephrectomies. All procedures were completed by LESS techniques with the use of the TriPort and a 2-mm needlescopic port and grasper for aid in retraction during hilar dissection and extraction. The specimen was placed in a bag for extraction just before vascular transection in all but one case. Mean warm ischemia time was 6.2 minutes while providing

a median length of harvested renal artery of 3.3 cm, 4 cm of renal vein, and 15 cm of ureter. No intraoperative complications occurred; each allograft functioned immediately on transplantation. Donor visual analog pain scale scores were all 0 of 10 after 2 weeks of follow-up.

Another population that traditionally has received only well-established treatments involves surgery in children. The initial pediatric urologic applications of LESS were reported by Kaouk and Palmer[29] in three adolescents undergoing unilateral LESS varicocelectomy. The Uni-X port was used in all cases with bent instruments to provide triangulation. Operative time was less than 1 hour in all cases and all patients were discharged on the same day as surgery.

Most investigators have remained even more careful and selective in applying LESS techniques for oncologic conditions. Ponsky and colleagues[15] reported single-access radical nephrectomy for a renal tumor with intact specimen extraction. The authors placed three standard laparoscopic ports through a GelPort that was seated in a 7-cm paramedian incision. Standard laparoscopic instruments were used for dissection and total operative time was 96 minutes with 10 mL blood loss. The patient was discharged on postoperative day 2 without complication.

Goel and Kaouk[30] reported their experience with single-port access renal cryoablation in six patients with a mean tumor size of 2.6 cm. This group favored the use of the Uni-X system with bent and articulating instruments being used to carry out the necessary dissection. The single port was placed transumbilically in two transperitoneal cases and at the tip of the twelfth rib in the remaining four retroperitoneoscopic procedures. A laparoscopic ultrasound probe for real-time ice ball monitoring was introduced next to the single port through the same incision. For smaller tumors a single cryoprobe was introduced through the single port. For larger tumors additional probes were placed percutaneously. Mean operative time was 170 minutes and mean hospital stay was 2.3 days. One patient required transfusion and a 1-week hospital stay for respiratory difficulty.

Laparoscopic partial nephrectomy remains a technically demanding procedure under the best of circumstances. To date, there have been two series reported that describe the use of LESS surgery in partial nephrectomy. Aron and colleagues[31] reported successful LESS partial nephrectomy in four patients using the TriPort. In all cases a 2-mm grasper was used through a separate entry to assist in suture closure of the

Table 2
Summary of current urologic laparoendoscopic single-site surgery series

First Author	Year	Number of Patients	Procedures	OR Time (min)	Hospital Stay (d)	Complications	Analgesic Use (Morphine Equivalents)
Raman	2007	3	Nephrectomy (N = 3)	133	2	None	—
Kaouk	2007	10	Renal cryotherapy (N = 4); Kidney biopsy (N = 1); Radical nephrectomy (N = 1); Radical prostatectomy (N = 4)	150	2.8 and 2	1	—
Rane	2008	5	Simple nephrectomy (N = 2)	—	—	None	—
			Right orchidectomy (N = 1)	—	—	None	—
			Left ureterolithotomy (N = 1)	—	—	None	—
			Left orchidopexy, appendectomy (N = 1)	—	—	None	—
Kaouk	2008	5	Sacrocolpopexy	150	2	None	—
Ponsky	2008	1	Radical nephrectomy	96	2	None	34.3
Gill	2008	4	Donor nephrectomy	242	—	—	34.8
Goel	2008	6	Renal cryotherapy	170	2.3	1	—
Aron	2008	5	Partial nephrectomy	270 (median)	3 (median)	1	—
Cadeddu	2008	11	Nephrectomy	122 (median)	2 (median)	None	8
Kaouk	2009	7	Partial nephrectomy (2 performed robotically)	163	3.3	1 focally positive margin	—
Desai[a]	2009	100	Simple nephrectomy (N = 13)	145	2		64
			Radical nephrectomy (N = 4)	208	3.5	Bleeding from gonadal vein, clipped	—
			Donor nephrectomy (N = 17)	230	2.9	Corneal abrasion, dyskinesia from antiemetics	23

Partial nephrectomy (N = 6)	271	7.2	1 postoperative bleed required angioembolization	28
Renal cyst excision (N = 1)	60	1	None	—
Nephrpureterectomy (N = 2)	90	5	None	—
Pyeloplasty (2 performed robotically) (N = 16)	236	2	None	28
Ureteroneocystostomy (N = 2)	210	2	None	—
Ileal interposition (N = 3)	330	4	1 anastomotic leak required nephrostomy tube	—
Simple prostatectomy (1 performed robotically) (N = 32)	113	3	1 mortality in Jehovah's Witness from hemorrhage; 2 postoperative bleeds required surgical intervention; 4 postoperative bleeds required transfusion alone; 1 bowel injury required exploration, 1 urinary tract infection	29
Transvesical mesh sling removal (N = 1)	100	1	None	—
Adrenalectomy (N = 1)	150	3	1 renal vein injury repaired leading to renal vein thrombosis requiring long-term anticoagulation (patent at 3-month follow-up)	—
Hysterectomy (N = 1)	120	2	None	—

a Includes patients in series from references[16,29,31] also by Desai published in 2007 and 2008.

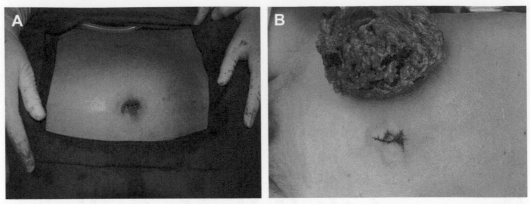

Fig. 3. (*A*) Postoperative appearance of surgical incision following LESS simple nephrectomy with morsellation of the specimen. Note the incision is hidden completely within the umbilicus. (*B*) Postoperative appearance of surgical incision and specimen following LESS radical nephrectomy with intact extraction of the specimen. Notice the incision extends slightly outside of the borders of the umbilicus.

renal defect. An additional patient required the placement of an extra 5-mm port. Median tumor size was 3 cm (range, 1–5.9 cm). The median operating time was 270 minutes and median estimated blood loss was 150 mL. The median warm ischemia time was 20 minutes (range, 11–29 minutes). Median hospital stay was 3 days. One patient had postoperative hemorrhage and

pulmonary embolism. Subsequently, Kaouk and Goel[32] reported on their experience with seven LESS partial nephrectomies. This series included the use of robotic assistance in two cases. One patient required conversion to conventional laparoscopy with the placement of additional ports for control of bleeding after tumor resection. The only complication reported was a focally positive

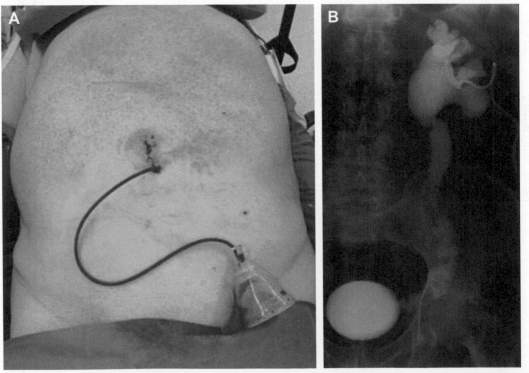

Fig. 4. Postoperative cosmetic appearance (*A*) and radiographic appearance (*B*) of cystogram following LESS ileal ureter creation. Note that the umbilical incision has been extended slightly to allow for extracorporeal harvest of the ileal segment and performance of the bowel anastomosis.

margin on final pathology, which was initially read as negative on intraoperative frozen section.

LESS radical prostatectomy has been reported for the treatment of prostate cancer in carefully selected patients. With the need for both precise dissection and reconstructive techniques, this has been undertaken only by those surgeons with sufficient skill and experience to perform these technically challenging cases. Kaouk and colleagues[33] reported their initial LESS radical prostatectomy experience in four patients who were all clinical stage T1c, had no prior pelvic surgery, and had a body mass index less than or equal to 35. Mean total operative time was 285 minutes (200 minutes for prostate excision and 66 minutes for vesicourethral anastomosis). Of the four patients, two had positive margins and one developed a rectourethral fistula 2 months postoperatively. Barret and colleagues[34] reported on both their cadaveric and live clinical experience with LESS radical prostatectomy. They performed a LESS radical prostatectomy in a cadaveric model using a combination of both standard laparoscopic instrumentation and articulating instruments noting that although the articulating instruments were helpful at times during the case, the standard instrumentation was equally necessary. They also performed a robotic-assisted LESS radical prostatectomy in a live patient. Estimated blood loss was 500 mL while achieving bilateral nerve preservation with negative surgical margins.

Raman and colleagues[13] reported the first comparative study between laparoscopic and LESS applications. The investigators compared 11 LESS nephrectomies with 22 standard laparoscopic nephrectomies. The groups were matched at a 2:1 ratio for patient age, surgical indication, and tumor size. The authors reported similar outcomes between the two groups in terms of operative time (122 versus 125 minutes); percent decrease from preoperative hemoglobin; analgesic use; length of stay; and complication rate. Indeed, further prospective randomized comparative analyses incorporating quality of life investigations are needed to identify benefits of LESS procedures.

The largest series compiled in the LESS experience is reported by Desai and colleagues.[35] They report their experience with 100 LESS procedures including a relatively heterogeneous group of procedures including nephrectomies (N = 40; simple, partial, radical, and donor); nephroureterectomy (N = 2); renal cyst excision (N = 1); pyeloplasty (N = 16); ureteroneocystostomy (N = 2); ileal ureter (N = 3); adrenalectomy (N = 1); hysterectomy (N = 1); transvesical simple prostatectomy (N = 32); and mesh sling removal (N = 1). This series demonstrates the breadth of possible procedures that can be performed with these techniques.

With the advent of any new technology there is often skepticism regarding the rapidity with which the technique is adopted. In a multi-institutional review of three high-volume centers, the authors have found that only 11.6% of over 1250 upper tract laparoscopic cases performed over the past 2 years at these centers were attempted using LESS techniques despite the surgeons' familiarity with the skill sets and instrumentation for both conventional and LESS laparoscopy. Of these, only 6.8% required conversion to a standard laparoscopic technique with the placement of additional ports safely to complete the procedure. This suggests that the early pioneers in the field have been careful in their patient selection and have been cognizant of their own limitations during this early phase of development of the techniques.

NOVEL APPROACHES

LESS surgery has been primarily applied to standard laparoscopic procedures within the peritoneal cavity. With the newer access devices being developed, novel approaches to procedures have been proposed. Transvesical procedures including simple and radical prostatectomy[36] and ureteral reimplantation[37] have been performed in the past by a combination of conventional robotic and laparoscopic techniques. The complexity of these cases has been prohibitive and often related to the need for multiple access points within the bladder. To simplify the access to the bladder Desai and colleagues[38] have described a single-port transvesical enucleation of the prostate procedure that takes advantage of the potential working space within the bladder by the use of a pneumovesicum. This as an example of transluminal surgery made possible by the development of single-incision access devices.

FUTURE DIRECTIONS

Through the development of such groups as the Urologic NOTES working groups and the LESS-CAR consortium, the future of LESS surgery is being well documented and promoted. LESSCAR has proposed the creation of a LESS registry to monitor and coordinate the collection of clinical data as they become available. They would be in a position to design and oversee the development and execution of prospective randomized trials needed to determine the effectiveness and potential benefits of such new techniques.

By creating these organizations, leaders in the field can formulate teaching platforms and curricula for the formal application of the techniques in a safe and efficacious manner. By doing so, they not only ensure the success of the providers, but of the technique itself. This has been and will continue to be a critical step in the success of not only LESS surgery, but other newly developing techniques across medical disciplines.

REFERENCES

1. Wheeless CR Jr. An inexpensive laparoscopy system for female sterilization. Am J Obstet Gynecol 1975;123(7):727–33.
2. Buess G, Kipfmuller K, Hack D, et al. Technique of transanal endoscopic microsurgery. Surg Endosc 1988;2(2):71–5.
3. Box G, Averch T, Cadeddu J, et al. Nomenclature of natural orifice translumenal endoscopic surgery (NOTES) and laparoendoscopic single-site surgery (LESS) procedures in urology. J Endourol 2008; 22(11):2575–81.
4. Junker H. [Laparoscopic tubal ligation by the single puncture technique (author's transl)]. Geburtshilfe Frauenheilkd 1974;34(11):952–5 [German].
5. Mehta PV. Laparoscopic sterilizations (16,803) without vaginal manipulation. Int J Gynaecol Obstet 1982;20(4):323–5.
6. Milliken I, Fitzpatrick M, Subramaniam R. Single-port laparoscopic insertion of peritoneal dialysis catheters in children. J Pediatr Urol 2006;2(4):308–11.
7. Hirano D, Minei S, Yamaguchi K, et al. Retroperitoneoscopic adrenalectomy for adrenal tumors via a single large port. J Endourol 2005;19(7):788–92.
8. Canes D, Desai MM, Aron M, et al. Transumbilical single-port surgery: evolution and current status. Eur Urol 2008;54(5):1020–9.
9. Rao GV, Reddy DN, Banerjee R. NOTES: human experience. Gastrointest Endosc Clin N Am 2008; 18(2):361–70.
10. Gettman MT, Lotan Y, Napper CA, et al. Transvaginal laparoscopic nephrectomy: development and feasibility in the porcine model. Urology 2002;59(3): 446–50.
11. Clayman RV, Box GN, Abraham JB, et al. Rapid communication: transvaginal single-port NOTES nephrectomy: initial laboratory experience. J Endourol 2007;21(6):640–4.
12. Raman JD, Bensalah K, Bagrodia A, et al. Laboratory and clinical development of single keyhole umbilical nephrectomy. Urology 2007;70(6):1039–42.
13. Raman JD, Bagrodia A, Cadeddu JA. Single-incision, umbilical laparoscopic versus conventional laparoscopic nephrectomy: a comparison of perioperative outcomes and short-term measures of convalescence. Eur Urol 2008; in press.

14. Tracy CR, Raman JD, Cadeddu JA, et al. Laparoendoscopic single-site surgery in urology: where have we been and where are we heading? Nat Clin Pract Urol 2008;5(10):561–8.
15. Ponsky LE, Cherullo EE, Sawyer M, et al. Single access site laparoscopic radical nephrectomy: initial clinical experience. J Endourol 2008;22(4):663–6.
16. Desai MM, Rao PP, Aron M, et al. Scarless single port transumbilical nephrectomy and pyeloplasty: first clinical report. BJU Int 2008;101(1):83–8.
17. Rane A, Rao P, Rao P. Single-port-access nephrectomy and other laparoscopic urologic procedures using a novel laparoscopic port (R-port). Urology 2008;72(2):260–3.
18. Kaouk JH, Haber GP, Goel RK, et al. Single-port laparoscopic surgery in urology: initial experience. Urology 2008;71(1):3–6.
19. Raman JD, Cadeddu JA, Rao P, et al. Single-incision laparoscopic surgery: initial urological experience and comparison with natural-orifice transluminal endoscopic surgery. BJU Int 2008;101(12):1493–6.
20. Park S, Bergs RA, Eberhart R, et al. Trocar-less instrumentation for laparoscopy: magnetic positioning of intra-abdominal camera and retractor. Ann Surg 2007;245(3):379–84.
21. Zeltser IS, Bergs R, Fernandez R, et al. Single trocar laparoscopic nephrectomy using magnetic anchoring and guidance system in the porcine model. J Urol 2007;178(1):288–91.
22. Caddedu JD, Fernandez R, Desai MM, et al. Novel magnetically guided intra-abdominal camera to facilitate laparoendoscopic single site surgery: initial human experience. Surgical Endoscopy 2009; in press.
23. Kaouk JH, Goel RK, Haber GP, et al. Robotic single-port transumbilical surgery in humans: initial report. BJU Int 2008;71:3–6.
24. Desai MM, Aron M, Gill IS, et al. Flexible robotic retrograde renoscopy: description of novel robotic device and preliminary laboratory experience. Urology 2008;72(1):42–6.
25. Rentschler ME, Dumpert J, Platt SR, et al. Mobile in vivo biopsy and camera robot. Stud Health Technol Inform 2006;119:449–54.
26. Lehman AC, Dumpert J, Wood NA, et al. Natural orifice cholecystectomy using a miniature robot. Surg Endosc 2009;23(2):260–6.
27. Desai MM, Stein R, Rao P, et al. Embryonic natural orifice transumbilical endoscopic surgery (E-NOTES) for advanced reconstruction: initial experience. Urology 2009;73(1):182–7.
28. Gill IS, Canes D, Aron M, et al. Single port transumbilical (E-NOTES) donor nephrectomy. J Urol 2008; 180(2):637–41.
29. Kaouk JH, Palmer JS. Single-port laparoscopic surgery: initial experience in children for varicocelectomy. BJU Int 2008;102(1):97–9.

30. Goel RK, Kaouk JH. Single port access renal cryoablation (SPARC): a new approach. Eur Urol 2008; 53(6):1204–9.
31. Aron M, Canes D, Desai MM, et al. Transumbilical single-port laparoscopic partial nephrectomy. BJU Int 2008;103:516–21.
32. Kaouk JH, Goel RK. Single-port laparoscopic and robotic partial nephrectomy. Eur Urol 2009; in press.
33. Kaouk JH, Goel RK, Haber GP, et al. Single-port laparoscopic radical prostatectomy. Urology 2008; 72(6):1190–3.
34. Barret E, Sanchez-Salas R, Kasraeian A, et al. A transition to laparoendoscopic single-site surgery (less) radical prostatectomy: human cadaver experimental and initial clinical experience. J Endourol 2009; in press.
35. Desai MM, Berger A, Brandina R, et al. Laparoendoscopic single site (LESS) surgery: initial 100 patients. Urology 2009; in press.
36. Desai MM, Aron M, Berger A, et al. Transvesical robotic radical prostatectomy. BJU Int 2008; 102(11):1666–9.
37. Gill IS, Ponsky LE, Desai M, et al. Laparoscopic cross-trigonal Cohen ureteroneocystostomy: novel technique. J Urol 2001;166(5):1811–4.
38. Desai MM, Aron M, Canes D, et al. Single-port transvesical simple prostatectomy: initial clinical report. Urology 2008;72(5):960–5.

Technological Advances in Robotic-Assisted Laparoscopic Surgery

Gerald Y. Tan, MBChB, MRCSEd, MMed, FAMS[a,c],
Raj K. Goel, MD, FRCSC[b], Jihad H. Kaouk, MD[b],
Ashutosh K. Tewari, MD, MCh[a,*]

KEYWORDS

- Robot • Single-port • NOTES • Haptics • Simulator
- Laparoscopic • Navigation • Telestration

This article is not certified for AMA PRA Category 1 Credit™ because product brand names are included in the educational content. The Accreditation Council for Continuing Medical Education requires the use of generic names and or drug/product classes as the required nomenclature for therapeutic options in continuing medical education.

For more information, please go to www.accme.org and review the Standards of Commercial Support.

Despite its relative infancy, laparoscopic surgery has radically transformed the landscape of operative urology. The advent of surgical robotics at the turn of the new millennium heralded a quantum leap forward for minimally invasive urologists, who first used it successfully for performing robotic-assisted radical prostatectomy. Since then, there has been an unprecedented explosion in the use of robotics in other aspects of oncologic and reconstructive urologic procedures, with more than 55,000 radical prostatectomies performed with da Vinci® (Intuitive Surgical, Inc., Sunnyvale, California) robotic assistance in the United States in 2007[1] and more than 70,000 performed worldwide in 2008 (unpublished data, Intuitive Surgical, Inc., 2008). The increasing popularity of robotic-assisted laparoscopic surgery seems to be mirrored in Europe and other parts of the world, and in the arenas of cardiothoracic, gynecologic, and general surgery.[2–4]

Propelling this zeitgeist for surgical robotics have been exciting advances in robotic technologies and their potential applications in urologic surgery. This article therefore serves as a timely review of these promising innovations to date and discusses likely future directions for our craft as the practice of surgery becomes increasingly robotic-assisted and computer-aided.

Dr. Tewari has received a research grant from Intuitive Surgical, Inc. Dr. Tan receives financial support from the Ferdinand C. Valentine Fellowship in Urologic Research, New York Academy of Medicine and the Medical Research Fellowship, National Medical Research Council, Singapore. Dr. Kaouk serves as a proctor for Intuitive Surgical Inc.

[a] Brady Foundation Department of Urology, Weill Medical College of Cornell University, New York Presbyterian Hospital, 525 East 68th Street, Starr 900, New York, NY 10065, USA
[b] Glickman Urological and Kidney Institute, Cleveland Clinic Foundation, 9500 Euclid Avenue, Cleveland, OH 44195, USA
[c] Department of Urology, Tan Tock Seng Hospital, 11 Jalan Tan Tock Seng, Singapore 308433, Singapore
* Corresponding author.
E-mail address: ashtewarimd@gmail.com (A.K. Tewari).

Urol Clin N Am 36 (2009) 237–249
doi:10.1016/j.ucl.2009.02.010

EVOLUTION OF UROLOGIC ROBOTIC SYSTEMS AND CURRENT STATE OF THE ART

Urologic robotic systems used in recent years have essentially comprised a computer with real-time imaging capability linked to various effector units for execution of specific tasks. Off-line (ie, fixed path) robots are automated systems that execute precise movements within specified confines based on preprogrammed imaging studies obtained before surgery, operating independently without requiring active input from the surgeon.[5] These include (1) robots for prostate access, such as the ProBot (prototype by a team from Imperial College, London–not commercially available and not manufactured), a robotic resection device with 7 *df*, and various robotic prostate biopsy systems,[6–8] and (2) renal access systems, such as the PAKY-RCM and Acubot robots (prototypes developed by Stoianovici et al at URobotics Laboratory, Johns Hopkins Medical Institute, Baltimore, Maryland), for precise percutaneous access to the kidney.[9,10]

Conversely, on-line robotic systems are designed to replicate the surgeon's movements in real time in the operative field with improved tremor-free precision and scale adjustment when applicable. These surgeon-directed robots may be broadly divided into endoscope manipulators and master-slave systems. Endoscopic manipulators, such as the Automated Endoscopic System for Optimal Positioning (AESOP; Intuitive Surgical Inc.) and Naviot (Hitachi Hybrid Network Co., Ltd., Yokohama, Japan) systems, have the benefits of being less expensive, smaller, and easier to set up with stable adjustable positioning, but their usefulness remains limited in complex operations.[5] Master-slave systems, such as the now obsolete Zeus (originally manufactured by Computer Motion, Inc., Goleta, California) and the da Vinci® system, comprise a computerized surgical console connected to an endoscopic manipulator with two or three robotic arms for instrument manipulation. Precise digital control of surgical instruments through the console eliminates movement tremors and allows motion scaling, wherein the surgeon's movements may be amplified or dampened.

The most commercially successful robotic system to date has been the da Vinci® system,[11] with more than 1000 systems currently installed in hospitals worldwide. From its inception, the benefits of the da Vinci® system over conventional laparoscopy were readily apparent: superior ergonomics; optical magnification of the operative field within direct control of the console surgeon; and enhanced dexterity, precision, and control of operative movements. Comprising a patient-side cart with three or four robotic manipulator arms connected to a master console, the da Vinci's binocular images obtained by means of the laparoscopic camera lens (0° or 30°) are integrated by the computer to provide a composite three-dimensional (3D) image when viewed by means of the immersive stereo viewer at the console. The patented robotic instruments also have additional articulating joints (EndoWrist; Intuitive Surgical, Inc.) that permit 7 *df* of movement, empowering the minimally invasive surgeon to perform intracorporeal suturing and dissection intuitively and effortlessly.

Its current state-of-the-art version, the da Vinci® S HD Surgical System (Intuitive Surgical, Inc.), integrates 3D high-definition vision capability with the existing robotic platform, providing twice the effective viewing resolution with improved clarity and detail of tissue planes (**Fig. 1**). Its digital zoom function reduces interference between the endoscope and instruments, and the integrated touch-screen monitor permits telestration for improved proctoring and team communication. In addition, the TilePro® (Intuitive Surgical, Inc.) multi-image stereo viewer enables simultaneous display of multiple video inputs in the surgeon console, integrating display of the patient's ultrasound, CT, and MRI images. Extended-reach instruments are also now available for multiquadrant access, with a 50% increase in pitch and yaw range of motion and four times the working volume.[12] Fewer cable connections between components has also helped to shorten setup time, and a high-speed fiberoptic connection in the surgical platform offers the potential for remote telementoring.

Despite these technical innovations, there still exist some limitations. First, the da Vinci® S HD Surgical System is unable to provide haptic feedback for the console surgeon, who must necessarily base his or her intraoperative decisions on visual cues encountered during surgical dissection. Second, the large size of the robot presents some challenges to the operating staff when docking and repositioning the robot during complex procedures. Third, there remains a lack of simulator technologies available to surgeons and residents desiring familiarity with the robotic console, with their options currently limited to attending training courses that are mostly didactic in nature. Finally, the high cost of this technology may limit or slow the adoption of robotic-assisted laparoscopic surgery on a larger scale internationally.

Against this background, we now review some exciting technological advances that promise to redress some of these technical issues and bring the practice of robotic surgery into the mainstream.

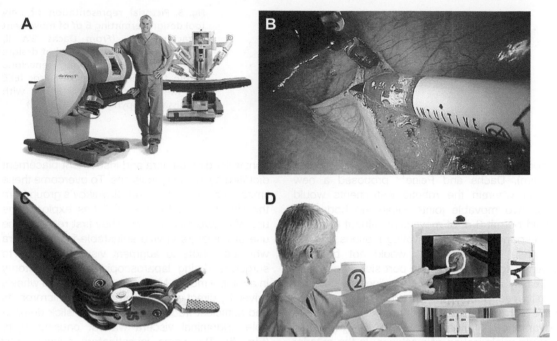

Fig. 1. (*A*) Surgeon console, patient cart, and robotic arms of the da Vinci® S HD Surgical System. (*B*) High-resolution 3D real-time images of the operative field as seen through the immersive viewer. (*C*) EndoWrist capable of 7 *df* of movement. (*D*) Interactive Tilepro® integrated touch-screen video display allows telestration and proctoring during live surgery, with multi-input display of a patient's preoperative clinical data and images. (*Courtesy of Intuitive Surgical, Inc., Sunnyvale, CA; with permission.*)

MINIATURIZATION OF ROBOTIC PLATFORM

The current design of the da Vinci's robotic cart is based on the traditional laparoscopic platform, wherein straight rigid instruments are used intracorporeally through small incisions by the surgeon maneuvering the instrument handles outside the patient's body. As a result, the current da Vinci® system occupies significant overhead over the sterile field, presenting spatial challenges for the patient-side assistants to overcome to operate dexterously alongside the robotic arms and cart.

In contrast, the Laprotek system (EndoVia, Inc., Norwood, Massachusetts, subsequently taken over by Hansen Medical, Inc., Mountain View, California) comprises slave instrument "motor packs" that are mechanically mounted on the existing bed rails of the operating table. The movements from these motors are then transmitted to the surgical instruments by means of stainless-steel cables. Whereas the da Vinci® system directs its straight instruments by moving their back handles through a 3D cone, the Laprotek system uses a curved guide tube to position its instruments intracorporeally. Its design occupies significantly less space in the sterile field, reducing collisions between the robotic instruments and camera (**Fig. 2**). Although not commercially available, it has been projected to cost significantly less than the da Vinci® system.

Working on the premise that the motion outside the patient should be confined to a line rather than

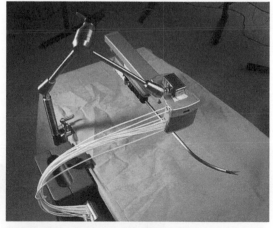

Fig. 2. Photograph of the Laprotek mainframe and guide tube. The stainless-steel guide tube controls upward and downward movement of the instrument, whereas the back end pivots about the incision. The arrow indicates the surgical port site position. (*From* Rentschler ME, Platt SR, Berg K, et al. Miniature in vivo robots for remote and harsh environments. IEEE Trans Inf Technol Biomed 2008;12:66–75; with permission.)

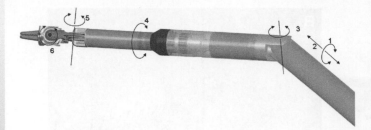

Fig. 3. Pictorial representation of new tool design permitting 6 *df* of movement intracorporeally. (*From* Dachs GW II, Peine WJ. A novel surgical robot design: minimizing the operating envelope within the sterile field. Conf Proc IEEE Eng Med Biol Soc 2006;1:1505–8; with permission. Copyright © 2006 IEEE.)

a cone (da Vinci® system) or a plane (Laprotek system), Dachs and Peine[13] proposed a new design wherein the robotic instruments would have two movable joints within the body that would permit 6 *df* of movement without requiring corresponding external pivoting motions (**Fig. 3**). Because the instruments would not be constrained to pivot about the port side, they could be easily mounted on a streamlined mechanical arm that supports its linear track to deliver comparable intracorporeal dexterity and precision. The advantages of their proposed design would include minimization of machinery in the exterior working envelope, giving surgical assistants more room to operate, and elimination of instrument collisions attributable to suboptimal port placement (**Fig. 4**).

MOBILE MINIATURIZED IN VIVO ROBOTS

Despite improvements in high-definition real-time clarity of tissue architecture and a wider field of view with the da Vinci® S HD Surgical System, the surgeon's visual and operative fields remain

constrained by camera and instrument placement dictated by the entry incisions. To overcome these limitations, Rentschler and Oleynikov's group from the University of Nebraska[2,14] has explored the use of in vivo microrobots. They first reported the use of miniature in vivo adjustable-focus camera wheeled robots to augment visual feedback to surgeons during laparoscopic cholecystectomy in a canine model. Mounted on two helical wheels driven by direct current motors, these microrobots had sufficient traction to move over slick deformable abdominal viscera without causing injury (**Fig. 5**). The same investigators subsequently designed a fixed-base pan-and-tilt camera robot that permitted forward tilting at an angle of 45°. Comprising tripod legs that were spring-loadable and could be abducted during insertion through the laparoscopic port, this microrobot could then be guided into a desired intra-abdominal position with laparoscopic instruments, offering surgeons alternate views of the organs being operated on to that obtained by means of the laparoscopic camera.[15] Joseph and colleagues[16] recently

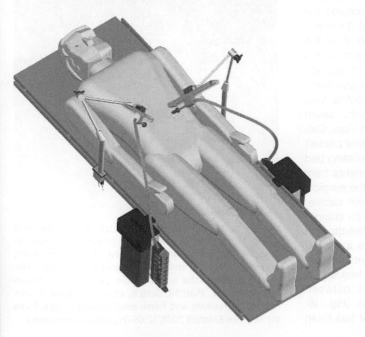

Fig. 4. Envisioned design of robotic setup as proposed by Dachs and Peine. (*From* Dachs GW II, Peine WJ. A novel surgical robot design: minimizing the operating envelope within the sterile field. Conf Proc IEEE Eng Med Biol Soc 2006; 1:1505–8; with permission. Copyright © 2006 IEEE.)

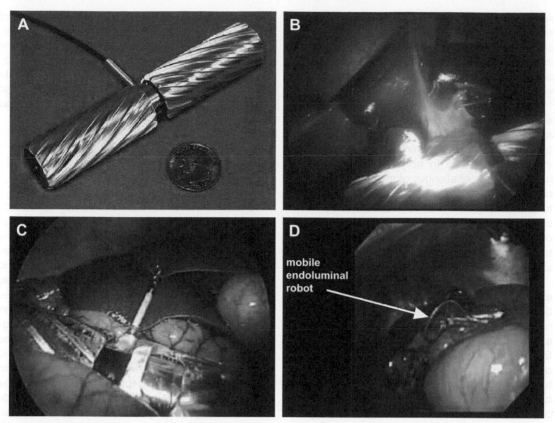

Fig. 5. (*A*) Mobile adjustable-focus robotic camera (MARC) prototype designed by researchers at the University of Nebraska. (*B*) Intracorporeal view of the MARC during porcine cholecystectomy, (*C*) Mobile in vivo robot executes liver biopsy. (*D*) Same robot performs peritoneoscopy. (*From* Oleynikov D. Robotic surgery. Surg Clin North Am 2008;88:1121–30; with permission.)

reported their collaborative experience with these prototypes in performing laparoscopic prostatectomy and laparoscopic nephrectomy in a canine model. Rentschler and colleagues[17] also demonstrated their use in guiding a surgically naive crew member to perform the steps of a laparoscopic appendectomy in a harsh environment by means of remote telementoring. Albeit successful, technical drawbacks encountered during these operations included the need for a separate controller to maneuver the robot into position; significant hindrance attributable to the tethered design for the robot's continuous power; and lack of a self-cleaning mechanism for the camera lens positioned between the helical wheels, which resulted in obscured images from direct contact with intra-abdominal organs and fluids.

The feasibility of using multiple miniature in vivo robots for bettering spatial orientation while facilitating tasks was recently reported by Lehman and colleagues.[18] They used three robots—a peritoneum-mounted camera robot, a lighting robot, and a retraction robot—together with a conventional upper gastrointestinal endoscope to augment the scope of natural orifice transluminal endoscopic surgery (NOTES) procedures in a porcine model.

Although still in their early stages, these and other feasibility studies[19–21] have demonstrated significant potential for eventual development of wireless robotic sensors to provide composite all-round real-time images and robotic manipulators that would obviate the need for multiple incision sites for instrument access.

ADVANCES IN ENDOSCOPIC NAVIGATION SYSTEMS

In performing laparoscopic urologic procedures with da Vinci® assistance, surgeons rely on visual cues instead of tactile feedback to achieve comparable outcomes to those reported for traditional open surgery. Suture tension, for example, has been dictated by the degree of deformation on the respective tissue. Imaging technologies based on virtual and augmented reality have evolved to provide real-time navigational guidance for the surgeon to perform image-guided surgery.

Augmented reality may be defined as the integration of computer-generated images (from reconstructed preoperative MRI, CT, or ultrasound images) to live video or other real-time images, such as ultrasound, allowing visualization of visceral anatomy and surrounding structures.[22]

The initial experience of such image-guided surgery in neurosurgery, maxillofacial surgery, and orthopedics was based on integrating images over fixed bony landmarks.[23–25] Attempts to extrapolate its use in abdominal surgery have highlighted the challenges of imaging viscera that constantly shifts and undergoes deformation: (1) to find constant intra-abdominal reference points and (2) to merge preoperative images over constantly shifting soft tissue anatomy attributable to breathing, heartbeat, patient movement, and surgical instrumentation.[22,26]

Ukimura and Gill[27] recently described their experience of using a color-coded zonal navigation system to perform laparoscopic partial nephrectomy. Such a system affords the surgeon a 3D visual surgical roadmap based on preoperative CT images to identify safe resection margins during surgery by giving different colors to the tumor and its adjacent tissues. Ukimura and his colleagues[28–30] further reported the use of intraoperative transrectal 3D ultrasonography to guide the course of laparoscopic nerve-sparing radical prostatectomy.

Attempts at incorporating conventional fluoroscopy during robotic procedures have been hindered by spatial difficulties of reconciling the sizable overhead footprint of the fluoroscopic and da Vinci® systems over the sterile field. In addition, fluoroscopy only provides cursory images of calcified or radiopaque structures, with limited soft tissue information; the need for operating staff to wear heavy protective gowns to protect them from collateral radiation exposure is an unattractive prospect during complex laparoscopic procedures; and the anterior-posterior images afforded by fluoroscopy leave many "blind spots" during surgical dissection.[31]

The TilePro® system uses a "picture in picture" viewer in the da Vinci® surgeon's console to toggle among images from various sources. Bhayani and Snow[32] recently described their experience with this system to assimilate images from preoperative CT or MRI scans, real-time ultrasonographic images, and 3D images viewed through the da Vinci® surgeon console during robotic-assisted laparoscopic partial and radical nephrectomy. In 2 of 17 partial nephrectomies, superselective arterial control was possible using Doppler information fed into the surgical console during tumor resection. Although providing invaluable information

during surgery, the images were static and not superimposable to the mobile operative field. Although the TilePro® system has increased the availability of anatomic images available to the console surgeon during surgery, the ultimate direction would certainly be to integrate these images in real time onto the operative field as seen through the immersive viewer.

ROBOTIC NATURAL ORIFICE TRANSLUMINAL ENDOSCOPIC SURGERY AND SINGLE-PORT SURGERY

NOTES has made significant advancements since its inception in the late 1990s. Using a natural orifice to conceal surgery has not been a new concept to urology, because transurethral procedures, including cystoscopy, prostatectomy, and ureteroscopy, have been routinely performed through a natural orifice for several decades now. Previous limitations in equipment and technique had daunted minimally invasive surgeons from attempting intraperitoneal procedures through a natural orifice, however. Gettman and colleagues[33] successfully performed the first transvaginal NOTES nephrectomy in a porcine model, using conventional laparoscopic equipment through a single abdominal 5-mm trocar. Single-port NOTES access through transvaginal,[34] transgastric,[35] transvesical,[36,37] and even transcolonic[38,39] routes has now been reported. Nonetheless, NOTES procedures remain limited by the degree of mobility and stability afforded by current endoscopic technologies.

Building on their experience with single-port laparoscopic urologic surgery, Kaouk and his colleagues from the Cleveland Clinic[40–42] recently pioneered the use of the da Vinci® system for natural orifice procedures, first in the porcine model[43] and subsequently in humans.[44] The first technical constraint their group encountered was to overcome the critical distance between robotic arms required for uninterrupted maneuverability during surgery. Second, traditional transabdominal placement of robotic trocars creates a fulcrum at the fascial level, allowing the robotic system to recognize a pivot around which the robotic arm can rotate. Altering the ideal location of this fulcrum and constricting port placement potentially predispose to inadvertent tissue injury and restricted movement.

Despite these limitations, configuring the robotic arms in unorthodox positions provided an opportunity to explore the potential of robotics in NOTES. Box and colleagues[39] successfully completed a robotic NOTES porcine nephrectomy by placing the robotic scope through a single abdominal trocar site while the right and left arms of the robot were placed transvaginally and transcolonically, respectively. Given the configuration, the robotic camera required manual control, whereas the robotic arms were manipulated by the surgeon at the console. The porcine nephrectomy was completed uneventfully despite the expected clashing of robotic arms externally. In contrast, Kaouk and colleagues placed the robotic camera lens and one arm through the umbilicus, with the other robotic arm inserted through the vagina, permitting successful completion of more than 30 robotic NOTES procedures to date. The arm configuration provided for greater articulation and closely mimicked internal triangulation as appreciated during standard laparoscopy. In all, robotic NOTES dismembered pyeloplasty, partial nephrectomy, and completion nephrectomy were successfully performed.[43]

Immense interest recently in laparoscopic single-port surgery has also witnessed the emergence of urologic procedures being accomplished through a single multichannel port.[45–48] As in NOTES, critical analysis of surgical technique identified limitations of the da Vinci® system in instrumentation and dissecting capabilities in such a confined space, chiefly that the proximity of robotic arms through a single multichannel port would invariably lead to external clashing. Attempting novel modifications to port and robotic instrument configuration, Kaouk and colleagues[44] reported the first successful series of single-port robotic procedures in humans, including radical prostatectomy, dismembered pyeloplasty, and radical nephrectomy. A salient highlight of these procedures was the improved facility for intracorporeal dissecting and suturing. During urethral-vesical anastomosis and ureteropelvic anastomosis, a continuous running suture creating a watertight closure was possible because of greater instrument articulation and rigidity.

ADVANCES IN FLEXIBLE ROBOTICS

Abbott and colleagues[49] from Purdue University have been working to develop an endoluminal robotic system (ERS) comprising a camera lens with two adjacent robotic instruments, each having at least 6 df plus an end-effector gripping action. The first-generation design, the ViaCath system (EndoVia Medical, Norwood, Massachusetts), was fashioned on the Laprotek master console with haptic interfaces and flexible robotic instruments that run alongside a standard gastroscope or colonoscope. The key components of these robotic instruments are a mechanical coupler to the position arm, a flexible shaft, and

an articulating tip with an end effector delivering a total of 7 df within the scope's visual field (**Fig. 6**). The early results in an in vivo porcine model revealed various technical difficulties, chiefly difficulty in intubating the patient and positioning the instruments at the desired site, the instruments catching on tissue during deployment, and the limited lateral force produced by the instruments being insufficient for effectively executing the intended procedures on gastrointestinal tissue. To redress these limitations, the investigators have proposed a second-generation flexible ERS and instruments to improve kinematic instrument control and reduce inherent friction to boost the force available for instrument actuation and manipulation.

Apart from laparoscopic and intraperitoneal procedures, flexible robotic systems have also been applied during ureterorenoscopy. A novel device created by Hansen Medical, Inc. incorporates a robotic console to manipulate and control the deflection of a flexible ureteroscope (**Fig. 7**). Using this novel remote system, retrograde ureterorenoscopy was successfully performed in a swine model.[50,51] The increasing range of motion and stability of the platform parallel that of laparoscopic robotic systems. Further refinements in the product may ease the learning curve required during flexible upper tract ureterorenoscopy.

ADVANCES IN HAPTICS

Despite affording the surgeon improved operative dexterity and optical magnification, the current da Vinci® system is unable to deliver the element of haptics. Haptics has been categorized by Okamura[52] as being kinesthetic (involving forces and positions of the muscles and joints) or cutaneous (tactile, related to skin), encompassing the spectrum of force, distributed pressure, temperature, vibrations, and texture. The sense of touch has long been considered essential in limiting inadvertent tissue injury during surgical procedures. Haptics in robotics has demonstrable benefits in reducing tissue injury and reducing suture breakage while maintaining respectable operative time in the hands of an experienced surgeon.[53–57]

Attempts at developing sensory information from the robotic end effectors are cursory at this time and are largely focused on force-feedback systems. Although successfully used in various engineering situations, the translation of current commercial force-feedback sensors to live surgery has been hampered by constraints in size, design, cost, compatibility, and ability to withstand conventional sterilization procedures.

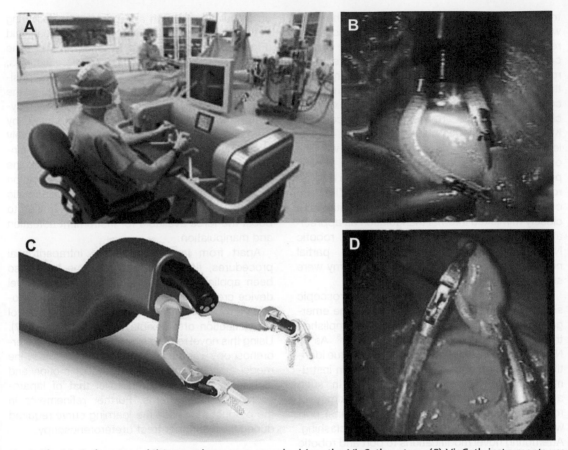

Fig. 6. The ViaCath system. (*A*) Laprotek surgeon console drives the ViaCath system. (*B*) ViaCath instruments use a double-flex section design at the distal tip for articulation. (*C*) Articulated overtube facilitates introduction of the flexible endoscope with its two highly articulated instruments. (*D*) In vivo visualization of abdominal viscera in a porcine model. (*From* Abbott DJ, Becke C, Rothstein RI, et al. Design of an endolumenal NOTES robotic system. In: Proceedings of the IEEE/RSJ International Conference on Intelligent Robots and Systems. San Diego, CA: October 29-November 2, 2007. p. 412; with permission.)

Preliminary evidence that haptic feedback with robotics is possible has emerged, wherein specialized grippers are attached to the jaws of existing robotic instruments to deliver haptic feedback.[57,58] Redesigning robotic instruments to integrate force-sensing capability has also been reported but has not been met with much enthusiasm, given the recurrent prohibitive costs of disposing of these surgical expendables after each case in current practice.

Robotic haptic technology has also found new use in the arena of disaster and emergency medicine.[59] Robotics used for hazardous waste identification and removal has removed individuals from danger by means of direct exposure. These "hazbot" platforms with haptics have demonstrated greater reproducibility and ease of use with novice manipulators. Comparative evaluation between standard robotic systems and more refined humanistic platforms may propel robotics to a new level to improve surgeon ability further.

ADVANCES IN SIMULATOR TRAINING PLATFORMS FOR ROBOTICS

Another significant hurdle in assimilating robotics into the vanguard of mainstream urologic surgery involves the training of robotic-naive surgeons with no prior experience at the robotic console. The high costs of purchasing and housing a dedicated dry laboratory "training" da Vinci® system and the cost of surgical expendables used during training cases in wet laboratories often mean that console experience obtained at various hands-on courses is limited and fleetingly transient. In addition, heightened expectations from patients undergoing robotic surgery, medicolegal implications of accountability of attending surgeons, and demands from hospital administrators to turn

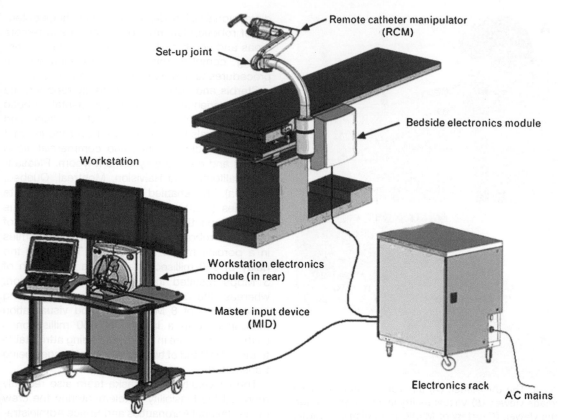

Fig. 7. Pictorial illustration of the flexible robotic catheter-control system. AC, alternating current. (*Courtesy of Hansen Medical, Mountain View, CA; © 2009 Hansen Inc. Used with permission.*)

around robotic procedures have resulted in limited opportunities for urology residents to gain operative maturity at the console.

The dV-Trainer (MIMIC Technologies, Inc., Seattle, Washington) has been developed in collaboration with Intuitive Surgical, Inc. as a solution to some of these current obstacles in surgical training.[60,61] It consists of a master console with finger-cuff telemanipulators connected to a binocular 3D visual output that aims to reproduce the look and feel of the da Vinci® console. The program encompasses exercises in EndoWrist manipulation, camera control, clutching, object transfer and placement, needle handling, needle driving, knot tying, and suturing. The cable-driven system also provides haptic feedback for the trainee as he or she executes surgical movements spatially (**Fig. 8**). Among 15 subjects with varying experience with robotic surgery, Lendvay and colleagues[62] reported significant reduction of total task time, economy of motion, and time the telemanipulators spent outside of the center of the platform's workspace in the experienced group compared with the novice group.

Researchers at the University of Nebraska are also working to produce a da Vinci®-compatible virtual reality simulator, using kinematic data from the da Vinci® console through LabVIEW (National Instruments, Austin, Texas) to drive simulation software (Cyberbotics, Ltd., Lausanne, Switzerland).[63,64] Medical Education Technologies, Inc. (Sarasota, Florida) has also made an attempt to produce a robotic surgery simulator for its SurgicalSIM package,[65] although the reception to this has yet to be reported.

ADVANCES IN REMOTE ROBOTIC SURGERY

In 2001, Marescaux and colleagues[66] reported the first experience of performing transatlantic robotic-assisted laparoscopic cholecystectomies in six pigs and one human, with the surgeon based in New York and the Zeus system installed in Strasbourg, France. Anvari and colleagues[67] subsequently reported their experience of 21 telerobotic laparoscopic operations between St. Joseph's Hospital in Hamilton, Ontario, Canada and North Bay General Hospital 400 km north of Hamilton. Through an IP-VPN (15 Mbps of bandwidth)

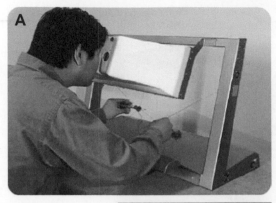

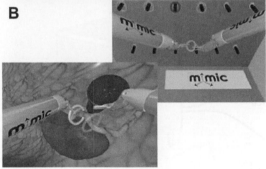

Fig. 8. The dV-Trainer. (*A*) Binocular console with 3D image viewer. (*B*) Virtual reality images seen through the viewer. (*Courtesy of* MIMIC Technologies, Seattle, WA; with permission.)

network that linked the Zeus robotic console in the teaching institute with the three arms of the Zeus TS System (Computer Motion Inc., Santa Barbara, California) in the rural hospital, the surgeons were able to operate together with the same surgical footprint, with overall latency at 135 to 140 milliseconds.[67] Their experience, albeit with two-

dimensional vision, demonstrated the huge potential of robotic platforms to deliver care in remote areas and combat situations, in addition to telestrating complex robotic-assisted laparoscopic procedures to surgeons on the learning curve.

Sterbis and colleagues[68] recently reported the first experience with transcontinental robotic surgery using the da Vinci® system. Video and robotic signals were transmitted over the Internet using nondedicated lines and commercial video coding and decoding systems (Plycom, Pleasanton, California and Haivision, Montreal, Quebec, Canada). This enabled surgeons at two separate consoles (1300 and 2400 miles away from the robot, respectively) to control different parts of the same robot to complete four nephrectomies in a porcine model successfully. The round-trip delay of 900 milliseconds using a bandwidth of 3 Mbps resulted in intermittently poor vision, whereas the second console surgeon using a bandwidth of 8 Mbps had good visualization throughout with a latency of 450 milliseconds (with the difference in bandwidth being attributable to the 3D instead of two-dimensional images being transmitted).

The University of Nebraska team also recently reported the feasibility of telementoring the crew of the National Aeronautics and Space Administration (NASA) Extreme Environment Mission Operations (NEEMO) 9 mission in executing the steps of a laparoscopic appendectomy using these in vivo microrobots.[17] In this study, the crew member was telementored by means of video conferencing software after viewing a 30-second video describing the steps of the appendectomy and successfully dissected, stapled, and removed the appendix (**Fig. 9**). Lum and colleagues[69] from the

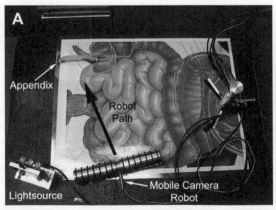

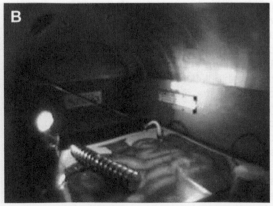

Fig. 9. (*A*) Setup for telementoring of the surgically naive crew of the NEEMO 9 mission to perform a simple appendectomy. (*B*) Real-time visual feedback of the appendectomy by means of the mobile robot's adjustable camera. (*From* Rentschler ME, Platt SR, Berg K, et al. Miniature in vivo robots for remote and harsh environments. IEEE Trans Inf Technol Biomed 2008;12:66–75; with permission.)

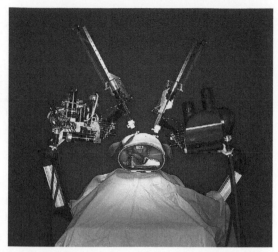

Fig. 10. The RAVEN robot designed at the University of Washington. (*From* Oleynikov D. Robotic surgery. Surg Clin North Am 2008;88:1121–30; with permission.)

University of Washington also reported their experience with the RAVEN robot (prototype designed by Dr. Blake Hannaford and his team from the Biorobotics Laboratory, Department of Electrical Engineering, University of Washington, Seattle, Washington–not yet commercially available), a prototype smaller in size than the da Vinci® system with the capability of being mounted on the patient and operated in harsh and remote environments (**Fig. 10**). Bell and colleagues[70] from the same institute also reported on their experience with a brain-computer interface that allows a person to control a humanoid robot directly using noninvasive brain signals from the scalp through electroencephalography. In that study, a partially autonomous robot was able to perform complex tasks like walking to specific locations and picking up specific objects under direction from nine different users.

As rapid advances in Internet technologies for swifter and more secure transmission of data couple the developments in surgical robotics, it is foreseeable that robotic telestration and remote surgery are likely to become commonplace practices in the not too distant future, possibly even with hands-off control of advanced robotic instruments.

SUMMARY

The advent of novel robotic and compatible technologies has occurred at a breathtaking pace in the past decade, mirroring the rapid adoption of robotic surgery among urologists and their patients worldwide. The current da Vinci® S HD System represents the state of the art, incorporating several new features that have made surgery more ergonomic and interactive for console surgeons and their patient-side assistants. Early trials of microelectrical mechanical systems devices have been encouraging, and the next step would be to refine these technologies further for empowering the surgeon with augmented real-time visualization of tissue and intracorporeal dexterity, possibly even through a single port. Virtual reality simulator training packages compatible with the da Vinci® system are going to be commercially available soon, giving robotically naive surgeons a much needed bridge for gaining familiarity and confidence at the console before live surgery. Image-guided surgery should also become increasingly more popular as technologies develop to overcome the current limitations of working with deformable mobile viscera. Developments in data and image transmission over Internet protocols and satellite platforms may soon allow remote telestration of complex robotic operations, obviating the need for surgeons to be physically present to perform or mentor such operations and delivering improved patient care to those living in remote or hazardous environments. These promising innovations look set to usher in a new era in operative urology in the near future, and the authors look forward with immense interest to how this article may be deemed archaic in a few years.

ACKNOWLEDGMENTS

The authors thank the management of Intuitive Surgical, Inc. (Sunnyvale, California) and MIMIC Technologies (Seattle, Washington) for their invaluable constructive input and use of their illustrations for this article.

REFERENCES

1. Su L. Role of robotics in modern urologic practice. Curr Opin Urol 2009;19:63–4.
2. Oleynikov D. Robotic surgery. Surg Clin North Am 2008;88:1121–30.
3. Stoianovici D. Robotic surgery. World J Urol 2000; 18:289–95.
4. Camarillo DB, Krummel TM, Salisbury K. Robotic technology in surgery: past, present and future. Am J Surg 2004;188:2S–15S.
5. Sim HG, Yip SKH, Cheng CWS. Equipment and technology in surgical robotics. World J Urol 2006; 24:128–35.
6. Harris SJ, Arambula-Cosio F, Mei Q, et al. The Probot—an active robot for prostate resection. Proc Inst Mech Eng [H] 1997;211:317–25.

7. Rovetta A, Sala R. Execution of robot-assisted biopsies within the clinical context. J Image Guid Surg 1995;1:280–7.

8. Hempel E, Fischer H, Gumb L, et al. An MRI-compatible surgical robot for precise radiological interventions. Comput Aided Surg 2003;8:180–91.

9. Cadeddu JA, Bzotek A, Schreiner S, et al. A robotic system for percutaneous renal access. J Urol 1997; 158:1589–93.

10. Cleary K, Melzer A, Watson V, et al. Interventional robotic systems: applications and technology state-of-the-art. Minim Invasive Ther Allied Technol 2006;15:101–13.

11. Mozer P, Troccaz J, Stoianovici D. Urologic robots and future directions. Curr Opin Urol 2009;19:114–9.

12. Available at: www.intuitivesurgical.com/products/davincissurgicalsystem. Accessed March 23, 2009.

13. Dachs GW II, Peine WJ. A novel surgical robot design: minimizing the operating envelope within the sterile field. Conf Proc IEEE Eng Med Biol Soc 2006;1:1505–8.

14. Rentschler ME, Dumpert J, Platt SR, et al. Mobile in vivo camera robots provide sole visual feedback for abdominal exploration and cholecystectomy. Surg Endosc 2006;20:135–8.

15. Rentschler ME, Oleynikov D. Recent in vivo surgical robot and mechanism developments. Surg Endosc 2007;21:1477–81.

16. Joseph JV, Oleynikov D, Rentschler ME, et al. Microrobot assisted laparoscopic urological surgery in a canine model. J Urol 2008;180:2202–5.

17. Rentschler ME, Platt SR, Berg K, et al. Miniature in vivo robots for remote and harsh environments. IEEE Trans Inf Technol Biomed 2008;12:66–75.

18. Lehman AC, Berg KA, Dumpert J, et al. Surgery with cooperative robots. Comput Aided Surg 2008;13: 95–105.

19. Hawks JA, Rentschler ME, Redden L, et al. Towards an in vivo wireless mobile robot for surgical assistance. Stud Health Technol Inform 2008;132:153–8.

20. Rentschler ME, Dumpert J, Platt SR, et al. Mobile in vivo biopsy and camera robot. Stud Health Technol Inform 2006;119:449–54.

21. Rentschler ME, Dumpert J, platt SR, et al. Natural orifice surgery with an endoluminal mobile robot. Surg Endosc 2007;21:1212–5.

22. Teber D, Baumhauer M, Guven EO, et al. Robotic and imaging in urological surgery. Curr Opin Urol 2009;19:108–13.

23. Fox WC, Warzyniak S, Chandler WF. Intraoperative acquisition of three-dimensional imaging for frameless stereotactic guidance during transsphenoidal pituitary surgery using the Arcadis Orbic System. J Neurosurg 2008;108:746–50.

24. Tian Z, Lu W, Wang T, et al. Application of a robotic telemanipulation system in stereotactic surgery. Stereotact Funct Neurosurg 2008;86:54–61.

25. Paul HA, Bargner WL, Mittelstadt B, et al. Development of a surgical robot for cementless hip arthroplasty. Clin Orthop 1992;285:57–66.

26. Baumhauer M, Feuerstein M, Meinzer HP, et al. Navigation in endoscopic soft tissue surgery: perspectives and limitations. J Endourol 2008;22:751–66.

27. Ukimura O, Gill IS. Imaging assisted endoscopic surgery: Cleveland Clinic experience. J Endourol 2008;22:803–10.

28. Ukimura O, Magi-Galluzzi C, Gill IS. Real-time transrectal ultrasound guidance during laparoscopic radical prostatectomy: impact on surgical margins. J Urol 2006;175:1304–10.

29. Ukimura O, Gill IS. Real-time transrectal ultrasound guidance during nerve-sparing laparoscopic radical prostatectomy: pictorial essay. J Urol 2006;175: 1311–9.

30. Ukimura O, Ahlering TE, Gill IS. Transrectal ultrasound-guided, energy-free, nerve-sparing laparoscopic radical prostatectomy. J Endourol 2008;22: 1993–5.

31. Afthinos JN, Latif MJ, Bhora FY, et al. What technical barriers exist for real time fluoroscopic and video image overlay in robotic surgery? Int J Med Robot 2008;4:368–72.

32. Bhayani SB, Snow DC. Novel dynamic information integration during da Vinci robotic partial nephrectomy and radical nephrectomy. Journal of Robotic Surgery 2008;2:67–9.

33. Gettman MT, Lotan Y, Napper CA, et al. Transvaginal laparoscopic nephrectomy: development and feasibility in the porcine model. Urology 2002;59:446–50.

34. Clayman RV, Box GN, Abraham JB, et al. Rapid communication: transvaginal single-port NOTES nephrectomy: initial laboratory experience. J Endourol 2007;21:640–4.

35. Kalloo AN, Singh VK, Jagannath SB, et al. Flexible transgastric peritoneoscopy: a novel approach to diagnostic and therapeutic interventions in the peritoneal cavity. Gastrointest Endosc 2004;60:114–7.

36. Lima E, Rolanda C, Pego JM, et al. Transvesical endoscopic peritoneoscopy: a novel 5mm port for intra-abdominal scarless surgery. J Urol 2006;176: 802–5.

37. Desai MM, Aron M, Berger A, et al. Transvesical robotic radical prostatectomy. BJU Int 2008;102: 1666–9.

38. Pai RD, Fong DG, Bundga ME, et al. Transcolonic endoscopic cholecystectomy: a NOTES survival study in a porcine model (with video). Gastrointest Endosc 2006;64:428–34.

39. Box GN, Lee HJ, Santos RJ, et al. Rapid communication: robot-assisted NOTES nephrectomy: initial report. J Endourol 2008;22:503–8.

40. Kaouk JH, Haber GP, Goel RK, et al. Single-port laparoscopic surgery in urology: initial experience. Urology 2008;71:3–6.

41. Kaouk JH, Goel RK, Haber GP, et al. Single-port laparoscopic radical prostatectomy. Urology 2008; 72:1190–3.
42. Kaouk JH, Palmer JS. Single-port laparoscopic surgery: initial experience in children for varicocoelectomy. BJU Int 2008;102:97–9.
43. Haber GP, Crouzet S, Kamoi K, et al. Robotic NOTES (natural orifice transluminal endoscopic surgery) in reconstructive urology: initial laboratory experience. Urology 2008;71:996–1000.
44. Kaouk JH, Goel RK, Haber GP, et al. Robotic single-port transumbilical surgery in humans: initial report. BJU Int 2009;103:366–9.
45. Aron M, Canes D, Desai MM, et al. Transumbilical single port laparoscopic partial nephrectomy. BJU Int 2009;103:516–21.
46. Desai MM, Rao PP, Aron M, et al. Scarless single port transumbilical nephrectomy and pyeloplasty: first clinical report. BJU Int 2008;83:101–88.
47. Gill IS, Canes D, Aron M, et al. Single port transumbilical (E-NOTES) donor nephrectomy. J Urol 2008; 180:637–41.
48. Canes D, Desai MM, Aron M, et al. Transumbilical single-port surgery: evolution and current status. Eur Urol 2008;54:1020–9.
49. Abbott DJ, Becke C, Rothstein RI, et al. Design of an endoluminal NOTES robotic system. Proceedings of 2007 IEEE/RSJ International Conference on Intelligent Robots and systems. October 29-November 2, 2007; San Diego, CA. p. 410–6.
50. Aron M, Haber GP, Desai MM, et al. Flexible robotics: a new paradigm. Curr Opin Urol 2007;17:151–5.
51. Desai MM, Aron M, Gill IS, et al. Flexible retrograde renoscopy: description of novel robotic device and preliminary laboratory experience. Urology 2008; 72:42–6.
52. Okamura AM. Haptic feedback in robot-assisted minimally invasive surgery. Curr Opin Urol 2009;19:102–7.
53. Mahvash M. Novel approach for modeling separating forces between deformable bodies. IEEE Trans Inf Technol Biomed 2006;10:618–26.
54. Mahvash M, Hayward V. High fidelity haptic synthesis of contact with deformable bodies. IEEE Comput Graph Appl 2004;24:48–55.
55. Mahvash M, Voo LM, Kim D, et al. Modeling the forces of cutting with scissors. IEEE Trans Biomed Eng 2008;55:848–56.
56. Weiss H, Ortmaier T, Maass H, et al. A virtual reality based haptic surgical training system. Comput Aided Surg 2003;8:269–72.
57. Wagner CR, Howe RD. Force feedback benefit depends on experience in multiple degree of freedom robotic surgery. IEEE Trans Robot 2007;23:1235–40.
58. Rizun P, Gunn D, Cox B, et al. Mechatronic design for haptic forceps for robotic surgery. Int J Med Robot 2006;2:341–9.
59. Jurmain JC, Blancero AJ, Geiling JA, et al. Hazbot: development of a telemanipulator robot with haptics for emergency response. Am J Disaster Med 2008; 3:87–97.
60. Available at: http://www.mimic.ws/products/MIMIC-dV-Trainer-Brochure.pdf.
61. Sweet RM, McDougall EM. Simulation and computer-animated devices: the new minimally invasive skills training paradigm. Urol Clin North Am 2008;35:519–31.
62. Lendvay TS, Casale P, Sweet R, et al. Initial validation of a virtual-reality robotic simulator. Journal of Robotic Surgery 2008;2:145–9.
63. Katsavelis D, Siu KC, Brown-Clerk B, et al. Validated robotic laparoscopic surgical training in a virtual-reality environment. Surg Endosc 2009;23:66–73.
64. Brown-Clerk B, Siu KC, Katsavelis D, et al. Validating advanced robotic-assisted laparoscopic training task in virtual reality. Stud Health Technol Inform 2008;132:45–9.
65. Available at: http://www.meti.com/products_ss_rss.htm.
66. Marescaux J, Leroy J, Gagner M, et al. Transatlantic robot-assisted telesurgery. Nature 2001;413:379–80.
67. Anvari M, McKinley C, Stein H. Establishment of the world's first telerobotic remote surgical service: for provision of advanced laparoscopic surgery in a rural community. Ann Surg 2005;241:460–4.
68. Sterbis JR, Hanly EJ, Herman BC, et al. Transcontinental telesurgical nephrectomy using the da Vinci robot in a porcine model. Urology 2008;71:971–3.
69. Lum MJH, Rosen J, King H, Telesurgery via unmanned aerial vehicle (UAV) with a field deployable surgical robot. In: Proceedings of Medicine Meets Virtual Reality (MMVR15), Long Beach (CA), 2007. p. 313–5
70. Bell CJ, Shenoy P, Chaladhorn R, et al. Control of a humanoid robot by a non-invasive brain-computer interface in humans. J Neural Eng 2008;5:214–20.

Miniature In Vivo Robotics and Novel Robotic Surgical Platforms

Bhavin C. Shah, MD[a], Shelby L. Buettner, BS[a],
Amy C. Lehman, MS[b], Shane M. Farritor, PhD[b],
Dmitry Oleynikov, MD, FACS[c],*

KEYWORDS

- Miniature robots • In vivo robots • Robotic surgery
- Novel technology • Natural orifice surgery

This article is not certified for AMA PRA Category 1 Credit™ because product brand names are included in the educational content. The Accreditation Council for Continuing Medical Education requires the use of generic names and or drug/product classes as the required nomenclature for therapeutic options in continuing medical education.

For more information, please go to www.accme.org and review the Standards of Commercial Support.

Laparoscopy reduces surgical invasiveness, and thus leads to a shortened recovery period and better cosmesis by decreasing the size of incisions within the abdominal wall. Today, long rigid instruments inserted into the peritoneal cavity through small incisions limit the surgeon's range of motion, and thus the complexity of the procedures that can be performed. The advent of robotic surgical systems, such as the da Vinci Surgical System (dVSS; Intuitive Surgical, Inc., Sunnyvale, California), has revolutionized laparoscopic surgery. The addition of stereoscopic three-dimensional visualization, tremor abolition, increased dexterity, and motion scaling to robotic surgical systems has allowed the surgeon to perform complex tasks using only laparoscopic techniques. In addition to the loss of haptic feedback, the cameras currently used in robotic surgical systems have a limited view, relying on a fixed-port system that is constrained to 4 *df*. Current robots are bulky and require significant space allocation in an already crowded operating suite. Furthermore, there is a significant delay between the formulation of an idea, its development, and the commercialization of surgical robotic products. Robotic surgery, still in its infancy, should inevitably progress as several new concepts are brought to fruition.

Novel robotic surgical systems are being developed that address the aforementioned visualization and manipulation limitations; however, many of these systems remain constrained by the entry incisions. Alternatively, miniature in vivo robots are being developed that are inserted entirely into the peritoneal cavity for laparoscopic and natural orifice transluminal endoscopic surgical

This work was supported by the Telemedicine and Advanced Technology Research Center.

[a] Minimally Invasive and Robotic Surgery, University of Nebraska Medical Center, 983280 Nebraska Medical Center, Omaha, NE 68198–3280, USA

[b] Department of Mechanical Engineering, University of Nebraska, Lincoln, NE 68588–0656, USA

[c] Center for Advanced Surgical Technology, University of Nebraska Medical Center, 983280 Nebraska Medical Center, Omaha, NE 68198–3280, USA

* Corresponding author.

E-mail address: doleynik@unmc.edu (D. Oleynikov).

(NOTES) procedures. These robots can provide vision and task assistance without the constraints of the entry port incision while reducing the number of incisions required for laparoscopic procedures. Miniature robots are easily deployed in a myriad of environments. These robotic surgical systems are smaller, smarter, and less expensive. Easily deployable robots, tailored for specific operations, can be manipulated by telepresence and remote access. Miniature camera robots and microrobots should be able to provide a mobile viewing platform. This article discusses the current state of miniature robotics and novel robotic surgical platforms and the development of future robotic technology.

PRESENT COMMERCIAL SYSTEMS AND COMMON LIMITATIONS

The dVSS was the first surgical robotics system cleared by the US Food and Drug Administration (FDA) for use in general and urologic laparoscopic surgery.[1] The system has three-dimensional visualization of the operating field, 7° range of motion, tremor elimination, and provision of comfortable postural seating for the operating surgeon.[2] These advantages allow surgeons improved hand-like distal tip dexterity, tremor reduction, and correction of motion reversal and motion scaling, which ultimately provide enhanced precision. Urologists have widely accepted its use in prostate surgery. Studies have shown that robotic prostatectomy is safe and effective in men who have prostate cancer.[3]

Surgeons using such robots lack haptic feedback during operations, are unable to switch instruments or tailor the operating field view during the procedure, are inhibited by the large size of the robot, and cannot justify the high cost of the technology.[4] Much effort is being directed toward the development of next-generation robots with improved mobility and sensing and reduced complexity and cost. Today, research focused on the development of a master-slave telerobotic system, with enhanced dexterity and sensing using millimeter-scale robotic manipulators, can be found.[5] Intelligent microsurgical instruments are also being developed to filter involuntary hand motion in hand-held instruments. A full prototype of this device has demonstrated a reduction in tremor oscillations by as much as 50%.[6,7] Other work focuses on developing smaller telerobotic surgical systems with improved haptics.[8,9] Many surgical robotic developments have focused on mitigating and circumventing the incisional limitations of minimally invasive surgery; however, such devices continue to be constrained by the fulcrum effect.

MINIATURE IN VIVO ROBOT PLATFORM FOR LAPAROSCOPY AND NATURAL ORIFICE TRANSLUMINAL ENDOSCOPIC SURGICAL PROCEDURES

Miniature in vivo robots have been designed to assist surgeons during laparoscopic surgery by providing an enhanced view of the surgical environment from multiple angles and improving movement by means of dexterous manipulators unconstrained by the abdominal wall fulcrum effect. Miniature robots that are inserted completely into the peritoneal cavity can overcome some of the limitations of current surgical robotic systems, such as the dVSS, by restoring lost *df*. The miniature in vivo robots developed by the authors' research group can be classified as having a fixed-base or mobile platform.

MINIATURE ROBOT FAMILY
Imaging Robots

The authors have created two types of imaging robots: the pan-and-tilt camera robot and the imaging robot. The 15-mm diameter pan-and-tilt camera robot, made of an aluminum body, was initially fabricated for standard laparoscopic use (**Fig. 1**) and tested in a porcine in vivo environment.[10] This robot allows for rotation of approximately two independent axes, allowing it to pan 360° and tilt 45°. Increased rotation enhances visualization and depth perception of the abdominal cavity in surgical procedures. Independent motors actuate the robot's tilting lever and provide the panning motion. The entire assembly rests on a small ball bearing that is attached to the base and is externally controlled by a joystick. The platform legs are attached at the base and are abducted by torsion springs after abdominal entry. Light-emitting diodes (LEDs)

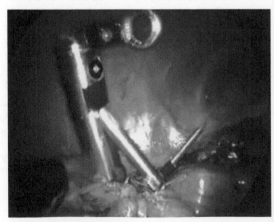

Fig. 1. Pan-and-tilt imaging robot.

provide illumination. The initial prototype was tethered for power; however, wireless prototypes are currently being developed.

The pan-and-tilt camera robot has been used to assist a standard laparoscopic cholecystectomy in a porcine model and a laparoscopic nephrectomy and prostatectomy in a canine model. In a nonsurvival porcine model experiment, a miniature camera imaging robot with a fixed-base platform was inserted through small abdominal incisions into the insufflated abdominal cavity. The placement of an additional trocar and laparoscopic instrument insertion were then viewed and guided using miniature robotic cameras. The miniature robots provided auxiliary visual feedback to the surgeon, giving an enhanced field of view from various orientations during a laparoscopic cholecystectomy. The robots were initially positioned by the surgeon and were reoriented, without requiring additional abdominal incisions, as needed throughout the procedure. The miniature robots provided additional camera angles that augmented surgical visualization and improved orientation.[10–12]

The imaging robot consists of an inner housing containing the lens and focusing mechanism, two white LEDs for lighting, and a permanent magnet direct current (DC) micromotor for rotating the inner housing within the clear outer housing (**Fig. 2**). This robot is 12 mm in diameter and designed to be inserted into the insufflated abdominal cavity through a standard trocar during laparoscopy or by endoscopic approach in NOTES procedures. Each end of the imaging robot is fitted with a magnetic cap. The robot is held to the peritoneum on the abdominal wall using the interaction of magnets housed in the robot with an external magnetic handle (see **Fig. 2**). The handle can be moved along the exterior surface of the abdomen for gross positioning and panning of the robot. The imaging robot's video feedback is displayed on a standard monitor in the operating room. Miniature imaging robots provide the surgeon with better depth perception, improve patient safety, and enable effective planning and execution of surgical procedures.

Lighting Robot

The lighting robot is similar to the imaging robot and is held to the inner anterior abdominal wall through magnetic attraction between the magnetic end caps and the magnets housed on an external handle. The clear outer tube houses six white LEDs. As with the imaging robot, this lighting robot can be inserted through a standard trocar during laparoscopic surgery or endoscopically in NOTES procedures (**Fig. 3**).

Modular Crawler or Mobile Endoluminal Robot

The mobile in vivo robot, or modular crawler, is composed of two independently driven wheels that enable forward, reverse, and turning motions within the abdominal cavity. A tail that collapses into the wheel tread for insertion through the trocar is used to prevent counterrotation. A 6-mm diameter permanent magnet DC micromotor is attached to each wheel using bearings and spur gears (**Fig. 4**). The robot also carries an adjustable-focus image sensor that provides real-time video feedback to the surgeon.

Multiple miniature robots can be placed inside the peritoneal cavity unrestrained by the small diameter of the natural orifice. Such robots, when equipped with stereoscopic imaging, could provide much needed depth perception while allowing triangulation between the image plane and the motion of the instruments. Mobile miniature robots provide a remotely controlled platform for vision and surgical task assistance, which is

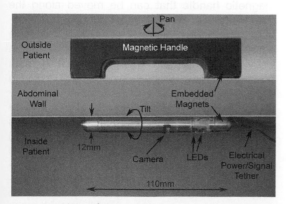

Fig. 2. Imaging robot.

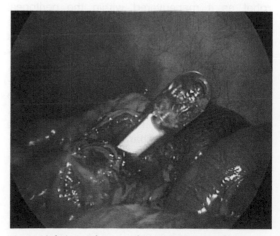

Fig. 3. Lighting robot used in NOTES procedure.

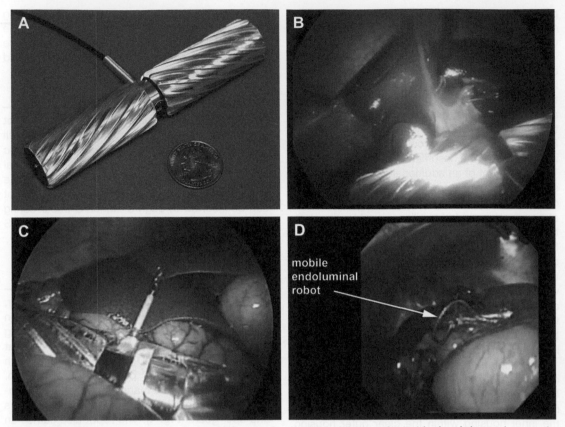

Fig. 4. (*A*) Mobile endoluminal robot or modular crawler. (*B–D*) Modular crawler inside the abdomen in a porcine model performing liver biopsies.

a feasible system, as was successfully demonstrated in a porcine model.[13] A mobile camera robot was introduced through the esophageal opening and inserted into the stomach through a sterile overtube using a standard upper endoscope. The robot explored the gastric cavity before advancing into the peritoneal cavity through a transgastric incision. Once fully inserted, an endoscope was advanced to view the mobile robot as it maneuvered within the peritoneal cavity. The robot was then retracted into the gastric cavity, and the transgastric incision was closed. The ability to navigate the peritoneal cavity without external restraint was advantageous, especially when using several robots simultaneously. These robots have the capability to traverse the abdominal cavity in all directions, obtain liver biopsies in porcine models (see **Fig. 4**), and provide enhanced imaging in operations, including nephrectomy and prostatectomy, as previously performed in canine models.

University of Nebraska AB1 Robot

A multiarmed dexterous miniature in vivo robot with stereovision capabilities has been developed

to provide the surgeon with a stable repositionable platform for visualization and tissue manipulation while performing NOTES procedures in the peritoneal cavity.[14] The basic design of the robot, shown in **Fig. 5**, consists of two "arms" each connected to a central "body" by a rotational "shoulder" joint. Each arm consists of an upper arm and a lower arm fitted with forceps or a cautery end effector. The body of the robot is held to the upper abdominal wall using magnets housed in the body of the robot and an external magnetic handle that can be moved along the outer surface of the abdomen throughout a procedure to reposition the robot internally. This handle enables the surgeon to position the robot to obtain alternative views and workspaces within each quadrant of the peritoneal cavity without requiring an additional incision or a retroflexed configuration. This NOTES-compatible robot has successfully aided in the completion of various operations, including cholecystectomy (**Fig. 6**) and small bowel dissection, in nonsurvivable porcine model experiments. The robot was inserted into the peritoneal cavity through an endoscopic gastrotomy and magnetically secured to the anterior abdominal wall.[14] Using video

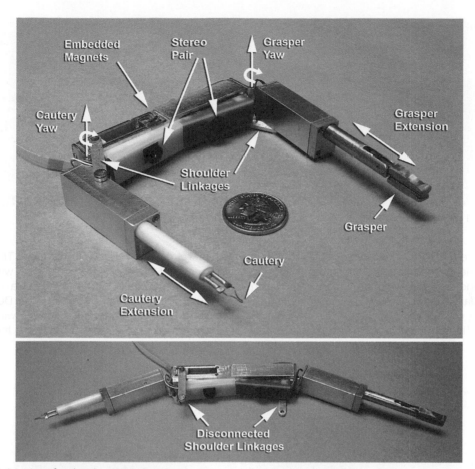

Fig. 5. University of Nebraska AB1 robot.

feedback from on-board cameras, the authors explored the peritoneal cavity, identified the target small bowel for manipulation, and positioned the robot to provide a suitable workspace for visualization and tissue manipulation. A small bowel dissection was then performed (**Fig. 7**). The forceps arm was extended toward the small bowel and was used to grasp the tissue. The arm was then retracted to provide access to the tissue for the cautery arm. The shoulder of the cautery arm was rotated, and the lower arm was extended to cauterize the small bowel. The robot provided flexibility for entrance through a gastrotomy and stability for visualization and dexterity, similar to that of routine laparoscopy, without abdominal wall incisions. This multiarmed dexterous miniature in vivo robot can potentially be used as a platform for urologic procedures, such as prostatectomy and nephrectomy, by means of a NOTES or laparoscopic approach.

Cooperative Robots

The insertion of multiple instruments is limited by the size of the natural orifice and the need to be entirely flexible for insertion through the complex geometry of the natural lumen. In a nonsurvivable in vivo procedure in a porcine model, the feasibility of multiple miniature robots in improving spatial orientation and providing task assistance was demonstrated.[15] This cooperative procedure

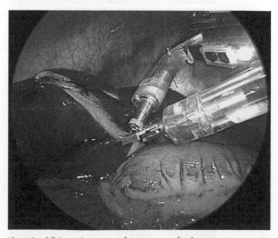

Fig. 6. AB1 robot performs a cholecystectomy in a porcine model.

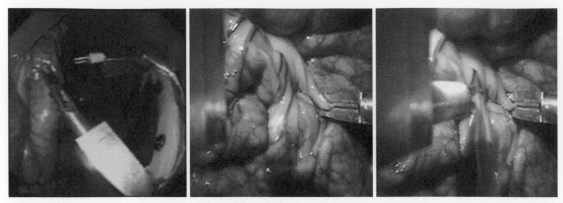

Fig. 7. AB1 robot performs small bowel dissection in a porcine model.

used three miniature in vivo robots, including a peritoneum-mounted imaging robot, a lighting robot, and a retraction robot, in cooperation with a standard upper endoscope to demonstrate various capabilities for NOTES procedures (**Fig. 8**). The retraction robot is designed to enable tissue retraction in NOTES procedures. This robot consists of an external housing with two embedded magnets for fixation and a tethered grasping device. A permanent magnet DC motor coupled with a drum is contained within the external housing. As the motor rotates, the tether

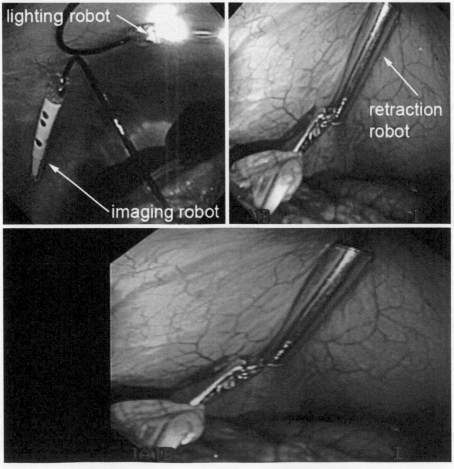

Fig. 8. Cooperative robots: imaging, retraction, and lighting robots used together.

is wound and unwound around the drum to elevate and lower the grasping device. The ability of this mobile platform robot to provide task assistance has been demonstrated through the successful biopsy of three samples of liver tissue.[16] The onboard camera provides visualization to locate the biopsy site accurately, and the mobile platform enables the robot to traverse the peritoneal cavity to the location site. Endoscopic or laparoscopic instruments are presently being used to actuate this grasper device to the perfect location. In the future, this task should be accomplished using a cooperative robot.

The peritoneum-mounted imaging robot provides a stable, repositionable, and adjustable focus imaging platform for minimally invasive surgery.

A nonsurvivable NOTES procedure was performed in a porcine model using the imaging, lighting, and retraction robots in cooperation with a standard upper gastrointestinal endoscope that was inserted by means of a gastrotomy into the peritoneal cavity. Once inserted, each robot was independently secured and positioned along the upper abdominal wall using external magnetic handles. The imaging robot's video feedback guided the exploration of the peritoneal cavity and provided visualization for endoscopic manipulation of the bowel and gallbladder (**Fig. 9**). The retraction robot provided endoscopic access to the surgical target. This procedure demonstrated the feasibility of providing a stable repositionable platform for NOTES procedures using multiple miniature in vivo robots with various capabilities. The stable image and additional lighting allowed the surgeon to visualize and manipulate tissues effectively within the peritoneal cavity for this NOTES procedure. The use of miniature in vivo cooperative robots represents a paradigm shift in robot-assisted surgery. The creation of a family of small robotic instruments, the ultimate objective of the authors' work, that can be inserted into the abdominal cavity during surgery and remotely controlled should enhance the capabilities of the surgeon, reduce costs, and improve patient care.

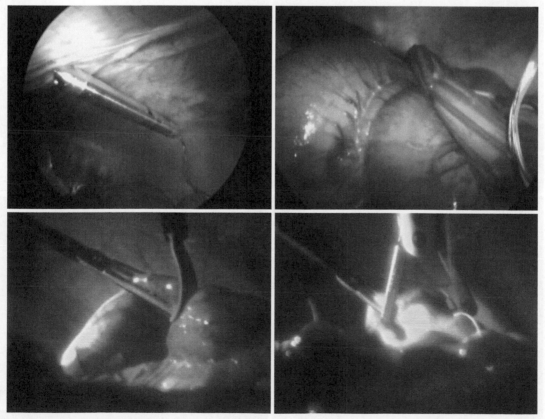

Fig. 9. Cooperative robots: modular crawler and lighting robots inserted by means of NOTES gastrostomy assist in bowel dissection.

Miniature Robots in Urology

The first use of miniature robots in urologic surgery involved the cooperative pilot use of the pan-and-tilt robot and mobile-camera robot used in conjunction with a standard endoscope in two canine models.[17] Video images provided by the microrobot were fed to separate monitors. The cameras were inserted in the abdomen and were used to view the abdominal wall, assist with proper trocar placement, and perform the procedure. The microrobots assisted with trocar placement planning and positioning and were used to assist in the completion of a laparoscopic prostatectomy (**Fig. 10**) and laparoscopic nephrectomy (**Fig. 11**) in two canine models. A supraumbilical 15-mm midline port was used to insert the microrobot cameras inside the abdominal cavity. One microrobot was used at a time. Additional ports were placed to facilitate a laparoscopic radical prostatectomy and nephrectomy. Conventional laparoscopic instruments were used to perform the procedures. The microrobot camera views provided the surgeon with an additional frame of reference that is unavailable when using a standard endoscope. These successful miniature camera devices were capable of providing additional views of the surgical field. The pan-and-tilt robot provides a 360° view of the abdomen while the surgeon maintains a view of the surgical field through the standard laparoscope. The crawler prototype was advanced to specific locations and provided posterior views of organs that are typically impossible to see when using current laparoscopic or robotic cameras that rely solely on a stationary viewing platform. This study demonstrated that small microrobot cameras can be inserted into the abdominal cavity to assist with laparoscopic prostatectomy and nephrectomy. Miniature robots may aid with the visualization and manipulation of the surgical field, eliminating the need for multiple port placement.

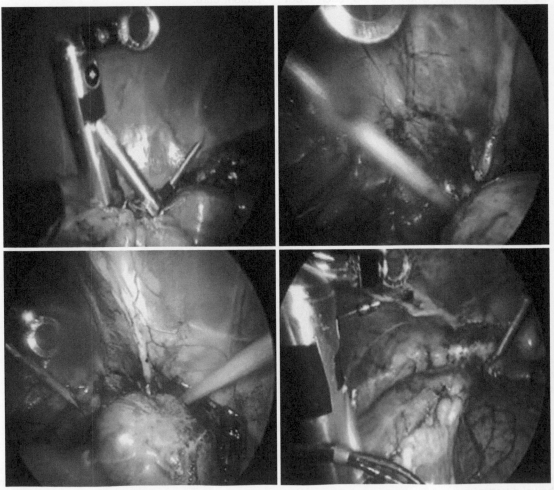

Fig. 10. Pan-and-tilt imaging robot is used to assist in laparoscopic prostatectomy in a canine model.

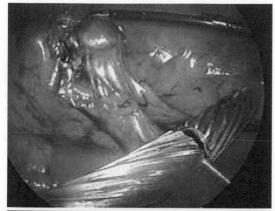

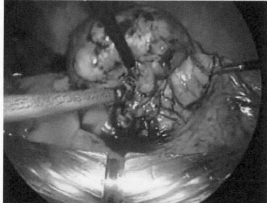

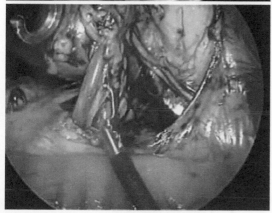

Fig. 11. Modular crawler assists in imaging from various angles in laparoscopic nephrectomy in a canine model.

Such robots could potentially be equipped with sensors to provide feedback from the abdomen or surgical site, further enhancing the benefits of robotic use in urologic procedures.

SINGLE-PORT LAPAROSCOPIC SURGERY

Since the initial report of single-port nephrectomy in 2007, urologists have successfully performed various procedures with laparoendoscopic single-site surgery (LESS), primarily attributable to the refinement and modification of laparoscopic instrumentation. In the Cleveland Clinic experience[18] of four patients undergoing single-port transumbilical live donor nephrectomy, donor vascular and tissue dissection could be performed with ease, and the donor's kidney was retrieved transumbilically without any extraumbilical skin incision. As with all laparoscopic surgery, adequate visualization of the operative field is essential during LESS. The R-Port system (ASC, Wicklow, Ireland) can accommodate a standard 12-mm laparoscope or a smaller 5-mm deflectable-tip video laparoscope (Olympus, Orangeburg, New York), whereas the Uni-X (Pnavel Systems, Cleveland, Ohio) requires a flexible laparoscope of 5 or 10 mm. Park and colleagues[19] have developed a "transabdominal magnetic anchoring and guidance system" (MAGS), which can be used to control an intra-abdominal laparoscope and multiple working instruments introduced through a single 1.5-cm port. Once passed into the abdomen, instruments are affixed to the abdominal wall using external magnetic anchors. The MAGS currently incorporates an internal camera system, two types of passive tissue retractors, and a robotic arm cauterizer.[20] By fixing internal instruments to external magnetic anchors, the platform allows for unrestricted intra-abdominal movement of surgical instruments, creating several potential benefits of LESS, while maintaining an operative perspective similar to that of standard laparoscopy. This system has the added benefit of allowing the surgeon to reposition instruments during surgery without additional incisions, a benefit not realized by any other LESS technology. The MAGS, together with an endoscope, has successfully been used in transgastric, transcolonic, and transvaginal non-survivable cholecystectomies in porcine models. LESS is problematic with regard to imaging, instrumentation, and dexterity. The authors' miniature imaging and retraction robots can be positioned by magnetic or remote control guidance and provide enhanced imaging and retraction for single-port laparoscopic procedures.

TELESURGERY

Robotics provides the unique possibility of separating the surgeon from the patient. This separation can range from a meter to thousands of miles. Telesurgery, along with telementoring, has now been determined feasible in several environments. The feasibility of telesurgery was shown by Marescaux and colleagues[21] in 2001, when the group performed a transatlantic cholecystectomy. Telesurgery has also been used in Canada to train surgeons in rural areas from a specialized laparoscopy hospital.[22] Continued research is required to prove its recurrent efficacy, its cost-effectiveness,[23] and the achievability of satellite connection use.[24] The possibility of tele-surgery can be realized with miniature wireless surgical robots. In the future, such miniature robots may be used in a similar fashion for diagnosis and treatment from a distant access site.

LIMITATIONS OF PRESENT MINIATURE ROBOTS

These microrobot prototypes have limitations, including the need for a separate operator to maneuver the joystick and guide the robot to a particular location.[17] The prototype robots used in the authors' experiment are tethered for power, which can be a significant impediment. Although tether-free prototypes have been developed, these technologies are still in their infancy. Today's prototypes lack a self-cleansing and anti-fogging mechanism, which is necessary because of lens condensation or contact with blood or

abdominal organs. The authors' pan-and-tilt prototype relies on the operator to place it in a specific desired location. It is less prone to contact with moisture from abdominal organs, because the camera is placed on top of the cylinder. The crawler prototype is capable of moving inside the abdomen using the joystick; its lens becomes dirty easily because of its location between the moving wheels. Without such a mechanism and further improvement in the optical system, the added views provided may, in some cases, be of limited use compared with views provided by currently available high-definition monitors or the three-dimensional view of the dVSS.

ROBOTICS IN FLEXIBLE ENDOSCOPY

Current flexible scopes have several deficiencies making their use unlikely in human NOTES procedures. A flexible endoscopy platform for natural orifice surgery with robotic actuation and

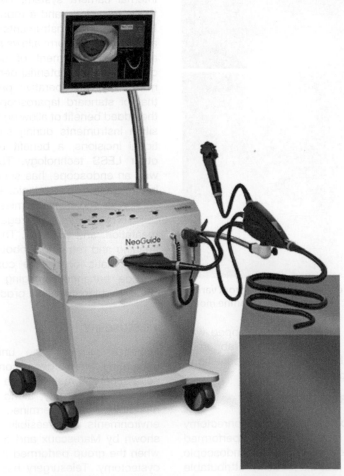

Fig. 12. Neoguide colonoscope. (*Courtesy of* NeoGuide Systems, Inc., San Jose, CA; with permission.)

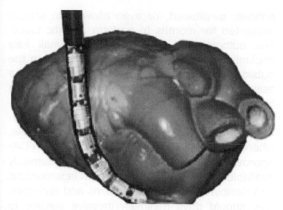

Fig. 13. i-Snake.

visualization enhancement is the next advancement for NOTES procedures. Work has been performed to develop an endoluminal robotic system for providing visualization and dexterous instrumentation for the performance of endoluminal surgery.[25] A first-generation teleoperated robot for endoluminal surgery, the ViaCath System, has been developed by EndoVia Medical (Norwood, Massachusetts). The device consists of a master console with haptic interfaces, slave drive mechanisms, and two flexible instruments located alongside a standard endoscope instrument that, with its positioning arm, provides 7 *df*. Several end effectors have been developed specifically for this device, including a needle holder, grasper, scissors, and electrocautery knife. This computer-assisted catheter system is targeted for endoscopic therapeutic use for colonic

mucosal resection, treatment of gastroesophageal reflux disease, transgastric surgery, obesity surgery, and colectomy. It allows the endoscopist or surgeon to manipulate catheter instruments precisely within the patient and perform tasks, including dissection and suturing.

OTHER ROBOTIC PLATFORMS
Neoguide

Unlike conventional scopes, the NeoGuide colonoscope (NeoGuide Systems Inc., San Jose, California), a computer-assisted colonoscopy system, is built out of multiple segments that can be actively controlled (**Fig. 12**). As the NeoGuide scope is inserted, the system automatically creates a three-dimensional map of the colon and then directs these segments to follow the path taken by the tip, thus avoiding looping of the scope.[26] NeoGuide expects its proprietary robotic endoscopic technology, which was originally developed for application in colonoscopy and is approved by the US FDA, to provide unparalleled access to the abdominal and thoracic cavities and a stable force-bearing platform from which surgical tasks can be performed.

i-Snake

Sir Ara Darzi, Health Minister, surgeon, and Co-Director of the Hamlyn Center for Robotic Surgery at the Imperial College London, has recently experimented with the i-Snake (**Fig. 13**), a mechanical prototype that enters the body through the mouth or other natural orifice, to

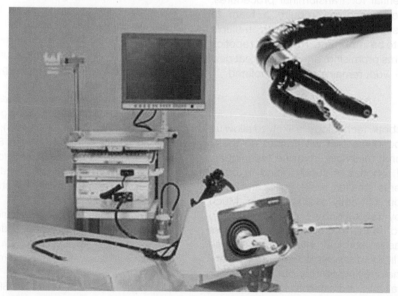

Fig. 14. Endosamurai.

perform surgery in animal models. The i-Snake has enhanced imaging and sensing capabilities, coupled with accessibility and sensitivity, that enable more complex diagnostic and therapeutic procedures than are currently possible.[27,28]

Endosamurai

The Endosamurai[29] is a video gastroscope developed by Olympus Medical Systems Corporation (Center Valley, Pennsylvania) that combines distal end arms with two working channels and a third channel for retraction (**Fig. 14**). Using this device, a surgeon can operate with true triangulation and three instruments at a time.

AN IDEAL NATURAL ORIFICE TRANSLUMINAL ENDOSCOPIC SURGICAL PLATFORM

An ideal NOTES platform should have a compact size of less than 20 mm, variable flexible steerability, reconfigurable instrumentation (a minimum of three ports), and quick tool exchangeability.[30] For simple transgastric procedures, such as peritoneoscopy or specimen retrieval, a multitasking platform may be unnecessary. A multitasking platform[31] is critical in the development of NOTES procedures, however. Many important maneuvers for tissue manipulation, such as aggressive grasping for traction and countertraction and division of structures, are difficult to perform even with a two-channel endoscope. The flexibility of the endoscope, which is advantageous for traversing the gut lumen, is a disadvantage when applying force to tissue, because it is difficult to push and pull simultaneously. Fixation and endoscope stiffening are essential for transluminal procedures. Because these procedures require a team to manipulate instruments, devices with multiple ports are likely to be important. The role of robotics in this area seems promising, although a great deal of foundational work remains to be completed.

SUMMARY

In the future, robotic technology is likely to allow us to perform procedures that we cannot do today with conventional minimally invasive techniques. The benefit of robotics is surely going to be to make instruments smaller, more agile, and more precise than our currently available tools. Much as laparoscopy revolutionized general surgery, robotics should, in the future, usher in the era of minimally invasive surgical intervention. These robots are not likely to resemble the giant conventional robots that we know today but, instead, are likely to be small and dedicated to specific procedures. They may be inserted through small

orifices, swallowed, or even allowed to remain implanted for months to perform specific tasks. The authors' research shows that small fully implantable robots can be manipulated from the outside with much less force and trauma to the tissues, allowing for more precision and delicate handling of surgical fields.

The evolution of miniature robots is in a developmental stage and is being tested in animal models, whereas the dVSS remains the only US FDA-approved therapeutic robotic system currently available. In the next 20 years, newer laparoscopic and flexible endoscopic platforms and technologies should drive minimally invasive surgery to increased computer interface, automation, and mechanical assistance and further away from traditional open surgery, ultimately improving patient outcomes.

REFERENCES

1. Perez A, Zinner M, Ashley S, et al. What is the value of telerobotic technology in gastrointestinal surgery? Surg Endosc 2003;17:811–3.
2. Intuitive Surgical. Available at: www.intuitivesurgical.com. 2004. Accessed March 19, 2008.
3. Pasticier G, Rietbergen JB, Guillonneau B, et al. Robotically assisted laparoscopic radical prostatectomy: feasibility study in men. Eur Urol 2001;40(1):70–4.
4. Hanly EJ, Zand J, Bachman SL, et al. Value of the SAGES learning center in introducing new technology. Surg Endosc 2005;19(4):477–83.
5. Cavusoglu MC, Williams W, Tendick F, et al. Robotics for telesurgery: second generation Berkeley/UCSF laparoscopic telesurgical workstation and looking towards the future applications. Industrial Robot: An International Journal 2003;30(1):22–9.
6. Choi DY, Riviere CN. Flexure-based manipulator for active handheld microsurgical instrument. Engineering in Medicine and Biology Society 2005; 5085–8.
7. Riviere C, Ang W, Khosla P. Toward active tremor canceling in handheld microsurgical instruments. IEEE Trans Rob Autom 2003;15(5):793–800.
8. Rosen J, Lum M, Trimble D, et al. Spherical mechanism analysis of a surgical robot for minimally invasive surgery—analytical and experimental approaches. Studies in Health Technology and Informatics 2005;111:422–8.
9. Rosen J, Hannaford B, MacFarlane M, et al. Force controlled and teleoperated endoscopic grasper for minimally invasive surgery—experimental performance evaluation. IEEE Trans Biomed Eng 1999;46: 1212–21.
10. Rentschler ME, Dumpert J, Platt SR, et al. Mobile in vivo camera robots provide sole visual feedback for

abdominal exploration and cholecystectomy. Surg Endosc 2006;20(1):135–8.

11. Rentschler ME, Hadzialic A, Dumpert J, et al. In vivo robots for laparoscopic surgery. Studies in Health Technology and Informatics 2004;98:316–22.

12. Oleynikov D, Rentschler M, Hadzialic A, et al. Miniature robots can assist in laparoscopic cholecystectomy. Surg Endosc 2005;9(4):473–6.

13. Rentschler ME, Dumpert J, Platt SR, et al. Natural orifice surgery with an endoluminal mobile robot. Surg Endosc 2007;21(7):1212–5.

14. Lehman AC, Dumpert J, Wood NA, et al. Natural orifice translumenal endoscopic surgery with a miniature in vivo surgical robot. Presented at the 2008 Annual Meeting of the Society of American Gastrointestinal and Endoscopic Surgeons, Philadelphia, April 9–12, 2008.

15. Lehman AC, Berg KA, Dumpert J, et al. Surgery with cooperative robots. Comput Aided Surg 2008;13: 95–105.

16. Rentschler M, Dumpert J, Platt S, et al. An in vivo mobile robot for surgical vision and task assistance. ASME J Med Devices 2007;1(1):23–9.

17. Jean V Joseph, Dimitry Oleynikov, et al. Microrobot assisted laparoscopic urological surgery in a canine model. J Urol 2008;180:2202–5.

18. Gill IS, Canes D, Aron M, et al. Single port transumbilical (E-NOTES) donor nephrectomy. J Urol 2008; 180(2):637–41 [discussion: 641] Epub 2008 Jun 12.

19. Park S, Bergs RA, Eberhart R, et al. Trocar-less instrumentation for laparoscopy: magnetic positioning of intra-abdominal camera and retractor. Ann Surg 2007;245:379–84.

20. Zeltser IS, Bergs R, Fernandez R, et al. Single trocar laparoscopic nephrectomy using magnetic anchoring and guidance system in the porcine model. J Urol 2007;178:288–91.

21. Anvari M, McKinlet C, Stein H. Establishment of the world's first telerobotic remote surgical service: for provision of advanced laparoscopic surgery in a rural community. Ann Surg 2004;241:460–4.

22. Sebajang H, Trudeau P, Dougall A, et al. The role of telementoring and telerobotic assistance in the provision of laparoscopic colorectal surgery in rural areas. Surg Endosc 2006;20(9):1389–93.

23. Rayman R, Croome K, Galbraith N, et al. Long-distance robotic surgery: a feasibility study for care in remote environments. Int J Med Robot 2006;2:216–24.

24. Rayman R, Croome K, Galbraith N, et al. Robotic telesurgery: a real-world comparison of ground and satellite-based Internet performance. Int J Med Robot 2007;3:111–6.

25. Abbott DJ, Becke C, Rothstein RI, et al. Design of an endolumenal NOTES robotic system. In: Proceedings of the IEEE/RSJ International Conference on Intelligent Robots and Systems. San Diego, CA, October 29–November 2, 2007; p. 410–6.

26. Available at: http://sanjose.bizjournals.com/sanjose/stories/2008/01/14/story7.html. Accessed November 17, 2008.

27. Darzi A. Available at: http://news.bbc.co.uk/2/hi/health/7155635.stm. Accessed November 17, 2008.

28. Darzi A. Medical tech: robotic snake surgery. Available at: http://www.techradar.com/news/world-of-tech/medical-nanotech-robotic-snakes-transform-surgery-481719. Accessed November 17, 2008.

29. Ikeda K, Taziri H. NOTES update DDW 2008—NOTES-related research reported at DDW 2008. Digestive Internal Medicine 2008;23(10):1477–80 [Japanese]. Available at: http://www.nmckk.jp/japanese/html/books/S2310_1477-1480.pdf. Accessed November 17, 2007.

30. Swanstorm L, Rothstein, et al. Development of a multitasking platform. Presentation at Natural Orifice Surgery Consortium for Assessment and Research (NOSCAR) conference 2006. Available at: http://www.noscar.org/presentations.html#. Accessed November 14, 2008.

31. Rattner D, Kalloo A, ASGE/SAGES Working Group. ASGE/SAGES working group on natural orifice translumenal endoscopic surgery. October 2005. Surg Endosc 2006;20:329–33.

Advances in Bioadhesives, Tissue Sealants, and Hemostatic Agents

Jeffery C. Wheat, MD, J. Stuart Wolf, Jr., MD*

KEYWORDS

- Bioadhesives • Sealants • Hemostats • Fibrin • Thrombin

This article is not certified for AMA PRA Category 1 Credit™ because product brand names are included in the educational content. The Accreditation Council for Continuing Medical Education requires the use of generic names and or drug/product classes as the required nomenclature for therapeutic options in continuing medical education.

For more information, please go to www.accme.org and review the Standards of Commercial Support.

The past two decades have witnessed a substantial growth in the use of bioadhesives, tissue sealants, and hemostatic agents across all disciplines of surgical practice. This growth has been encouraged by two major trends in surgical practice: an expansion of minimally invasive surgery and increasingly complex reconstructive procedures. Minimally invasive surgical techniques are more limited than open surgical ones in their capacity to obtain hemostasis, and hemostatic agents can help make up the deficit. Similarly, the outcomes of complex reconstructive procedures can be enhanced by bioadhesives and tissue sealants. The greatest applications of these agents, however, are when these two trends are combined, for minimally invasive complex reconstructive surgery. These procedures have been made possible in large part through the development of novel materials that help control blood loss and promote tissue healing.

Typically, the use of a specific bioadhesive, tissue sealant, or hemostatic agent has been based on the personal experience and training of individual physicians, and in many cases these applications are off-label. Despite their widespread use, there remains significant confusion regarding the appropriate indications for the use of individual agents. This article discusses the unique features, mechanism of action, safety profile, and several applications of the agents most commonly used in urologic practice. This article is not intended to be an exhaustive summary of all reported urologic uses of bioadhesives, tissue sealants, and hemostatic agents. Instead, it describes the evidence for a set of prototypical applications to guide the reader in the appropriate selection of a particular product based on a specific clinical situation.

ENZYMATIC HEMOSTASIS
Hemostasis and Thrombosis

Thrombus formation and hemostasis in the setting of vascular injury requires two separate

Dr. Wolf acknowledges that he is a consultant for Terumo Corporation and Gyrus-ACMI. Neither company makes any product related to the subject matter of this article. Dr. Wheat has no disclosures.

Department of Urology, University of Michigan Medical Center, 1500 East Medical Center Drive, 3875 Taubman Center, Ann Arbor, MI 48109-5330, USA

* Corresponding author.

E-mail address: wolfs@umich.edu (J.S. Wolf).

Urol Clin N Am 36 (2009) 265–275

doi:10.1016/j.ucl.2009.02.002

components[1]: plasma clotting factors to generate fibrin and platelets to form a hemostatic plug. The coagulation cascade consists of a tightly regulated set of enzymes, which results in the cleavage of prothrombin into its active form, thrombin. Thrombin ultimately causes enzymatic cleavage of soluble plasma fibrinogen into fibrin monomers. The fibrin then forms cross-linked polymers through enzymatic interactions with factor XIII. This cross-linked polymer is insoluble and forms a framework to which platelets can activate and adhere, forming a hemostatic plug.[1] This process is shown schematically in **Fig. 1**. There are several conditions, both acquired and inherited, which cause the coagulation cascade to be deficient. Examples of acquired conditions include hypothermia, consumptive coagulopathy, and pharmacologic anticoagulation. Inherited conditions include both qualitative (von Willebrand disease) and quantitative defects (hemophilia) in coagulation factors.

The goal of all enzymatic hemostatic agents is to mimic the final step of the coagulation cascade in which fibrinogen is cleaved by thrombin to form a fibrin clot. This bypasses the complicated sequential activation of multiple coagulation factors and allows for the delivery of active end products to the site of action allowing for efficient, localized coagulation. Fibrinogen or thrombin are ideally delivered to the site of injury by topical administration for two reasons: first, direct application to the site of injury allows for supraphysiologic concentration of specific prothrombotic agents producing the largest therapeutic effect in controlling hemorrhage; second, local application reduces the risk of unintended prothrombotic complications potentially seen with systemic administration of prothrombotic agents.

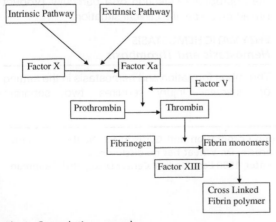

Fig. 1. Coagulation cascade.

Fibrin Sealants

All commercially available fibrin sealant preparations consist of two major components: thrombin and fibrinogen. The supraphysiologic concentration of fibrinogen in these preparations (15–25 times higher than in the circulating plasma) allows for rapid and predictable clot formation.[2] The two components are then delivered using a dual-chambered delivery system allowing each to be applied simultaneously. Specific preparations may also include antifibrinolytics, which act to preserve the clot against enzymatic degradation.

Currently, there are two commercially available fibrin sealant products in the United States: Tisseel (Baxter Health Care, Deerfield, Illinois) and Evicel (Johnson and Johnson, West Somerville, New Jersey). Both products include human donor fibrinogen and thrombin, but they differ in their mechanism of antifibrinolysis. Tisseel contains the antifibrinolytic aprotinin. This was originally derived from bovine lung, but current formulations contain a completely synthetic aprotinin[3] because of concerns regarding allergic reactions to bovine proteins. Aprotinin is a serine protease inhibitor that limits fibrinolysis through inhibition of plasmin, kallikrein, and trypsin.[4] Evicel does not use any specific antifibrinolytic; rather, plasminogen (the enzyme responsible for enzymatic cleavage of fibrin polymers) is removed through chromatographic filtering eliminating the need for an additional antifibrinolytic. All fibrin sealants are contraindicated for intravascular use, because the combination of fibrinogen and thrombin can induce systemic thrombosis. Fibrin sealants work best when applied to a dry (bloodless) surgical field, which is in contrast to thrombin-based hemostatic agents (see later).

The major safety concern regarding commercially available allogenic fibrin sealants relates to their use of donor plasma for obtaining fibrinogen and thrombin, with the associated risk of viral transmission. Following screening of donor plasma for hepatitis B and C and HIV, all available human-derived products undergo treatment to inactivate potential viral particles. In the case of Tisseel, this includes two-step vapor heating at 60°C and 80°C for both fibrinogen and thrombin. For Evicel, this includes solvent detergent treatment followed by pasteurization (fibrinogen) or nanofiltration (thrombin). There have been no documented cases of viral transmission from fibrin sealants from Food and Drug Administration (FDA)–approved agents, so it seems that the viral inactivation procedures are effective.

Nonetheless, in response to the concerns over infectious disease transmission, products have been developed that use autologous blood to derive thrombin and fibrinogen. Currently, there are two FDA-approved methods for obtaining autologous fibrin sealant. The first is Vitagel (Orthovita, Malvern, Pennsylvania), which is composed of microfibrillar bovine collagen and thrombin. This is combined with approximately 10 mL of the patient's own plasma as a source of fibrinogen, which can be prepared in approximately 5 to 7 minutes intraoperatively. The resulting collagen and fibrin scaffold is then absorbed in approximately 30 days. Although this product does not use any allogenic human components, it does use bovine collagen and thrombin, and it should not be used in patients with allergic reactions to bovine products.[5]

The other method for generating autologous fibrin sealant uses blood bank devices that concentrate thrombin and fibrinogen from a patient's own plasma. This system, marketed as CryoSeal (Thermogenesis, Rancho Cordova, California), requires 60 minutes to produce fibrin sealant, but the sealant can be stored frozen at $-18°C$ for up to 1 year.[6] The CryoSeal system uses approximately 400 mL of autologous plasma,[7] whereas the VivoStat system (VivoStat A/S, Denmark, not currently available in the United States) uses similar technology but requires only 120 mL of plasma and requires approximately 30 minutes to prepare.[7,8] Although the fibrin and thrombin concentration is significantly lower in the clots formed from CryoSeal and VivoStat systems compared with Tisseel,[7,9] maximum clot strength was similar between CryoSeal-derived fibrin sealant and Tisseel.[9] A limitation of the CryoSeal system is that because it uses a patient's own coagulation factors, it is contraindicated in patients with acquired or inherited coagulation disorders, or a recent history of anticoagulation.

The first reports of the use of fibrin sealants for hemostasis in renal parenchymal injuries was described in the setting of renal trauma by Kram and colleagues.[10] In their series of 14 patients with penetrating renal trauma, they noted that fibrin glue was able to prevent hemorrhage and urinary leak in all patients with no complicating infections, urinary fistulae, rebleeding episodes, or urinary obstruction. Fibrin sealants can also be useful in iatrogenic trauma. Canby-Hagino and colleagues[11] described two patients who suffered splenic injuries during laparoscopic partial nephrectomy (LPN) treated with fibrin sealant. In both cases, bleeding was able to be controlled and splenectomy was avoided. Several reports have documented the efficacy of fibrin sealants in obtaining hemostasis during partial nephrectomy. Levinson and colleagues[12] reported no

hematoma or abscess formation in seven patients undergoing open partial nephrectomy. The use of hemostatic agents during LPN becomes even more important because achieving hemostasis though the use of direct pressure can be difficult or impossible (except for hand-assisted techniques). Pruthi and colleagues[13] found that in 15 patients undergoing LPN, application of fibrin sealant following argon beam electrocautery was successful in obtaining hemostasis in all cases. Johnston and colleagues[14] found that when the collecting system or renal sinus was entered during LPN, fibrin sealant (plus a gelatin sponge, see later) resulted in significantly higher rates of hemorrhage or urine leak compared with sutured bolster. They concluded that although fibrin glue alone is acceptable for closure of superficial LPN parenchymal defects, sutured bolster is recommended when there is collecting system or renal sinus entry. **Fig. 2** shows fibrin glue applied to a porcine LPN defect. Schips and colleagues[8] have reported the successful use of autologous fibrin sealant for hemostasis in 10 patients undergoing LPN using the VivoStat system. Although the results of these studies are difficult to compare because of the lack of adequate control groups and the use of additional hemostatic methods in addition to fibrin glue (eg, argon beam coagulator, bipolar cautery, and mechanical hemostatic materials), the results do suggest that fibrin sealant is useful in obtaining hemostasis in the setting of superficial LPN, and as an adjunct in closure with sutured bolster when the collecting system or renal sinus is entered.

In addition to its role in hemostasis, fibrin sealants have the ability to induce fibroblast cellular migration and growth factor induction[15–17] making them ideal for use as a urinary tract sealant where a water-tight seal is required.

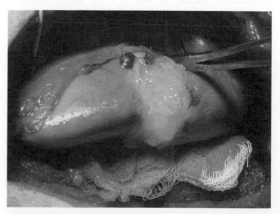

Fig. 2. Fibrin glue applied to a partial nephrectomy defect in a porcine model.

Initial animal experiments demonstrated that the use of fibrin sealant to close a pyeloplasty was superior to laser tissue welding in terms of leak pressure, histologic appearance, flow characteristics, and operative time.[18,19] Subsequently, Eden and colleagues[20] performed the first series of laparoscopic pyeloplasty using fibrin glue in eight patients. In this study, sutures were placed to approximate the two edges and fibrin glue was used to complete the anastomosis. The investigators found that operative time was decreased compared with historic controls (142 versus 193 minutes) and all anastomoses were patent on diuretic renography at 1 to 2 years follow-up.

Fibrin sealant has been used in both simple and radical retropubic prostatectomy. In simple prostatectomy, Morey and colleagues[21] applied fibrin sealant to the prostatic capsule of five patients allowing for a drain-free closure without apparent adverse effects. Diner and colleagues[22] showed that fibrin sealant applied following radical retropubic prostatectomy significantly decreased the drain output compared with controls ($P<.001$). The small sample size in these cohorts and recent evidence that routine pelvic drainage may not be necessary at all[23] suggest, however, that these studies were underpowered to detect small differences between the groups. Further evidence from large, randomized trials is required before it can be concluded that fibrin sealant provides appreciable reduction of anastomotic leakage in the setting of prostatectomy.

The sealant properties of fibrin glue can also be used to promote chronic wound healing by increasing tissue adherence, reducing dead space, inducing fibroblast migration and differentiation, and accelerating revascularization.[15,16,24,25] The first application of fibrin sealant to close a urinary fistula was in 1985 by Papadopoulos and colleagues[26] in an artificial vesicovaginal fistula in a rabbit model. In their study, sutured closure was associated with a 30% recurrence rate, whereas no recurrences were noted in the group closed with fibrin sealant. Since then there have been numerous small case reports of attempts at closure of urinary fistula using fibrin sealants, generally with favorable results[27–30] even in the setting of prior pelvic irradiation.[31] Evans and colleagues[32] reported their use of fibrin sealant in six patients (five males) with complex urinary fistulas. All patients in this group had successful repair of their fistula with a combination of fibrin sealant and surgical correction. In addition to closure of lower urinary tract fistulae, fibrin sealant has been used successfully to close a persistent nephrocutaneous fistula following partial nephrectomy.[33]

Thrombin

Thrombin acts through the enzymatic cleavage of fibrinogen to fibrin creating an insoluble clot to which platelets can adhere. The major difference between the commercially available thrombin preparations and fibrin sealants is the absence of fibrinogen in the former. Thrombin is most efficacious when there is blood present in the field to provide the necessary fibrinogen for enzymatic hemostasis. Three sources of thrombin have been used: (1) bovine, (2) human pooled plasma, and (3) recombinant. **Table 1** provides a list of commercially available thrombin agents. The efficacy of the various thrombin preparations has been compared in several randomized trials, although none was placebo controlled. No significant difference was noted between human plasma and bovine-derived thrombin in a phase III, double-blinded trial with greater than 90% of the subjects in each arm achieving hemostasis within 6 minutes.[34] Recombinant thrombin has been similarly compared with bovine-derived thrombin.[35] Again, this trial showed no difference in time to hemostasis between the recombinant group and the bovine group (95.4% versus 95.1% hemostasis within 10 minutes, respectively).

The safety concerns relating to the use of allogenic human blood products have been previously discussed. Another safety concern relates to the use of bovine-derived products. These products can induce allergic reactions, especially when used repeatedly in a single patient. In patients with known hypersensitivity to bovine products the use of products containing bovine proteins is contraindicated. Additionally, the antibodies formed following exposure to bovine thrombin (or factor V contaminants found in small amounts in bovine-derived thrombin preparations) can cross-react with human clotting factors and induce severe coagulopathy.[36–38] Recombinant thrombin has a significantly lower incidence of development of specific antiproduct antibodies compared with bovine thrombin (1.5% versus 18%, respectively).[35] Additionally, patients who formed antibovine thrombin antibodies were shown to have increased bleeding, thrombotic events, and abnormal activated partial thromboplastin time values compared with those who formed antirecombinant thrombin antibodies. The recent trend to replace bovine products with recombinant or human-derived proteins avoids this complication.

Although thrombin alone has been shown to be effective in hemostasis when blood is present in the surgical field (Thrombin-JMI PI), most studies

Table 1
List of commercially available bioadhesives, tissue sealants, and hemostatic agents currently available in the United States

Class	Brand Name	Manufacturer
Enzymatic agents		
Fibrin	Tissee	Baxter Health Care
	Evicel	Johnson & Johnson
	Vitagel	Orthovita
	CryoSeal	Thermogenesis Corporation
Thrombin		
Bovine	Thrombin-JMI	King Pharmaceuticals
Human	Evithrom	Johnson & Johnson
Recombinant	Recothrom	Zymogenetics
Gelatin matrix	FloSeal	Baxter Health Care
Cross-linking sealants		
Polyethylene glycol	CoSeal	Baxter Health Care
Albumin-gluteraldehyde	BioGlue	CryoLife
Cyanoacrylate	Dermabond	Johnson & Johnson
Mechanical Scaffold		
Porcine gelatin	Gelfoam	Pfizer
	Surgifoam/Surgifl	Johnson & Johnson
Collagen	Avitine	Davol
	Helistat/Helitene	Integra
	Instat/Ultrafoam	Johnson & Johnson
Oxidized cellulose	Surgicel	Johnson & Johnson
	Nu-Knit	
	Fibrillar	
	Original	

have used it in combination with an absorbable gelatin matrix.[34,35] FloSeal (Baxter Health Care, Deerfield, Illinois) uses a combination of human thrombin and bovine gelatin to provide a scaffold with both enzymatic and mechanical hemostatic properties.[39] The gelatin matrix granules swell by as much as 20% within 10 minutes when placed in contact with blood allowing for conformation to the shape of a wound, providing both mechanical tamponade and a scaffold for the resulting fibrin polymer. **Fig. 3** shows FloSeal applied to a partial nephrectomy defect in a porcine model. The matrix is biocompatible and is resorbed within 6 to 8 weeks. The question still remains, however, as to whether the enzymatic or mechanical properties provide most of the hemostatic function. Although there has not been a randomized, controlled trial comparing thrombin plus gelatin sponge, thrombin plus gelatin matrix, and gelatin matrix alone, comparison of individual trials shows roughly equivalent efficacy in terms of hemostasis at 10 minutes (97%, 96%, and 97%, respectively).[34,39,40]

The urologic applications of gelatin matrix thrombin agents (FloSeal) have been most extensively studied in LPN. In a porcine model, Desai and colleagues[41] found that application of

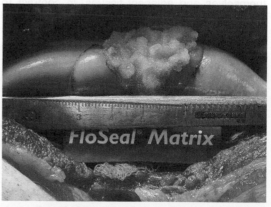

Fig. 3. FloSeal applied to a partial nephrectomy defect in a porcine model.

gelatin matrix following LPN resulted in complete hemostasis without the need for renal ischemia despite significant collecting system entry. Gill and colleagues[42] compared outcomes of patients who had FloSeal applied to the surgical defect before performing sutured renorrhaphy with those in which FloSeal was not used. They found that FloSeal application was associated with a decreased risk of overall complications (37% versus 16%; $P = .008$) and a trend toward fewer hemorrhagic events (12% versus 3%; $P = .08$).

The use of other topical thrombin-based hemostatic agents has not been well described in the urology literature. Typically, stand-alone topical thrombin agents are used in conjunction with an absorbable gelatin sponge to provide a scaffold. The reason for the popularity of FloSeal over other thrombin preparations with absorbable gelatin sponges may be the ease of application of a flowable preparation to an irregular surgical defect.

Although surgical exploration for high-grade renal trauma has classically resulted in nephrectomy, the availability of hemostatic agents has sparked interest in renal preservation for these injuries. Hick and colleagues[43] induced a complex upper pole renal injury in a porcine model and compared FloSeal with conventional sutured repair. They found that the use of FloSeal was associated with significantly reduced overall blood loss and time to hemostasis with no delayed bleeding or urine leak. Although these laboratory results are promising, the role of hemostatic agents for renal salvage therapy has not been investigated in human subjects.

CROSS-LINKING SEALANTS

Agents in this class form a barrier to leakage and bleeding through covalent polymerization between themselves and adjacent tissues. In contrast to fibrin-based sealants that act by the induction of clot formation, cross-linking sealants are completely synthetic and polymerize through nonenzymatic chemical reactions, which do not require the presence of blood or any components of the coagulation cascade.

Polyethylene Glycol–Based Sealants

Currently, two polyethylene glycol (PEG)–based tissue sealants are available. Duraseal (Covidien, Norwalk, Connecticut) is indicated for dural sealing and has no urologic applications. CoSeal (Baxter Health Care, Deerfield, Illinois), which is FDA approved for sealing vascular grafts, has been used for some urologic procedures.

CoSeal consists of two distinct PEG polymers and dilute solutions of hydrogen chloride and sodium phosphate-sodium carbonate.[44] When mixed, the two PEG molecules and solutions form a hydrogel that is adherent to tissues. CoSeal requires a relatively dry surgical field for application.

The main safety concern with CoSeal is related to expansion. Following application, CoSeal can swell up to 400% of its original size. Caution should be exercised when used in closed spaces or in contact with pressure-sensitive structures, such as nerves.

Most controlled clinical trials evaluating CoSeal have been related to vascular reconstruction. In a trial comparing CoSeal with Gelfoam plus thrombin in patients undergoing placement of prosthetic vascular grafts, there was equivalent hemostasis after 10 minutes. The median time to hemostasis was significantly shorter, however, in the CoSeal group (16 seconds versus 189 seconds; $P = .01$).[45]

Based on these results, several groups have evaluated the use of PEG-based sealants for partial nephrectomy. Park and colleagues[46] found that PEG-based hydrogel was effective as a hemostatic agent in a porcine partial nephrectomy model. Additionally, they showed that there was no detectable humoral or cell-mediated immune response to sealant after 2 weeks. In contrast, Bernie and colleagues[47] also used a porcine partial nephrectomy model to compare the risk of hemorrhage and urine leak between intracorporeal suturing, fibrin sealant, and PEG-based sealant. They found that the PEG-based sealant did not adhere well to the cut surface of the renal parenchyma or to the collecting system and had an increased risk of hemorrhage and urine leak compared with fibrin sealant. Only one study has evaluated PEG sealant in humans undergoing partial nephrectomy. Hidas and colleagues[48] showed decreased renal parenchymal loss of function following partial nephrectomy when tissue sealant (either glutaraldehyde or PEG-based) was used compared with suturing alone. This study grouped both sealants together, however, making it unclear if there was a difference between these two classes of agents.

Gluteraldehyde-Albumin–Based Sealants

Glutaraldehyde-albumin–based tissue sealants (BioGlue, Cryolife, Kennesaw, Georgia) consist of purified bovine serum albumin and glutaraldehyde, which when mixed, rapidly polymerizes and forms a covalent bond between it and proteins on the cell surface of adjacent tissues. BioGlue begins to polymerize within 20 seconds and reaches full strength within 2 minutes.[49] Similar to PEG-based sealants, it requires a dry surgical field to polymerize and control of surgical bleeding with sutures or bolsters may be necessary before application. Currently, BioGlue is FDA approved for use as an adjunct in hemostasis following closure of large blood vessels; however, several studies have indicated use in urologic applications.

Following polymerization, the hard matrix is quite adherent to tissues. Although this is generally effective in maintaining hemostasis, further tissue manipulation or placement of sutures can be difficult. BioGlue should only be applied at the conclusion of any reconstructive procedures, such as repair of a collecting system injury,[50] to minimize the risk of urinary obstruction.[51] Care should be taken to protect surrounding tissues from inadvertent application because removal of dried adhesive can cause tearing of tissues. Animal studies have demonstrated that direct application of BioGlue to exposed nerves can cause acute nerve injury, and application near exposed nerves should be avoided. Another safety concern relates to the toxicity of glutaraldehyde. After polymerization, a significant amount of glutaraldehyde is released locally and has been shown to be toxic to cultured cells.[52] Although these results have not been shown to have clinically significant adverse outcomes in humans, care should be taken to use the minimal amount required and to avoid excess application to adjacent tissues.

Two studies have evaluated the use of BioGlue for LPN. Nadler and colleagues[50] found that the mean blood loss was lower when BioGlue was applied compared with a sutured bolster alone (237 versus 419 mL). In this study, the adhesive was applied following placement of a sutured bolster consisting of FloSeal and Surgicel to achieve hemostasis. Hidas and colleagues[48] described the use of BioGlue in open partial nephrectomy in comparison with traditional suturing and found significantly reduced warm ischemia time (17 versus 26 minutes, respectively; $P = .002$) and mean blood loss (45 versus 112 mL, respectively; $P = .001$). There were no cases of urinary fistula in the BioGlue group, compared with two fistulas in the traditional suturing group.

The ability of BioGlue to link adjacent tissues forming a watertight seal makes it an ideal candidate for reinforcing vesicourethral anastomoses during radical prostatectomy. To test this hypothesis, Hruby and colleagues[53] compared a Bio-Glue-reinforced anastomosis with a standard running sutured anastomosis in a porcine model of laparoscopic radical nephrectomy. They found

that in addition to being challenging and time consuming to apply, BioGlue seemed to prevent complete tissue approximation thereby inhibiting proper wound healing leading to an increased risk of urinary extravasation. This led the authors to recommend that BioGlue not be used to reinforce vesicourethral anastomoses following radical prostatectomy.

Cyanoacrylate-Based Sealants

Although there are currently two FDA-approved cyanoacrylate-based sealants available (2-octyl cyanoacrylate marketed as Dermabond by Johnson and Johnson, and N-butyl 2-cyanoacrylate, marketed as Indermil by Covidien), their use is limited to skin closure. There have been a limited number of animal studies, however, demonstrating urologic tissue sealing applications. Marcovich and colleagues[54] showed that 2-octyl cyanoacrylate was superior to fibrin glue in the closure of a cystotomy in a porcine model. This formulation of cyanoacrylate is not biodegradable and could possibly act as a nidus for infection or calculus formation, limiting its urologic applications. In response to this, biodegradable cyanoacrylate glue was tested with respect to its tensile strength and inflammatory response.[55] Four weeks after cystotomy, all four porcine bladders were able to withstand a filling pressure of 200 mm Hg without rupture. In a rabbit model, the inflammatory response associated with this biodegradable glue was similar to a sutured closure and there was no evidence of calcification. Human studies of cyanoacrylate glues have been limited because of their lithogenic potential and inflammatory stimulation, which can result in infection and fistula formation.

MECHANICAL HEMOSTATIC MATERIALS

One of the oldest principles of surgical hemostasis is mechanical tamponade. This relies on direct pressure to tamponade surgical bleeding until such time as the body's own intrinsic clotting cascade can be activated to achieve durable hemostasis. Several products are available that provide a mechanical barrier to hemorrhage and a scaffold to which platelets can adhere stimulating the body's own coagulation mechanism.

Porcine Gelatin

Currently, two different porcine gelatin products are available: Gelfoam (Pfizer, New York, New York) and Surgifoam (Johnson and Johnson, West Somerville, New Jersey). Gelfoam is available as a compressed sponge (shown in **Fig. 4** used in a partial nephrectomy bed), whereas Surgifoam is supplied as both a sponge and as a flowable matrix (Surgiflo).[40,56,57] The flowable matrix form is the same as used in FloSeal; however, in Surgiflo, thrombin is omitted. There has been no clinical trial comparing the efficacy of flowable gelatin matrix with and without thrombin, although individual comparison of their ability to achieve hemostasis after 10 minutes shows no difference between flowable gelatin matrix with thrombin and flowable gelatin matrix alone (96% versus 97%, respectively). All of these products can be used either dry, with sterile saline, or in conjunction with topical thrombin. When applied dry, the sponge is able to absorb up to 45 times its weight in whole blood.[57] The mechanism of action is thought to be primarily supportive and mechanical; however, one of the original trials suggested that the hemostatic effect may be caused by the release of thromboplastins from platelets on entering the irregular matrix.[58] This may accelerate the coagulation process in addition to providing a mechanical scaffold for the clot to adhere. Following application, the gelatin sponge is completely absorbed within 4 to 6 weeks.

Most trials using porcine gelatin sponges for topical hemostasis have also included the use of enzymatic hemostatic agents making it difficult to evaluate their efficacy alone. The use of gelatin matrix with thrombin (FloSeal) has been discussed previously. Another successful strategy for partial nephrectomy is to place fibrin-soaked gelatin sponge, with or without a sutured bolster,[59] although no trials have been conducted to compare these techniques.

To prevent thermal injury to the neurovascular bundle during robot-assisted radical prostatectomy, Ahlering and colleagues[60] developed a cautery-free dissection of the vascular pedicles using FloSeal covered with a dry sheet of Gelfoam along the length of the pedicle after division with cold scissors. They reported that this is a feasible means to dissect the pedicles without excessive blood loss; however, potency data were not included and it is difficult to interpret the benefit of this approach.

Collagen-Based Mechanical Hemostats

Hemostatic collagen is derived from either bovine dermal collagen or bovine Achilles tendon. Several different products are available including Avitene® (Davol, Warwick, Rhode Island); Instat (Johnson and Johnson, West Somerville, New Jersey); and Helitene (Integra, Plainsboro, New Jersey). Hemostatic collagen products are supplied in foam, in sheets, and as a powder (Avitene shown in **Fig. 5**). As with other mechanical hemostatic agents, these products are able to provide a stable matrix for clot formation but have the additional feature of enhancing platelet aggregation, degranulation, and release of clotting factors further promoting clot formation. Although there are no reports of the use of collagen-based mechanical hemostats in partial nephrectomy, one group has described its use in obtaining hemostasis following percutaneous renal biopsy.[61]

Oxidized Cellulose

Oxidized cellulose is a plant-based product and is available in three different forms (Johnson and Johnson, West Somerville, New Jersey): (1) Surgicel Original, (2) Surgicel Nu-Knit, and (3) Surgicel Fibrillar. Surgicel Original is a perforated single thin sheet that is thin enough to allow continued visualization of sites of bleeding after application. Moreover, the thin sheet is able to conform to irregular surfaces. Surgicel Fibrillar has a cotton-sponge consistency and is able to be peeled off

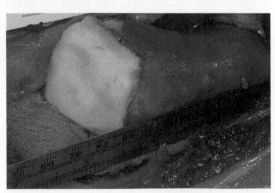

Fig. 4. Porcine gelatin sponge applied to a partial nephrectomy bed.

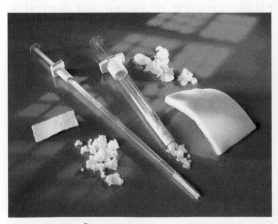

Fig. 5. Avitene® Microfibrillar Collagen Hemostat Sheets, Flour and Ultrafoam® collagen sponge. (*Courtesy of* Davol Inc., Warwick, RI; with permission.)

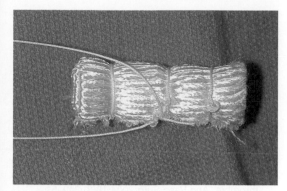

Fig. 6. Surgicel rolled bolster.

of the full sheet to conform to irregular surfaces. Surgicel Nu-Knit is a tightly knit thick fabric that has higher tensile strength, or can be rolled to fit within a surgical defect.[62]

Oxidized cellulose hemostats create a locally acidic environment and are antimicrobial.[63] Despite this antimicrobial activity, however, there does seem to be a significant local foreign-body reaction to oxidized cellulose with the formation of a granuloma at 21 days in a porcine model.[64] Although the clinical significance of this immune reaction is not known, it is well documented that the postoperative imaging of patients undergoing partial nephrectomy is often confusing with Surgicel bolsters being confused with both tumor recurrence[65] and abscess formation.[66]

The use of oxidized cellulose is well documented in both open and LPN during closure of the renal defect to prevent development of urinary fistula and hemorrhage.[67,68] Johnston and colleagues[69] evaluated seven different hemostatic techniques in a porcine LPN model. Although they found that most nonsuturing tissue sealants worked reasonably well for small resection beds, a rolled Surgicel Nu-Knit sutured bolster (**Fig. 6**) with FloSeal was the only technique able to achieve complete hemostasis in large surgical defects and should be used for tumors with greater than 5 mm depth of penetration.

SUMMARY

A variety of bioadhesives, tissue sealants, and hemostatic agents are available to surgeons today. This has allowed for a dramatic growth in the fields of laparoscopic and reconstructive urology with less morbidity and increased success. Currently, there is no perfect agent that is able to perform well in all surgical applications. Many agents are used in combination, and although this practice is clinically effective it limits the ability to discern the optimal properties of each

agent. A thorough knowledge of the safety, efficacy, cost, and biologic properties of these agents can help a surgeon select a product best suited to fit their needs, but individual operative experience remains a critical factor in determining successful outcomes.

REFERENCES

1. Schafer AI. Approach to the patient with bleeding and thrombosis. In: Goldman L, Ausiello D, editors. Cecil medicine. 23rd edition. Philadelphia: Saunders Elsevier; 2008. Chapter 178:1286–7.
2. Pursifull NF, Morey AF. Tissue glues and nonsuturing techniques. Curr Opin Urol 2007;17(6):396–401.
3. Package Insert. Tisseel, Baxter Health Care; 2007.
4. Evans LA, Morey AF. Current applications of fibrin sealant in urologic surgery. Int Braz J Urol 2006; 32(2):131–41.
5. Spotnitz WD, Burks S. Hemostats, sealants, and adhesives: components of the surgical toolbox. Transfusion 2008;48(7):1502–16.
6. Buchta C, Dettke M, Funovics PT, et al. Fibrin sealant produced by the CryoSeal FS System: product chemistry, material properties and possible preparation in the autologous preoperative setting. Vox Sang 2004;86(4):257–62.
7. Buchta C, Hedrich HC, Macher M, et al. Biochemical characterization of autologous fibrin sealants produced by CryoSeal and Vivostat in comparison to the homologous fibrin sealant product Tissucol/Tisseel. Biomaterials 2005;26(31):6233–41.
8. Schips L, Dalpiaz O, Cestari A, et al. Autologous fibrin glue using the Vivostat system for hemostasis in laparoscopic partial nephrectomy. Eur Urol 2006; 50(4):801–5.
9. Rock G, Neurath D, Semple E. Preparation and characterization of human thrombin for use in a fibrin glue. Transfus Med 2007;17(3):187–91.
10. Kram HB, Ocampo HP, Yamaguchi MP, et al. Fibrin glue in renal and ureteral trauma. Urology 1989; 33(3):215–8.
11. Canby-Hagino ED, Morey AF, Jatoi I, et al. Fibrin sealant treatment of splenic injury during open and laparoscopic left radical nephrectomy. J Urol 2000; 164(6):2004–5.
12. Levinson AK, Swanson DA, Johnson DE, et al. Fibrin glue for partial nephrectomy. Urology 1991;38(4): 314–6.
13. Pruthi RS, Chun J, Richman M. The use of a fibrin tissue sealant during laparoscopic partial nephrectomy. BJU Int 2004;93(6):813–7.
14. Johnston WK, Montgomery JS, Seifman BD, et al. Fibrin glue v sutured bolster: lessons learned during 100 laparoscopic partial nephrectomies. J Urol 2005;174(1):47–52.

15. Currie LJ, Sharpe JR, Martin R. The use of fibrin glue in skin grafts and tissue-engineered skin replacements: a review. Plast Reconstr Surg 2001;108(6): 1713–26.

16. Pandit AS, Feldman DS, Caulfield J. In vivo wound healing response to a modified degradable fibrin scaffold. J Biomater Appl 1998;12(3):222–36.

17. Lee MG, Jones D. Applications of fibrin sealant in surgery. Surg Innov 2005;12(3):203–13.

18. Eden CG, Coptcoat MJ. Assessment of alternative tissue approximation techniques for laparoscopy. Br J Urol 1996;78(2):234–42.

19. Wolf JS Jr, Soble JJ, Nakada SY, et al. Comparison of fibrin glue, laser weld, and mechanical suturing device for the laparoscopic closure of ureterotomy in a porcine model. J Urol 1997;157(4):1487–92.

20. Eden CG, Sultana SR, Murray KH, et al. Extraperitoneal laparoscopic dismembered fibrin-glued pyeloplasty: medium-term results. Br J Urol 1997;80(3): 382–9.

21. Morey AF, McDonough RC, Kizer WS, et al. Drain-free simple retropubic prostatectomy with fibrin sealant. J Urol 2002;168(2):627–9.

22. Diner EK, Patel SV, Kwart AM. Does fibrin sealant decrease immediate urinary leakage following radical retropubic prostatectomy? J Urol 2005; 173(4):1147–9.

23. Sharma S, Kim HL, Mohler JL. Routine pelvic drainage not required after open or robotic radical prostatectomy. Urology 2007;69(2):330–3.

24. Spotnitz WD, Falstrom JK, Rodeheaver GT. The role of sutures and fibrin sealant in wound healing. Surg Clin North Am 1997;77(3):651–69.

25. Bold EL, Wanamaker JR, Zins JE, et al. The use of fibrin glue in the healing of skin flaps. Am J Otol 1996;17(1):27–30.

26. Papadopoulos I, Schnapka B, Kelâmi A. Use of human fibrin glue in the closure of vesicovaginal fistulas. Urol Int 1985;40(3):141–4.

27. Shekarriz B, Stoller ML. The use of fibrin sealant in urology. J Urol 2002;167(3):1218–25.

28. Welp T, Bauer O, Diedrich K. Use of fibrin glue in vesico-vaginal fistulas after gynecologic treatment. Zentralbl Gynakol 1996;118(7):430–2.

29. Rossi D, Bladou F, Berthet B, et al. A simple alternative for the treatment of urinary fistulas: fibrin glue. Prog Urol 1991;1(3):445–8.

30. Tostain J. Conservative treatment of urogenital fistula following gynecological surgery: the value of fibrin glue. Acta Urol Belg 1992;60(3):27–33.

31. Morita T, Tokue A. Successful endoscopic closure of radiation induced vesicovaginal fistula with fibrin glue and bovine collagen. J Urol 1999;162(5):1689.

32. Evans LA, Ferguson KH, Foley JP, et al. Fibrin sealant for the management of genitourinary injuries, fistulas and surgical complications. J Urol 2003; 169(4):1360–2.

33. Bradford TJ, Wolf JS. Percutaneous injection of fibrin glue for persistent nephrocutaneous fistula after partial nephrectomy. Urology 2005;65(4):799.

34. Package insert. Evithrom, Johnson and Johnson; 2007.

35. Chapman WC, Singla N, Genyk Y, et al. A phase 3, randomized, double-blind comparative study of the efficacy and safety of topical recombinant human thrombin and bovine thrombin in surgical hemostasis. J Am Coll Surg 2007;205(2):256–65.

36. Sarfati MR, Dilorenzo DJ, Kraiss LW, et al. Severe coagulopathy following intraoperative use of topical thrombin. Ann Vasc Surg 2004;18(3):349–51.

37. Zehnder JL, Leung LL. Development of antibodies to thrombin and factor V with recurrent bleeding in a patient exposed to topical bovine thrombin. Blood 1990;76(10):2011–6.

38. Lawson JH, Lynn KA, Vanmatre RM, et al. Antihuman factor V antibodies after use of relatively pure bovine thrombin. Ann Thorac Surg 2005;79(3):1037–8.

39. Package insert. FloSeal, Baxter Health Care; 2005.

40. Package insert. Surgiflo, Johnson and Johnson; 2008.

41. Desai PJ, Maynes LJ, Zuppan C, et al. Hand-assisted laparoscopic partial nephrectomy in the porcine model using gelatin matrix hemostatic sealant without hilar occlusion. J Endourol 2005;19(5): 566–9.

42. Gill IS, Ramani AP, Spaliviero M, et al. Improved hemostasis during laparoscopic partial nephrectomy using gelatin matrix thrombin sealant. Urology 2005;65(3):463–6.

43. Hick EJ, Morey AF, Harris RA, et al. Gelatin matrix treatment of complex renal injuries in a porcine model. J Urol 2005;173(5):1801–4.

44. Package Insert. CoSeal, Baxter Health Care; 2006.

45. Glickman M, Gheissari A, Money S, et al. A polymeric sealant inhibits anastomotic suture hole bleeding more rapidly than Gelfoam/thrombin: results of a randomized controlled trial. Arch Surg 2002;137(3):326–31.

46. Park EL, Ulreich JB, Scott KM, et al. Evaluation of polyethylene glycol based hydrogel for tissue sealing after laparoscopic partial nephrectomy in a porcine model. J Urol 2004;172(6):2446–50.

47. Bernie JE, Ng J, Bargman V, et al. Evaluation of hydrogel tissue sealant in porcine laparoscopic partial-nephrectomy model. J Endourol 2005;19(9): 1122–6.

48. Hidas G, Kastin A, Mullerad M, et al. Sutureless nephron-sparing surgery: use of albumin glutaraldehyde tissue adhesive (BioGlue). Urology 2006;67(4): 697–700.

49. Package Insert. BioGlue, Cryolife. 2001.

50. Nadler RB, Loeb S, Rubenstein RA, et al. Use of BioGlue in laparoscopic partial nephrectomy. Urology 2006;68(2):416–8.

51. Msezane LP, Katz MH, Gofrit ON, et al. Hemostatic agents and instruments in laparoscopic renal surgery. J Endourol 2008;22(3):403–8.
52. Fürst W, Banerjee A. Release of glutaraldehyde from an albumin-glutaraldehyde tissue adhesive causes significant in vitro and in vivo toxicity. Ann Thorac Surg 2005;79(5):1522–8.
53. Hruby G, Marruffo F, Durak E, et al. Comparison of BioGlue reinforced and standard running sutured vesicourethral anastomoses. Urology 2006;68(6):1355–9.
54. Marcovich R, Williams AL, Rubin MA, et al. Comparison of 2-octyl cyanoacrylate adhesive, fibrin glue, and suturing for wound closure in the porcine urinary tract. Urology 2001;57(4):806–10.
55. Seifman BD, Rubin MA, Williams AL, et al. Use of absorbable cyanoacrylate glue to repair an open cystotomy. J Urol 2002;167(4):1872–5.
56. Package insert. Surgifoam, Johnson and Johnson; 2008.
57. Package insert. Gelfoam, Pfizer; 2007.
58. Jenkins HP, Senz EH, Owen H, et al. Present status of gelatin sponge for control of hemorrhage. JAMA 1946;132:124–32.
59. Wolf JS Jr, Seifman BD, Montie JE. Nephron sparing surgery for suspected malignancy: open surgery compared to laparoscopy with selective use of hand assistance. J Urol 2000;163(6):1659–64.
60. Ahlering TE, Eichel L, Chou D, et al. Feasibility study for robotic radical prostatectomy cautery-free neurovascular bundle preservation. Urology 2005;65(5):994–7.
61. Maturen KE, Nghiem HV, Caoili EM, et al. Renal mass core biopsy: accuracy and impact on clinical management. Am J Roentgenol 2007;188(2):563–70.
62. Package insert. Surgicel, Surgicel Fibrillar, and Surgicel Nu-Knit, Johnson and Johnson; 2005.
63. Spangler D, Rothenburger S, Nguyen K, et al. Vitro antimicrobial activity of oxidized regenerated cellulose against antibiotic-resistant microorganisms. Surg Infect 2003;4(3):255–62.
64. Sabino L, Andreoni C, Faria EF, et al. Evaluation of renal defect healing, hemostasis, and urinary fistula after laparoscopic partial nephrectomy with oxidized cellulose. J Endourol 2007;21(5):551–6.
65. Tolhurst SR, Rapp DE, Lyon MB, et al. Post-operative changes mimicking the radiographic appearance of recurrent renal cell carcinoma. Urol Int 2006;76(4):368–70.
66. Turley BR, Taupmann RE, Johnson PL. Postoperative abscess mimicked by Surgicel. Abdom Imaging 1994;19:345–6.
67. Novick AC, Derweesh I. Open partial nephrectomy for renal tumors: current status. BJU Int 2005;95:35–40.
68. Gill IS, Desai MM, Kaouk JH, et al. Laparoscopic partial nephrectomy for renal tumor: duplicating open surgical techniques. J Urol 2002;167:469–76.
69. Johnston WK, Kelel KM, Hollenbeck BK, et al. Acute integrity of closure for partial nephrectomy: comparison of 7 agents in a hypertensive porcine model. J Urol 2006;175(6):2307–11.

Index

Note: Page numbers of article titles are in **boldface** type.

Urol Clin N Am 36 (2009) 277–283
doi:10.1016/S0094-0143(09)00025-1

Moving?

Make sure your subscription moves with you!

To notify us of your new address, find your **Clinics Account Number** (located on your mailing label above your name), and contact customer service at:

E-mail: elspcs@elsevier.com

800-654-2452 (subscribers in the U.S. & Canada)
314-453-7041 (subscribers outside of the U.S. & Canada)

Fax number: 314-523-5170

Elsevier Periodicals Customer Service
11830 Westline Industrial Drive
St. Louis, MO 63146

*To ensure uninterrupted delivery of your subscription, please notify us at least 4 weeks in advance of move.

Printed and bound by CPI Group (UK) Ltd, Croydon, CR0 4YY

03/10/2024

01040353-0017